MCQs in Regional Anaesthesia and Pain Therapy

HERMAN SEHMBI

MBBS, MD

Clinical Fellow in Anaesthesia
Frimley Park Hospital
Surrey

and

USHMA JITENDRA SHAH

MBBS, DA, DNB

Clinical Fellow in Anaesthesia
Frimley Park Hospital
Surrey

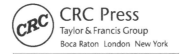

CRC Press
Taylor & Francis Group
Boca Raton London New York

CRC Press is an imprint of the
Taylor & Francis Group, an **informa** business

Radcliffe Publishing Ltd
33–41 Dallington Street
London
EC1V 0BB
United Kingdom

www.radcliffepublishing.com

Every effort has been made to ensure that the information in this book is accurate. This does not diminish the requirement to exercise clinical judgement, and neither the publisher nor the authors can accept any responsibility for its use in practice.

New research and clinical experience can result in changes in treatment and drug therapy. Users of the information in this book should therefore check the most recent product information on any drug they may prescribe to ensure they are complying with the manufacturer's recommendations concerning dosage, the method and duration of administration and contraindications.

British Library Cataloguing in Publication Data

A catalogue record for this book is available from the British Library.

ISBN-13: 978 184619 971 4

The paper used for the text pages of this book is FSC® certified. FSC (The Forest Stewardship Council®) is an international network to promote responsible management of the world's forests.

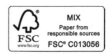

Typeset by Kate Broome, Auckland, New Zealand

Contents

Reviewers

Deepa Jadhav BMedSci, MBBS, FRCA, EDRA
Consultant in Anaesthesia
Frimley Park Hospital
Surrey

Madan Narayanan MBBS, MD, FRCA, FRARSCI, EDIC, EDRA
Consultant in Anaesthesia
Frimley Park Hospital
Surrey

Mohjir Baloch BSc, MBBS, MRCP, FRCA, FFPMRCA
Consultant in Anaesthesia and Chronic Pain
Frimley Park Hospital
Surrey

Suresh Kumar Jeyaraj MBBS, FCARCSI, EDRA
Specialty Doctor in Anaesthetics
Frimley Park Hospital
Surrey

Preface

A review book should have two purposes. Firstly, it should provide essential information in a concise manner, and secondly it should help to save time it would otherwise take to acquire the same knowledge. *MCQs in Regional Anaesthesia and Pain Therapy* has been an attempt in this direction. This review book targets trainees with an interest in regional anaesthesia, who may be taking any MCQ-based exam in the specialty.

As the vision for this book has been to serve both as a source of MCQ practice and a rapid review of the subject, we have divided this book into nine chapters and an appendix. These chapters provide a systematic approach to the topics, including relevant anatomy and physiology, techniques of nerve blockade, their indications, contraindications and complications. An effort has been made to include evidence-based questions where possible. Topics such as pain therapy and statistics have been covered as well. The book has over 125 tables and 95 illustrations to make understanding and learning easier. An appendix at the end includes miscellaneous information for rapid revision.

Rather than providing examinees with factual questions, we have framed almost all MCQs with intent to explain relevant concepts. We hope that the readers will find the questions challenging, explanations adequate and references as a source of further learning. Although we have written the book for trainees, we are quite sure that it will be useful for anyone who is an enthusiast in this field. *After all, a stimulated mind is an enlightened one!*

Herman Sehmbi
Ushma Jitendra Shah
May 2012

Acknowledgements

We would like to take this opportunity to thank all our teachers, without whose teaching and guidance we wouldn't be who we are. We also thank our consultants, who taught us the science and practice of regional anaesthesia. We thank our reviewers, who worked very hard to weed out errors from this guide. No book can see the light of day without the publishers. We are indebted to the team at Radcliffe Publishing for their guidance, effort and patience.

Above all, we dedicate this book to our parents. 'No words can express the gratitude, may we say: we love you.'

Recommended reading

Although no amount of reading can substitute insights gained by actual practice, it is important what we read when we are preparing for an exam. One should give adequate time to reading a standard textbook before exploring journals, websites and guidelines towards the end. A resource for MCQ practice is vital and should be started at the earliest.

We would recommend the following resources for preparation:

Textbooks

- Cousins MJ, Bridenbaugh PO, Carr DB, *et al. Cousins and Bridenbaugh's Neural Blockade in Clinical Anesthesia and Pain Medicine.* 4th ed. Philadelphia, PA: Lippincott Williams & Wilkins; 2008.
- Hadzic A. *Textbook of Regional Anesthesia and Acute Pain Management.* 1st ed. New York, NY: McGraw-Hill Medical; 2006.
- Mulroy MF, Bernards CM, McDonald SB, *et al. A Practical Approach to Regional Anesthesia.* 4th ed. Philadelphia, PA: Lippincott Williams & Wilkins; 2008.
- Neal JM, Rathmell JP. *Complications in Regional Anesthesia and Pain Medicine.* 1st ed. Philadelphia, PA: Saunders; 2006.

Journal

- *Regional Anesthesia and Pain Medicine (Reg Anesth Pain Med).* Philadelphia, PA: Lippincott Williams & Wilkins.

Websites

- American Society of Regional Anesthesia and Pain Medicine (www.asra.com)
- CSEN (www.csen.com/anesthesia)
- European Society of Regional Anaesthesia and Pain Therapy (www.esraeurope.org)
- New York School of Regional Anesthesia (www.nysora.com)

- Peripheral Regional Anaesthesia (www.nerveblocks.net)
- Regional Anaesthesia – United Kingdom (www.ra-uk.org)
- Regional for Trainees (www.regionalfortrainees.com)
- SonoSite (www.sonositeeducation.com)
- Ultrasound Guided Regional Anaesthesia (www.usgra.co.uk)
- Ultrasound Guided Regional Anaesthesia Web, Hong Kong (www.usgraweb.hk/en/Start.html)
- Ultrasound for Regional Anesthesia (www.usra.ca)

Guidelines

- National Institute for Health and Clinical Excellence. *Ultrasound-Guided Catheterisation of the Epidural Space: NICE guideline IPG249.* London: NIHCE; 2008. http://guidance.nice.org.uk/IPG249
- National Institute for Health and Clinical Excellence. *Guidance on the Use of Ultrasound Locating Devices for Placing Central Venous Catheter: NICE guideline TA49.* London: NIHCE; 2002. http://guidance.nice.org.uk/TA49
- National Institute for Health and Clinical Excellence. *Ultrasound Guided Regional Nerve Block: NICE guideline IPG285.* London: NIHCE; 2008. http://guidance.nice.org.uk/IPG285

American Society of Regional Anesthesia and Pain Medicine consensus statements (available at: www.asra.com/publications.php)

- *ASRA Practice Advisory on Local Anesthetic Systemic Toxicity*
- *The ASRA Evidence-Based Medicine Assessment of Ultrasound-Guided Regional Anesthesia and Pain Medicine: Executive Summary*
- *Regional Anesthesia in the Patient Receiving Antithrombotic or Thrombolytic Therapy: American Society of Regional Anesthesia and Pain Medicine Evidence-Based Guidelines (Third Edition)*
- *The American Society of Regional Anesthesia and Pain Medicine and the European Society of Regional Anaesthesia and Pain Therapy Joint Committee Recommendations for Education and Training in Ultrasound-Guided Regional Anesthesia*
- *ASRA Practice Advisory on Neurologic Complications in Regional Anesthesia and Pain Medicine*
- *Infectious Complications 2004*

1
The nerve

Questions

Distribution

Questions 1–8:   Nerve anatomy and physiology

Questions 9–11:   Local anaesthetic action

Choose one best answer for each of the following questions.

Q1   Which of the following statements regarding the development of neural structures is **correct**?
  a. The central nervous system is derived from ectoderm, whereas the peripheral nervous system is derived from mesoderm
  b. During their development, the upper limbs rotate medially but the lower limbs rotate laterally
  c. The median nerve is the only postaxial nerve below the shoulder
  d. The tibial nerve (preaxial) and common peroneal nerve (postaxial) lie enclosed within a single sheath

Q2   Which of the following statements is **incorrect**?
  a. Each neuron has only one axon
  b. Interneurons are bipolar
  c. Primary sensory neurons are unipolar
  d. Motor neurons are multipolar

Q3 Regarding nerve myelination, which of the following statements is **correct**?
a. Unmyelinated neurons lack Schwann cells
b. Schwann cells myelinate all neurons in the body
c. Oligodendrocytes myelinate the axons of the neurons in the central nervous system
d. Nodes of Ranvier allow for continuous and homogenous nerve conduction

Q4 Which of the following statements regarding the structural organisation of a peripheral nerve fibre is **incorrect**?
a. Endoneurium in the nerve fibres form the blood–nerve barrier
b. Individual nerve fibres are enclosed by endoneurium
c. Nerve fascicles are enclosed by perineurium
d. The entire nerve is enclosed within epineurium

Q5 Which of the following statements regarding peripheral nerves is **true**?
a. C fibres carry pain and proprioception
b. Thickly myelinated B fibres are postganglionic axons of the autonomic nervous system
c. Conduction velocity of Aδ fibres is 12–30 m/second
d. Thickness of Aβ fibres is 12–20 μm

Q6 Which of the following regarding the neuron action potential is **false**?
a. Resting membrane potential (RMP) is about –60 to –70 mV
b. Threshold potential is about –55 mV
c. During the depolarising phase, the K+ permeability rises, leading to an influx of K+ ions
d. During the repolarisation phase, opening of voltage-dependent K+ channels, cause a large outward K+ current rapidly restoring the axoplasm to its RMP

Q7 Regarding action potential, which is the **false** statement from the following?
a. During the absolute refractory period, it is not possible to stimulate a nerve
b. All membrane potentials are propagated
c. Because of margin of safety, 80% of Na+ channels must be blocked before conduction failure occurs
d. In disease or drugged axons, decremental impulse conduction is observed

Q8 What is the order of nerve blockade of different types of nerve fibres?
a. B > Aδ = C > Aγ > Aβ > Aα
b. B > Aδ > Aγ > Aβ > Aα > C
c. Aδ > Aγ > Aβ > Aα > B > C
d. C > B > Aδ > Aγ > Aβ > Aα

Q9 Which of the following statements regarding Na+ channels is **true**?
a. They consist of α, β and γ subunits
b. They cluster at the nodes of Ranvier
c. The β subunit has four domains, each having six membrane-spanning segments
d. Nerves have the same Na+ channel isoforms as muscles

Q10 Regarding action of local anaesthetic (LA) on NA+ channels, which of the following is **true**?
a. The affinity of LA for the inactivated state of the Na+ channel is higher than its resting state
b. At low frequencies of impulse firing, a phase- or use-dependent block is seen
c. The cationic form of LA acts on the Na+ channel from outside the axon
d. The unionised form acts from within the axon to inactivate the Na+ channel

Q11 Which of the following statements concerning LA-induced nerve blocks is **correct**?
a. The functional loss produced is proportional to impulse blockade
b. Minimum blocking concentration is the concentration of LA that blocks 50% of impulse conduction within a given nerve within a reasonable period of time
c. Differential block is observation of sensory preservation, despite complete motor loss
d. The anaesthesia induced by LA sweeps down the limb in a proximal to distal fashion

Answers

A1 D

▶ The nervous system (central and peripheral) is derived from the **ecto-derm**, but the vertebral column is **mesodermal** in origin.

▶ During their development, the limbs rotate in opposite directions; the upper limbs rotate **laterally** (placing extensors posterolaterally), while the lower limbs rotate **medially** (placing extensors anteromedially).

▶ The structures anterior to the bone or fascial plane or axis of the limb are termed **preaxial**, while the structures posterior to it are called **postaxial**. Hence the radial nerve is the only **postaxial nerve** below the shoulder (median and ulnar being preaxial).

▶ In the lower limb, tibial nerve (**preaxial**) and common peroneal nerve (**postaxial**) lie enclosed within a **single sheath**.

  • Hadzic A. *Textbook of Regional Anesthesia and Acute Pain Management*. 1st ed. New York, NY: McGraw-Hill Medical; 2006. pp. 23–42.

A2 B A typical neuron possesses a cell body (often called the soma), dendrites and an axon. Each neuron has only one axon, although it may have many dendrites. Neurons may be classified according to:

▶ **polarity**: unipolar (primary sensory neurons), bipolar (bipolar cell of the retina) or multipolar (cortical neurons, motor neurons, interneurons)

▶ **functionality**: sensory, motor, autonomic and so forth

▶ **direction**: afferent, efferent or interneurons

▶ **myelination**: myelinated or unmyelinated

▶ **characteristics of peripheral nerve fibres**: A (Aα, Aβ, Aγ, Aδ), B or C

▶ **neurotransmitters produced**: cholinergic, adrenergic, glutamatergic, GABAergic, dopaminergic, serotonergic and so forth.

A3 C

▶ **Myelin** is a dielectric (electrically insulating) material that forms a layer, the myelin sheath, usually around only the axon of a neuron. It is essential for the proper functioning of the nervous system.

- **Schwann cells** (a type of glial cell) supply the myelin for peripheral neurons, whereas **oligodendrocytes** myelinate the axons of the central nervous system.
- A and B fibres possess several layers of myelin. They have **nodes of Ranvier** resulting in a continuous but non-homogenous **saltatory conduction**.
- C fibres are the only unmyelinated fibres, as their Schwann cells do not form myelin. Their impulse conduction is **uniform** and homogenous.
  - Barrett KE, Barman SM, Boitano S, *et al. Ganong's Review of Medical Physiology*. 23rd ed. New York, NY: McGraw-Hill Medical. 2009. p. 82.

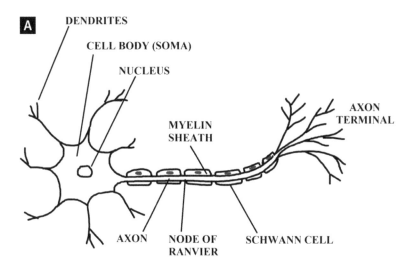

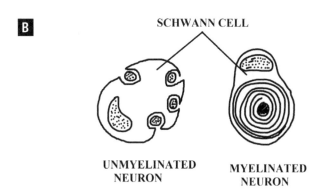

Figure 1.1 (A) Structure of a neuron; (B) Schwann cells

A4   A

> Within a nerve, each axon is surrounded by a layer of connective tissue called the **endoneurium**.
> The axons are bundled together into groups called **fascicles**, and each fascicle is wrapped in a layer of connective tissue called the **perineurium**. It forms the **blood–nerve barrier** and acts as a **diffusion barrier** to local anaesthetics.
> Finally, the entire nerve is wrapped in a layer of connective tissue called the **epineurium**. The space between fascicles is called the **interfascicular space**, while one within an individual fascicle is called the **intrafascicular space**.

It has been recently stated that an interfascicular injection may not cause neuronal injury, while an intrafascicular injection probably will. This is in opposition to the classic view that all intraneural injections lead to neuronal damage.

- Hadzic A. *Textbook of Regional Anesthesia and Acute Pain Management.* 1st ed. New York, NY: McGraw-Hill Medical; 2006. p. 81.
- Jeng CL, Rosenblatt MA. Intraneural injections and regional anesthesia: the known and the unknown. *Minerva Anestesiol.* 2011; **77**(1): 54–8.

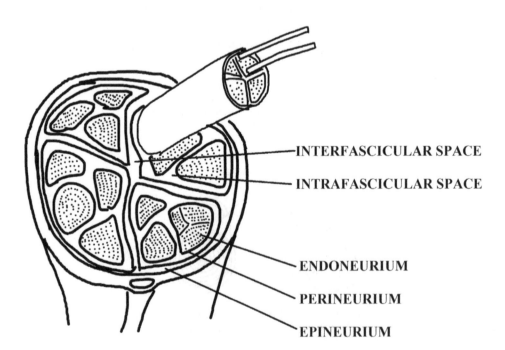

INTERFASCICULAR SPACE

INTRAFASCICULAR SPACE

ENDONEURIUM

PERINEURIUM

EPINEURIUM

Figure 1.2 Structure of a peripheral nerve

Table 1.1 Anatomical and physiological characteristics of peripheral nerves

Nerve type	Function	Diameter (μm)	Conduction velocity (ml second)	Myelin content	LA sensitivity
A fibres					
Aα	Motor	12–20	70–120	+ + +	+ +
Aβ	Touch, pressure	5–12	30–70	+ + +	+ +
Aγ	Proprioception, muscle tone	1–4	15–30	+ +	+ + +
Aδ	Pain, temperature	1–4	12–30	+ +	+ + +
B fibres	Preganglionic autonomic	1–3	3–15	+	+ +
C fibres	Postganglionic autonomic, pain, temperature, some mechanoreceptors	0.5–1	0.5–2	– –	+ (least)

A5   C The anatomical and physiological characteristics of peripheral nerves (**Erlanger and Gasser**) are as shown in Table 1.1.

- Barrett KE, Barman SM, Boitano S, *et al. Ganong's Review of Medical Physiology.* 23rd ed. New York, NY: McGraw-Hill Medical. 2008. p. 89.
- Cousins MJ, Bridenbaugh PO, Carr DB, *et al. Cousins and Bridenbaugh's Neural Blockade in Clinical Anesthesia and Pain Medicine.* 4th ed. Philadelphia, PA: Lippincott Williams & Wilkins; 2008. p. 35.

A6   C

▶ *The intracellular concentration* of K+ ions is 10 times greater than its extracellular concentration, and vice versa for Na+ ions. This difference is maintained by **Na+/K+ ATPase pump**. In a resting nerve cell membrane, a selective permeability to K+ exists, permitting net efflux of small number of K+ ions, resulting in negative resting membrane potential (RMP) of **–60 to –70 mV**, which is close to the equilibrium potential for K+ ions.

▶ Action potential is a **propagated impulse** caused by a rise of RMP to **threshold potential** (–55 mV) from a depolarising stimulus. During the **depolarising phase**, the Na+ permeability rises, leading to an influx of Na+ ions, and thus causing the RMP to become less negative. This is a brief event as the nerve enters the **repolarisation phase**. This is due

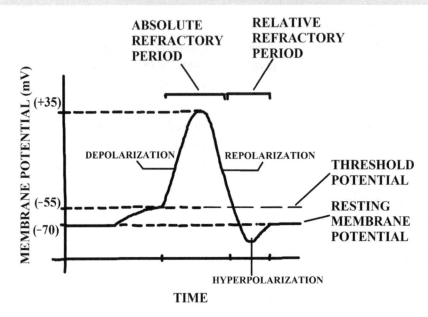

Figure 1.3 Action potential in a neuron

to slowing down of Na+ influx and opening of voltage-dependent K+ channels, causing a large outward K+ current rapidly restoring the axoplasm to its RMP or beyond it (**hyperpolarisation**). Finally the Na+/K+ ATPase pump restores the Na+ and K+ gradients across the membrane.

- Cousins MJ, Bridenbaugh PO, Carr DB, *et al. Cousins and Bridenbaugh's Neural Blockade in Clinical Anesthesia and Pain Medicine.* 4th ed. Philadelphia, PA: Lippincott Williams & Wilkins; 2008. p. 28.

A7   B

▶ A neuron is refractory to further stimulation during the rising and most of the falling phase of the action potential. This **refractory period** is divided into an **absolute refractory period** (from the time the firing level is reached until repolarisation is about one-third complete) and a **relative refractory period** (from this point to the start of afterdepolarisation).

▶ The nerve **cannot** be stimulated during this absolute refractory period, but during the relative refractory period, **stronger** (than normal) stimuli can cause excitation.

▶ On stimulation, once the threshold intensity is reached, a full-fledged action potential is produced. With a weaker (**subthreshold**) stimulus, the action potential **fails** to occur. The action potential follows the **'all or none' law**.

- The **current** flowing through the nerve is **5–10 times** that needed to depolarise it; this is called '**the margin of safety**' for impulse conduction. Because of this, **80%** of Na+ channels must be blocked before conduction failure occurs.
- Disease or drugs may **reduce membrane excitability**, resulting in lower action potential amplitude, slower rate of impulse depolarisation and slower conduction velocity. This is called **decremental impulse conduction**. When this exceeds the margin of safety, conduction failure occurs. *This underlies the clinical application of local anaesthetics (Na+ channel blockers) in regional anaesthesia.* It is considered that Na+ channels in at least **three successive nodes** of Ranvier should be blocked for axonal conduction to fail.
  - Barrett KE, Barman SM, Boitano S, *et al. Ganong's Review of Medical Physiology*. 23rd ed. New York, NY: McGraw-Hill Medical. 2009. pp. 85–6.
  - Cousins MJ, Bridenbaugh PO, Carr DB, *et al. Cousins and Bridenbaugh's Neural Blockade in Clinical Anesthesia and Pain Medicine*. 4th ed. Philadelphia, PA: Lippincott Williams & Wilkins; 2008. p. 29.

A8   A

- The sensitivity of nerve fibres to local anaesthetics depends on **both fibre type and size.**
- **Smaller fibres are blocked before larger fibres**, but an exception to this rule is B fibres (autonomic). The sequence of blockade is **B > Aδ = C > Aγ > Aβ > Aα.** Hence, sympathetic block appears before sensory block, which appears before motor block.
- The block reversal occurs in the **reverse manner** (i.e. Aα > Aβ > Aγ > Aδ = C > B). Therefore, motor block lasts the shortest time while the autonomic block lasts the longest.
  - Hadzic A. *Textbook of Regional Anesthesia and Acute Pain Management*. 1st ed. New York, NY: McGraw-Hill Medical; 2006. p. 159.

A9   B

- The Na+ channel is made up of two types of subunit: α (one) and β (one or two). The α subunit has four domains, each having six helical membrane-spanning segments.
- The α subunit contains a voltage sensor, an ion selectivity filter, gating structures and **P segment**, which forms the pore.
- Nine different isoforms of Na+ channels have been discovered, of which seven are in nerves; Na_v **1.4** is found in **skeletal muscles** and Na_v **1.5** is found in **cardiac muscles**.

❭ The Na+ channels are clustered around nodes of Ranvier and are essential for high-speed conduction.

❭ In **multiple sclerosis**, the **loss of clustering** underlies the electrophysiological consequences (decreased conduction velocity) and resultant manifestations.

   • Hadzic A. *Textbook of Regional Anesthesia and Acute Pain Management.* 1st ed. New York, NY: McGraw-Hill Medical; 2006. p. 109.

A10 A

❭ The Na+ channel exists in three states: **resting (R), open (O) and inactivated (I)**.

❭ The Na+ channel is in the resting state initially, but it assumes an open state on stimulation, resulting in Na+ influx intracellularly. This triggers the action potential. Subsequently, the channel is closed by assuming an inactivated state.

❭ **The LA has a higher affinity for the inactivated state than the resting state**, resulting in more Na+ channels in the inactivated state for a longer time. This increases the refractory period and limits the frequency with which a nerve can fire.

❭ At **higher frequencies** of impulse firing, a greater number of channels are in open as well as inactivated state; hence, the chance for LA binding is greater. This is called **phase- or use-dependent block**.

❭ Rate-dependent block of cardiac Na+ channels *in vivo* is the reason that hydrophobic LAs are more toxic than hydrophilic LAs.

❭ It is considered that the **unionised base** form of LA crosses the axon membrane and ionises intracellularly. This **cationic** form then acts from **within** the cell to inactivate the Na+ channel.

Note: the 1963 Nobel Prize in Physiology or Medicine was awarded to **Eccles, Huxley and Hodgkin** for their discoveries concerning the ionic mechanisms involved in excitation and inhibition in the peripheral and central portions of the nerve cell membrane.

   • Cousins MJ, Bridenbaugh PO, Carr DB, *et al. Cousins and Bridenbaugh's Neural Blockade in Clinical Anesthesia and Pain Medicine.* 4th ed. Philadelphia, PA: Lippincott Williams & Wilkins; 2008. pp. 29–31.
   • Mulroy MF, Bernards CM, McDonald SB, *et al. A Practical Approach to Regional Anesthesia.* 4th ed. Philadelphia, PA: Lippincott Williams & Wilkins; 2008. p. 8.

A11 D

▶ Though impulse conduction is vital for functioning of a peripheral nerve, its blockade is **not** proportional to functional loss produced. The minimum blocking concentration of LA is the lowest concentration of LA that blocks **all impulse conduction** within a nerve within a reasonable period of time (blockade of 50% fibres may result in limb movement and, more important, pain, which would be unacceptable clinically).

▶ **Differential block** is observation of motor preservation, despite complete sensory loss. This may be clinically employed in '**walking epidurals**'.

▶ The pharmacokinetics of LA in nerve block includes the following phases: **delivery, permeation of nerve sheath, induction and recovery**.

▶ In a given peripheral nerve, the outer fibres (mantle bundle) innervate the proximal structures while the inner fibres (core bundle) innervate the distal structures. LA diffuses down the **mantle to the core gradient**, with anaesthesia progressing in a **proximal to distal direction**. Because the vascularity of core fibres is higher, the recovery occurs in **distal to proximal direction**.

- Cousins MJ, Bridenbaugh PO, Carr DB, *et al. Cousins and Bridenbaugh's Neural Blockade in Clinical Anesthesia and Pain Medicine*. 4th ed. Philadelphia, PA: Lippincott Williams & Wilkins; 2008. pp. 35–40.
- Brunton LL, Lazo JS, Parker K. *Goodman and Gilman's The Pharmacological Basis of Therapeutics*. 11th ed. New York, NY: McGraw-Hill Medical. 2005. p. 381.

2

Pharmacology

Questions

Distribution

Questions 1–17: Local anaesthetics

Questions 18–24: Adjuvants

Questions 25–44: Analgesics (opioid and non-opioid)

Choose one best answer for each of the following questions.

Q1 Which of the following statements regarding the structure of local anaesthetic (LA) is **false**?
a. They consist of a hydrophobic aromatic ring and a hydrophilic tertiary amine group held by a hydrocarbon chain
b. All of them exist as a weak acid–base pair in solution except benzocaine
c. They are classified as esters or amides depending upon the type of linkage bond in the hydrocarbon chain
d. Cocaine is synthetically produced

Q2 Which of the following have LA-like properties?
a. Tetrodotoxin
b. Clonidine
c. Tricyclic antidepressants
d. All of the above

Q3 Which of the following is **true** regarding the ester and amide types of local anaesthetics?
a. Prilocaine is an amide-type LA
b. Esters have longer duration of action
c. Amides are generally less toxic
d. Allergic reactions to esters are rare

Q4 Which of the following statements regarding chirality is **incorrect**?
a. A chiral molecule is a type of molecule that lacks an internal plane of symmetry
b. Enantiomers are stereoisomers having a non-superimposable mirror image
c. Optical rotation (optical activity) is the turning of the plane of linearly polarised light about the direction of motion as the light travels through a substance
d. Enantiomers have similar optical activities but different physical and chemical properties

Q5 Regarding the physicochemical properties of LA, which of the following statements is **false**?
a. pKa is the pH at which half of the LA molecules are in the base form and other half are in the acid form
b. Lipid solubility is dependent on the size of the alkyl group on the tertiary amine and it increases with an increase in size of the tertiary amine
c. The partition coefficient of LA is the ratio of concentration of LA in a mix of an aqueous buffer and a hydrophobic lipid (octanol) after separation
d. More lipophilic LAs have higher protein binding, which is pH-dependent

Q6 Which of the following properties is **not** common among most local anaesthetics?
a. They are weak bases with pKa > 7.4
b. They are dispersed as acidic solutions of hydrochloride salts, providing increased lipid solubility
c. They exist in solution as an equilibrium mixture of unionised (lipid-soluble, free base) and ionised (water-soluble, cationic) forms
d. Body buffers raise pH and raise the amount of free base present

Q7 Which of the following statements regarding LA is **true**?
a. 2-Chloroprocaine is an amide anaesthetic
b. Lignocaine is a chiral molecule
c. Ropivacaine has a propyl group in its tertiary amine, while bupivacaine has a butyl group
d. Ropivacaine is a vasodilator

Q8 Which of the following statements regarding LA is **false**?
a. Ropivacaine produces more motor block than bupivacaine
b. Bupivacaine has a pKa of 8.1
c. Lignocaine has intermediate potency and duration of action
d. Prilocaine causes methaemoglobinaemia

Q9 Regarding onset of LA, which if the following statements is **incorrect**?
a. Proximity of injection to the nerve is the most important factor determining the onset of LA action
b. It is dose rather than concentration that determines the onset
c. More lipid-soluble drugs are more likely to partition, hence they have a slower onset
d. None of the above

Q10 Regarding duration of action of LA, which of the following statements is **correct**?
a. Block duration is largely dependent on the dose given
b. LAs with higher lipid solubility have longer duration of action
c. Higher protein binding increases duration of action
d. All of the above

Q11 Which of the following is **not** seen after the addition of adrenaline to LA?
a. Decrease in onset time
b. Increase in peak plasma concentration of local anaesthetic
c. Increase in the degree of sensory and motor block
d. Increase in the duration of block

Q12 Regarding pharmacokinetics of an injection of LA, which of the following statements is **correct**?

a. The pharmacological and clinical effects of LAs are the result of the drug absorption and its disposition

b. Disposition refers collectively to the process of drug distribution into and out of the tissues, and of drug elimination by metabolism and excretion

c. Local disposition of an injection drug involves both bulk flow and diffusion

d. All of the above

Q13 Regarding systemic absorption of LA, which of the following statements is **false**?

a. Systemic absorption of LA is chiefly responsible for its systemic toxicity (side effect)

b. Systemic absorption of more lipophilic drug (bupivacaine) is slower than less lipophilic drug (lignocaine)

c. The C_{max} (peak plasma concentration) is inversely proportional to the dose of LA injected

d. The addition of vasoconstrictor may decrease the C_{max}

Q14 Regarding systemic disposition of LA, which of the following statements is **false**?

a. The first capillary bed to be exposed to LA once it has entered the systemic circulation is lung

b. Protein binding of LA in blood is a non-saturable process

c. Ester LAs are rapidly cleared by plasma pseudocholinesterase

d. The clearance of lignocaine is dependent on both hepatic blood flow and enzyme activity

Q15 Which of the hepatic cytochrome enzymes is involved with hydroxylation of ropivacaine?

a. CYP1A2

b. CYP2D6

c. CYP3A4

d. CYP2C9

Q16 Which of the following statements regarding amide LA disposition in the given states is **incorrect**?
a. Clearance of LA increases with increasing age
b. In cardiovascular disease, LA clearance is impaired owing to decreased hepatic blood flow
c. In chronic hepatic disease, LA clearance is impaired because of decreased hepatic activity and blood flow
d. In renal disease, the disposition kinetics of LAs are largely unaffected

Q17 Regarding the pharmacokinetics and pharmacodynamics of LA in pregnancy, which of the following statements is **correct**?
a. Chlorprocaine is safer than lignocaine
b. Clearance of lignocaine is increased
c. Clearance of bupivacaine is decreased
d. All of the above

Q18 Which of the following is **not** used along with LAs as adjuncts in subarachnoid block?
a. Morphine
b. Adrenaline
c. Clonidine
d. Sodium bicarbonate

Q19 Regarding the use of opioids as adjuncts, which of the following statements is **false**?
a. They act through peripheral opioid receptors modulating afferent nociceptive stimuli
b. They have a synergistic action with LAs
c. Intrathecal morphine increases the risk of delayed respiratory depression
d. Epidural fentanyl as a bolus acts systemically, while infusion acts at spinal level

Q20 Which of the following statements concerning adrenaline use in neuraxial block is **true**?
a. It acts post-synaptically to impart analgesia
b. It may delay discharge in ambulatory settings
c. It increases mean blood pressure by vasoconstriction
d. It reduces cardiac output secondary to vasoconstriction

Q21 Which of the following statements about the use of clonidine in regional anaesthesia is **false**?
  a. It is unsuitable for ambulatory settings
  b. It acts through spinal mechanisms rather than acting systemically
  c. It reduces central sympathetic drive
  d. Sedation is the main side effect

Q22 Which of the following statements regarding carbonation of LAs is **false**?
  a. Alkalinisation raises pH close to pKa fastening onset
  b. It may intensify epidural anaesthesia
  c. Carbonation of ropivacaine results in faster onset
  d. Excessive carbonation may precipitate LA

Q23 Regarding adjuvant drugs in regional anaesthesia, which of the following is **false**?
  a. Epidurally administered liposomal morphine produces long-lasting analgesia when given with LAs
  b. Intrathecal neostigmine usage is limited by the severe nausea caused
  c. Intrathecal ketorolac has demonstrated antinociception
  d. Intrathecal midazolam offers analgesia when added to intrathecal bupivacaine

Q24 Concerning the adjuvants added to peripheral nerve blocks, which of the following is ineffective?
  a. Clonidine
  b. Buprenorphine
  c. Dexamethasone
  d. Ketorolac

Q25 Analgesics act by:
  a. Inhibition of inflammatory mediator actions
  b. Inhibition of nerve impulses
  c. Action on modulation and perception of pain
  d. All of the above

Q26 Which of the following statements regarding opioid receptors is **false**?
a. They are G-protein-coupled receptors
b. They are present peripherally as well
c. They have endogenous ligands
d. Sigma (σ) receptor is classified as an opioid subtype

Q27 Activation of opioid receptor by an opioid molecule produces:
a. Hyperpolarisation by K+ efflux
b. Inhibition of Ca+ influx, preventing neurotransmitter release
c. Inhibition of adenylate cyclase
d. All of the above

Q28 Which of the following is a partial agonist at the μ-(MOP) opioid receptor?
a. Fentanyl
b. Pethidine
c. Buprenorphine
d. Naloxone

Q29 Tolerance does **not** develop to which of the following side effects of opioids?
a. Itching
b. Respiratory depression
c. Urinary retention
d. Constipation

Q30 Which of the following analgesics has the least efficacy?
a. Codeine 60 mg
b. Diclofenac 100 mg
c. Ibuprofen 400 mg
d. Tramadol 100 mg

Q31 Which of the following drugs and their active metabolites provided here are **incorrectly** matched?
a. Morphine and morphine-6-glucuronide
b. Paracetamol and propacetamol
c. Codeine and morphine
d. Tramadol and M1 metabolite

Q32 Which of the following opioid doses is **not** equivalent to an oral dose of 30 mg morphine?
   a. 10 mg morphine if given intravenously
   b. 15 mg morphine if given intramuscularly
   c. 7.5 mg diamorphine if given subcutaneously
   d. 30 mg morphine if given subcutaneously

Q33 Regarding morphine, which of the following statements is **correct**?
   a. It is particularly effective in visceral pain
   b. Pruritis is due to histamine release
   c. Absorption through subcutaneous route is fast because of high lipid solubility
   d. Morphine-3-glucuronide is an active metabolite

Q34 Regarding the disposition of administered morphine, which of the following is **incorrect**?
   a. Lean body mass should be used to calculate dosage in individuals with a high body mass index value to avoid overdose
   b. Doses should be decreased in elderly patients to account for increased sensitivity and reduced lean mass
   c. Toxicity may be seen in renal failure, due to accumulation of morphine-6-glucuronide metabolite
   d. Higher doses are needed in liver failure to account for reduced formation of active metabolites

Q35 Regarding diamorphine, which of the following statements is **false**?
   a. It is twice as potent as morphine
   b. It is suitable for subcutaneous administration
   c. It has high abuse potential
   d. Given intrathecally, it can produce higher incidence of delayed respiratory depression, as it has two molecules of morphine

Q36 Which of the following statements regarding methadone is **correct**?
   a. It is used in opioid de-addiction therapy because it is shorter acting than morphine
   b. It is an opioid receptor antagonist
   c. It has a high first-pass metabolism
   d. It is useful in treatment of opioid-resistant chronic pain

Q37 Regarding codeine, which of the following statements is **false**?
a. It has good oral bioavailability
b. It is actually a prodrug
c. Its *O*-demethylation to morphine exhibits genetic polymorphism
d. Tramadol is a good choice in patients who do not have adequate analgesia with codeine

Q38 Regarding tramadol, which of the following statements is **false**?
a. It is not a controlled drug
b. It modulates the descending inhibitory pathway producing analgesia
c. Like other opioids, it can produce shivering
d. It intereacts with monoamine oxidase inhibitors, producing hypertensive crisis

Q39 Regarding the synthetic phenylpiperidine derivatives, which of the following statements is **correct**?
a. Pethidine has cholinergic properties
b. Fentanyl has lower respiratory depression when given intrathecally, because of its higher lipid solubility
c. Remifentanil's analgesia extends well into the post-operative period after discontinuation of intraoperative infusion
d. Alfentanil has a more rapid onset than fentanyl, because of higher pKa

Q40 Regarding naloxone, which of the following statements is **correct**?
a. It is used to reverse adverse effects of opioids without reversing analgesia
b. Its use in reversal of neonatal respiratory depression after maternal opioid use is remarkably safe
c. It is ideally given as a bolus followed by an infusion
d. It is used for opioid dependence

Q41 Which of the following statements regarding paracetamol is **incorrect**?
a. Intravenous formulation is more effective than oral
b. It inhibits peripheral prostaglandin synthesis
c. Overdose is treated by *N*-acetylcysteine
d. It is more effective than morphine when given with tramadol

Q42 Which of the following statements regarding NSAIDs is **correct**?
   a. They have low protein binding, which accounts for their analgesic efficacy
   b. They produce irreversible inhibition of cyclooxygenases
   c. They should always be avoided in asthmatics
   d. They reduce perioperative opioid consumption

Q43 Compared with non-selective cyclooxygenase inhibitors, selective cyclooxygenase-2 inhibitors display which of the following?
   a. Reduce gastrointestinal side effects
   b. Have better renal side-effect profile
   c. Offer cardioprotection
   d. Are more effective

Q44 A patient with allergy to fentanyl (severe hypotension) can be given which of the following opioids with close monitoring?
   a. Sufentanil
   b. Remifentanil
   c. Morphine
   d. Pethidine

Answers

A1   D Local anaesthetics (LAs) are **reversible Na+ channel blockers** used clinically to produce neuraxial anaesthesia (central or peripheral). The use of leaves of coca plant (*Erythroxylon coca*) for topical anaesthesia was known to Incas. In 1859, **Albert Niemann** isolated the chief alkaloid of coca, which he named 'cocaine'. In 1884, **Carl Koller** became the first to use cocaine for ophthalmic anaesthesia. The first synthetic LA was benzocaine (1900).

▶ The LA molecule consists of a **hydrophobic aromatic ring** and a **hydrophilic tertiary amine** group held by a hydrocarbon chain (with an **ester or amide** linkage), hence classified as **esters or amides**.

▶ Because the tertiary amine group can bind a proton to become a positively charged quaternary amine, all LAs exist as a **weak acid–base pair** in solution.

▶ This is most vital for LA action, as it is the **cationic** species that binds to the Na+ channel from inside the cell. **An exception to this is benzocaine, which lacks the tertiary amine.**

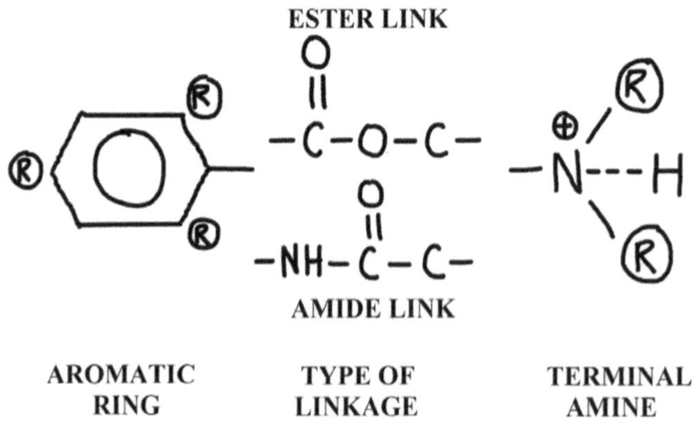

Figure 2.1 Structure of local anaesthetic molecule

- Hadzic A. *Textbook of Regional Anesthesia and Acute Pain Management*. 1st ed. New York, NY: McGraw-Hill Medical; 2006. p. 106.
- Mulroy MF, Bernards CM, McDonald SB, *et al. A Practical Approach to Regional Anesthesia*. 4th ed. Philadelphia, PA: Lippincott Williams & Wilkins; 2008. p. 1.

A2 D Many chemicals inhibit Na+ channels, including adrenergic agonists, tricyclic antidepressants, general anaesthetics, substance P inhibitors, menthol and nerve toxins (saxitoxin, scorpion toxin and tetrodotoxin). The nerve toxins block the Na+ channel from the **extracellular side**.
- Hadzic A. *Textbook of Regional Anesthesia and Acute Pain Management*. 1st ed. New York, NY: McGraw-Hill Medical; 2006. p. 112.

A3 A

Table 2.1 Differences between the two groups of local anaesthetics

Property	Esters	Amides
Bond in hydrocarbon chain	Ester type	Amide type
Metabolism	Plasma esterases	Hepatic enzyme N-dealkylation and hydroxylation
Potency	Generally less (except tetracaine)	Generally more
Synthesis	Were manufactured first	Were manufactured later
Allergic reactions	More common because of para-aminobenzoic acid (PABA)	Rare
Duration of action	Shorter	Longer
Toxicity	Generally less (except tetracaine and cocaine)	Generally more
Examples	Cocaine Benzocaine Procaine Tetracaine 2-Chlorprocaine	Lignocaine Mepivacaine Prilocaine Bupivacaine Ropivacaine Levobupivacaine

Note: the esters have a single 'i' in their names, while the amides have two 'i's.
- Mulroy MF, Bernards CM, McDonald SB, *et al. A Practical Approach to Regional Anesthesia*. 4th ed. Philadelphia, PA: Lippincott Williams & Wilkins; 2008. pp. 1–3.

A4 D

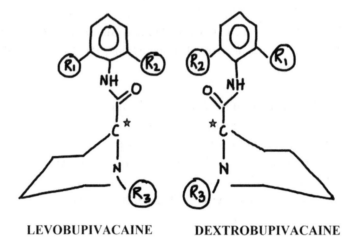

LEVOBUPIVACAINE   DEXTROBUPIVACAINE

Figure 2.2 Bupivacaine enantiomers (asterisks show asymmetric carbon atoms)

▶ Stereoisomerism describes those compounds which have the same molecular formula and chemical structure, but a different three-dimensional configuration. Stereoisomers may be **geometric or optical (enantiomers)**.

▶ Geometric isomerism or cis–trans isomerism describes the orientation of functional groups within the molecule. Such isomers typically contain double bonds or ring structures, where the rotation of bonds is greatly restricted.

▶ Optical isomers have **chiral** centres, such as a **quaternary nitrogen or carbon atom** surrounded by different chemical groups. Such a molecule is called a **chiral molecule**, as it lacks an internal plane of symmetry. As a result, these molecules have **non-superimposable mirror images**, imparting a particular type of stereoisomerism called **enantiomerism**. The non-superimposable mirror images depending on the configuration exist as R (rectus) and S (sinistra) isomers. Many substances in anaesthesia are chiral (volatile anaesthetics, ketamine, thiopental and local anaesthetics); however, few are **achiral** (sevoflurane, lignocaine, procaine, tetracaine).

▶ **Optical rotation (optical activity)** is the ability to turn the plane of **linearly polarised** light about the direction of motion as the light travels through a substance. Pure enantiomers may be dextrorotatory (d), (+) or levorotatory (l), (–). Based on the above two properties isomers can be referred to as R(+) and R(–) or S(+) and S(–) isomers.

▶ Racemic mixtures consist of equal amount of both enantiomers, and therefore do not rotate polarised light in either direction. Non-racemic mixtures have unequal amounts of two enantiomers. Pure enantiomers may have differences in absorption, distribution, potency, therapeutic action and most importantly toxicity profiles (ropivacaine and levo-bupivacaine).

- Cousins MJ, Bridenbaugh PO, Carr DB, *et al. Cousins and Bridenbaugh's Neural Blockade in Clinical Anesthesia and Pain Medicine*. 4th ed. Philadelphia, PA: Lippincott Williams & Wilkins; 2008. pp. 50–1.

A5   C The important physicochemical properties of LA are their **molecular weight (MW), pKa (ionisation), aqueous solubility, lipid solubility and protein binding**.

- ▶ **MW**: Addition of a butyl group to mepivacaine (MW 246) results in formation of bupivacaine (MW 288). This increase in molecular weight results in higher lipid solubility, i.e. partition coefficient (pKa), higher protein binding and higher potency.
- ▶ **pKa**: is the pH at which half the LA molecules are in the base form and half in the acid form. Most LAs have a pKa between 7.5 and 9.0 (weak bases). Because the LAs are supplied as unbuffered acidic solutions (salts of HCl) with pH of 3.5–5.0, the ionised form predominate. On injection into tissues (pH 7.4), the unionised form predominates and enters the cell to produce Na+ blockade. The closer the pKa to the extracellular pH (7.4), the higher the number of unionised forms available and the faster the onset of action. **Hence lignocaine with (pKa 7.7) has faster onset than bupivacaine (pKa 8.1)**.
- ▶ **Aqueous solubility**: It is the presence of the tertiary amine group that provides for ionisation and hence aqueous solubility. It is related directly to the extent of ionisation and inversely to its lipid solubility. **Benzocaine** lacks an ionisable amino group, and therefore has poor aqueous solubility, restricting it to only topical use.
- ▶ **Lipid solubility**: (sometimes wrongly called hydrophobicity) is dependent on the size of the alkyl group on tertiary amine increasing with its size. **It is directly proportional to LA potency, duration of action and toxicity. The distribution coefficient** of LA is the ratio of concentration of LA in a mix of an aqueous buffer and a hydrophobic lipid (octanol) after separation. The partition coefficient is the distribution coefficient at pH of 7.4 (octanol : buffer 7.4).
- ▶ **Protein binding**: In general, lipophilicity is **proportional** to protein binding. LA binds to both α1-acid glycoprotein and albumin, and this is **pH-dependent**, decreasing with acidosis increasing the amount of free drug in acidic environment. This lowers safety of LA in hypoproteinemic conditions like malnutrition, nephrotic syndrome and cirrhosis.

- Mulroy MF, Bernards CM, McDonald SB, *et al. A Practical Approach to Regional Anesthesia.* 4th ed. Philadelphia, PA: Lippincott Williams & Wilkins; 2008. pp. 1–4.

A6   B See Table 2.2 below

- Cousins MJ, Bridenbaugh PO, Carr DB, *et al. Cousins and Bridenbaugh's Neural Blockade in Clinical Anesthesia and Pain Medicine.* 4th ed. Philadelphia, PA: Lippincott Williams & Wilkins; 2008. p. 53.

A7   C

- ▶ 2-Chlorprocaine is a congener of procaine and thus an **ester**. It has low potency, a fast onset and short duration of action. It has been recently used for ambulatory surgeries under spinal anaesthesia.
- ▶ Most LAs are chiral, except lignocaine, procaine and tetracaine.
- ▶ Ropivacaine has a **propyl group** in its tertiary amine, while bupivacaine has a **butyl group**. This probably explains its lower potency, lower lipid solubility and lower toxicity than bupivacaine.
- ▶ All LAs are vasodilators (at high concentration), except cocaine and ropivacaine, which are **vasoconstrictors**.
  - Hadzic A. *Textbook of Regional Anesthesia and Acute Pain Management.* 1st ed. New York, NY: McGraw-Hill Medical; 2006. p. 123.
  - Mulroy MF, Bernards CM, McDonald SB, *et al. A Practical Approach to Regional Anesthesia.* 4th ed. Philadelphia, PA: Lippincott Williams & Wilkins; 2008. pp. 1–4.

Table 2.2 Common features of local anaesthetics

Property	*Implication*
Weak bases with pKa > 7.4	Free base has poor aqueous solubility
Available as **acidic solutions** (HCl salts)	Results in improved aqueous solubility
Exist in **equilibrium** of free base (unionised, lipid-soluble) and cationic (ionised, water-soluble)	This equilibrium can be shifted to either side by altering the pH of solution (hence adding HCO_3 to LA increases the availability of free base)
Body buffers raise pH	This raises the amount of free base present; the closer the pKa to the extracellular pH (7.4), the faster the onset of action
Free base (lipid-soluble) crosses neural membranes	Passes intracellularly to be ionised
Cationic moiety (water-soluble) is the active part	It blocks the Na+ channel from the inside

A8   A On the basis of their anaesthetic profile, LAs are classified as:
- **low** potency and short duration (procaine and 2-chlorprocaine)
- **intermediate** potency and duration (prilocaine, lignocaine and mepivacaine)
- **high** potency and long duration of action (tetracaine, etidocaine, bupivacaine and ropivacaine).

Table 2.3 Physicochemical properties of ester local anaesthetics

Agents	Chemical formula	Potency	pKa	Protein binding (%)	Onset	Duration
Cocaine	$C_{17}H_{21}NO_4$	N/A	8.6	92	Moderate	30–60 minutes
Benzocaine	$C_9H_{11}NO_2$	N/A	3.5	N/A	Moderate	30–60 minutes
Procaine	$C_{13}H_{20}N_2O_2$	1	8.9	6	Fast	30–60 minutes
Chlorprocaine	$C_{13}H_{19}ClN_2O_2$	1	8.7	N/A	Fast	30–60 minutes
Tetracaine	$C_{15}H_{24}N_2O_2$	8	8.5	75	Fast (spinal)	2–4 hours (spinal)

Table 2.4 Physiochemical properties of amide local anaesthetics

Agents	MW (kDa)	Chemical formula	Potency	pKa	Protein binding (%)	Onset	Duration (hours)
Prilocaine	220	$C_{13}H_{20}N_2O$	2	7.7	55	Fast	1–2
Lignocaine	234	$C_{14}H_{22}N_2O$	2	**7.7**	**65**	Fast	1–2
Mepivacaine	246	$C_{15}H_{22}N_2O$	2	7.6	78	Fast	2–3
Bupivacaine (butyl group)	**288**	$C_{18}H_{28}N_2O$	8	**8.1**	**95**	Moderate–slow	2–4
Etidocaine	276	$C_{17}H_{28}N_2O$	8	7.7	74	Moderate–slow	2–4
Ropivacaine (propyl group)	274	$C_{17}H_{26}N_2O$	4	**8.1**	**95**	Fast	2–4

Note: duration of LA action depends on the dose and the route of injection; ideally, the recommended doses should be block-specific.

- Cocaine is toxic and used topically in ophthalmic anaesthesia.
- Benzocaine and prilocaine may cause methaemoglobinaemia.
- Ropivacaine has a propyl group in its tertiary amine, while bupivacaine has a butyl group. It is less soluble, less potent and less toxic than bupivacaine. It produces less motor block as well. Mepivacaine, bupivacaine, ropivacaine and levobupivacaine share a **pipechol ring (2',6'-pipecoloxylidide)**.
  - Cousins MJ, Bridenbaugh PO, Carr DB, *et al. Cousins and Bridenbaugh's Neural Blockade in Clinical Anesthesia and Pain Medicine*. 4th ed. Philadelphia, PA: Lippincott Williams & Wilkins; 2008. pp. 97–8.
  - Mulroy MF, Bernards CM, McDonald SB, *et al. A Practical Approach to Regional Anesthesia*. 4th ed. Philadelphia, PA: Lippincott Williams & Wilkins; 2008. pp. 1–4.

A9 D

- Multiple **neuronal barriers** (epineurium, perineurium and endoneurium) must be crossed before LA can reach the nerve.
- The vasularity of the surrounding tissue, fascial layers and LA absorption by fat all have a detrimental effect on the delivery of LA to the nerve, and result in a decrease in onset. Hence, the **proximity** of injection to the nerve is the **most important factor** determining the onset of LA action.
- Importantly, it has been noted that the addition of **vasoconstrictors** and **hyaluronidase** may hasten the onset times.
- LA **dose** rather than the volume or concentration has been observed to affect the onset times.

  Lipophilic LAs are more likely to partition away from the hydrophilic extracellular fluid compartment into surrounding tissues and may bind to connective tissues rather than the nerve, and hence they have a slower onset. Clinically, bupivacaine (higher lipid solubility) has a slower onset than lignocaine (less lipid-soluble).
  - Mulroy MF, Bernards CM, McDonald SB, *et al. A Practical Approach to Regional Anesthesia*. 4th ed. Philadelphia, PA: Lippincott Williams & Wilkins; 2008. p. 11.

A10 D

- Block duration is largely dependent on the **drug clearance rate**.
- The **larger the dose given,** and the slower the metabolism and clearance, the greater the duration will be.
- **More lipid-soluble** LAs have longer duration of action because of slower clearance.

▶ At higher doses, LAs produce vasodilatation, enhancing their own clearance.

▶ Addition of **vasoconstrictors** may reduce clearance and enhance duration.

▶ Higher **protein binding** increases duration of action by virtue of lowering the free drug available for metabolism.

- Mulroy MF, Bernards CM, McDonald SB, *et al. A Practical Approach to Regional Anesthesia*. 4th ed. Philadelphia, PA: Lippincott Williams & Wilkins; 2008. p. 14.

A11 B

▶ The addition of vasoconstrictors such as adrenaline to LA acts by decreasing systemic absorption of the LA.

▶ This means more LA is available to act locally (on the peripheral nerve) **decreasing** onset time, but **improving** the degree of sensory and motor block, duration of the block and the area (extent) covered.

▶ The toxicity of LA may be reduced by lowering the peak plasma concentration, allowing administration of a greater dose.

▶ However, the effect of longer-acting LAs like bupivacaine may not be much affected.

- Cousins MJ, Bridenbaugh PO, Carr DB, *et al. Cousins and Bridenbaugh's Neural Blockade in Clinical Anesthesia and Pain Medicine*. 4th ed. Philadelphia, PA: Lippincott Williams & Wilkins; 2008. p. 101.

A12 D

▶ The pharmacological effects (neural blockade) and clinical effects (analgesia and anaesthesia) of LAs are the result of the drug absorption and its disposition. **Disposition** refers collectively to the process of **drug distribution** (into and out of the tissues) and **drug elimination** (by metabolism and excretion). An injection of LA undergoes **local disposition, systemic absorption and systemic disposition**.

▶ Local disposition of an injection drug pool near the nerve undergoes **neural tissue uptake**, non-neural tissue uptake, uptake by fat, and redistribution to cerebrospinal fluid (if neuraxial). This involves both bulk flow and diffusion. It is the neural tissue uptake that results in **neural blockade** (clinical effect).

- Cousins MJ, Bridenbaugh PO, Carr DB, *et al. Cousins and Bridenbaugh's Neural Blockade in Clinical Anesthesia and Pain Medicine*. 4th ed. Philadelphia, PA: Lippincott Williams & Wilkins; 2008. pp. 57–9.

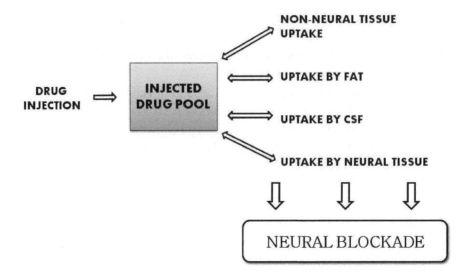

Figure 2.3 Local disposition of local anaesthetic

A13 C

Systemic absorption of LA is chiefly responsible for its **systemic toxicity (side effect)**. This is inferred from peak plasma concentration (C_{max}) and the time of its occurrence (T_{max}). This is not absolute, as the peak plasma concentration reflects the **net result** of systemic absorption and disposition.

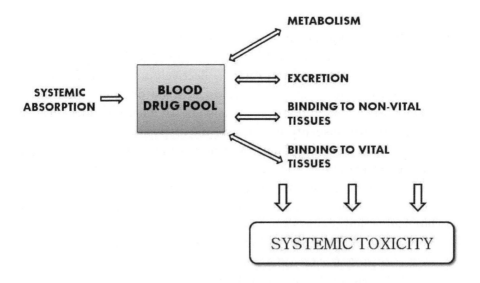

Figure 2.4 Systemic disposition of local anaesthetic

Table 2.5 Factors affecting systemic disposition of local anaesthetics

Property	Effect	Clinical relevance
Lipophilicity	Systemic absorption of longer-acting, more lipophilic agents is slower	Lignocaine absorption is faster, but bupivacaine is absorbed slowly into the circulation
Site of administration	Anatomical features such as vasularity and presence of tissues and fat that can bind LA influences disposition	*Intravascular > intrapleural > intercostal > caudal > epidural > brachial plexus > femoro-sciatic > subcutaneous > intra-articular > spinal*
Dosage	All other factors being constant, dose is the primary determinant of peak plasma concentrations after any route of injection	$C_{max} \propto$ dose given; therefore, **increased C_{max}**
Speed of injection	Accidental intravenous administration of LA may result in higher peak (C_{max}) with higher speed of injection	**Dose fractionation** may allow early detection of systemic toxicity
Vasocontrictor	Decrease rate of systemic absorption by reducing uptake	**Decreased C_{max}**
Depot formulations	Slow the release of local anaesthetic and hence its absorption	**Decreased C_{max}**

- Cousins MJ, Bridenbaugh PO, Carr DB, *et al. Cousins and Bridenbaugh's Neural Blockade in Clinical Anesthesia and Pain Medicine.* 4th ed. Philadelphia, PA: Lippincott Williams & Wilkins; 2008. pp. 59–72.

A14   B

❭ The systemic disposition of LA involves both its **distribution** (uptake by lung, plasma proteins and tissues) and its **elimination** (metabolism and excretion). Lung is the first capillary bed to be exposed to LA once it has entered the systemic circulation. This delays and reduces the exposure of brain and heart to LA.

❭ Protein binding of LA in blood is a **saturable process**. This implies that as the dose increases, the **fraction** of drug bound to plasma proteins **falls** (after saturation of all binding sites). Binding is of two types: high affinity and low capacity (α1-acid glycoprotein) and low affinity and high capacity (**albumin**). In **elevation** of the amount of α1-acid glycoprotein (cancer, inflammatory states, chronic pain, trauma, uraemia, postoperatively), binding capacity increases. However, with a **decline** in its level (pregnancy and neonates), this binding may be limited, resulting in a higher free fraction of LA.

▶ Ester LAs are rapidly cleared by plasma **pseudocholinesterase**. In hepatic and renal disease, a **decreased synthesis** of pseudocholinesterase may be responsible for its prolonged half-life. The erythrocyte esterase activity is preserved.

▶ The amides are metabolised in liver by *N*-dealkylation and hydroxylation. **Etidocaine** clearance is dependent mostly on liver blood flow, whereas that of **ropivacaine and bupivacaine** is dependent on hepatic enzymatic activity. The clearance of **lignocaine** is dependent on both hepatic blood flow and enzyme activity.

- Cousins MJ, Bridenbaugh PO, Carr DB, *et al. Cousins and Bridenbaugh's Neural Blockade in Clinical Anesthesia and Pain Medicine*. 4th ed. Philadelphia, PA: Lippincott Williams & Wilkins; 2008. pp. 72–80.

A15 **A** Amide LAs structurally have an alkyl chain, an aromatic ring and an amide bond between the two. They undergo *N*-**dealkylation, aromatic hydroxylation and amide hydrolysis** in liver.

▶ Lignocaine undergoes *N*-dealkylation by CYP3A4.

▶ Both bupivacaine and ropivacaine undergo *N*-dealkylation (CYP3A4) and hydroxylation (CYP1A2).

▶ Inhibitors of CYP3A4 (Itraconazole) reduce bupivacaine elimination while those of CYP1A2 (Fluvoxamine) reduced ropivacaine clearance.

▶ Inhibitors of CYP2D6 (beta blockers and H_2 antagonists) reduce hepatic blood flow and reduce metabolism of amide LA.

- Cousins MJ, Bridenbaugh PO, Carr DB, *et al. Cousins and Bridenbaugh's Neural Blockade in Clinical Anesthesia and Pain Medicine*. 4th ed. Philadelphia, PA: Lippincott Williams & Wilkins; 2008. p. 80.
- Hadzic A. *Textbook of Regional Anesthesia and Acute Pain Management*. 1st ed. New York, NY: McGraw-Hill Medical; 2006. p. 114.

A16   A

Table 2.6 Effects of patient variables on disposition of amide local anaesthetics

Physiological state	Pharmacokinetics	Reason	Implication
Foetus/age < 6 months	Reduced metabolism	Deficiency of CYP3A4	Use lower doses
Elderly	**Clearance of LA decreases with increasing age**	Reduced hepatic mass in elderly	Use lower doses
Obese	Terminal elimination half-life of lignocaine is prolonged	Increased volume of distribution rather than a decreased clearance	Dose according to **total body weight**
Cardiovascular disease	**High C$_{max}$ due to low volume of distribution and clearance**	Reduced hepatic blood flow and hepatocellular dysfunction	Use lower doses
Hepatic disease	**Prolonged half-life**	Reduced hepatic blood flow and hepatocellular dysfunction	Use lower doses
Renal disease	Disposition kinetics are **unaffected**	Amides are metabolised by liver	In **severe renal insufficiency**, clearance is halved and metabolites accumulate

Note: ester LAs are largely **unaffected** by hepatic disease, renal disease or pregnancy.

- Cousins MJ, Bridenbaugh PO, Carr DB, *et al. Cousins and Bridenbaugh's Neural Blockade in Clinical Anesthesia and Pain Medicine.* 4th ed. Philadelphia, PA: Lippincott Williams & Wilkins; 2008. pp. 80–2.

A17   D

- In pregnancy, though pseudocholinesterase levels may be decreased, the metabolism of **ester LA** is relatively preserved. Hence they have better toxicity profiles. Lignocaine is more dependent on hepatic blood flow, which is increased in pregnancy. This **increases its clearance**. **Bupivacaine** is more dependent on hepatic enzymatic activity, which is reduced in pregnancy, **reducing its clearance**.
- Pregnancy also increases **neural sensitivity** to LA. This has been

attributed to **progesterone**. However, progesterone has little effect on myocardial sensitivity to ropivacaine, as shown by in vitro studies.

- Cousins MJ, Bridenbaugh PO, Carr DB, *et al. Cousins and Bridenbaugh's Neural Blockade in Clinical Anesthesia and Pain Medicine.* 4th ed. Philadelphia, PA: Lippincott Williams & Wilkins; 2008. p. 81.
- Hadzic A. *Textbook of Regional Anesthesia and Acute Pain Management.* 1st ed. New York, NY: McGraw-Hill Medical; 2006. p. 124.

A18 D Various adjuncts have been used with local anaesthetics for either prolonging their actions or reducing side effects. They may be used for neuraxial (spinal or epidural) or peripheral nerve blocks.

Table 2.7 Adjuncts used in regional anaesthesia

Routes	Favoured	Have been used but not favoured
Spinal	Opioids (except cocaine and remifentanil)	Ketorolac
	Adrenalin and phenylephrine	Neostigmine
	Clonidine	Midazolam
Epidural	Opioids	Ketamine
	Vasoconstrictors	Neostigmine
	Clonidine	
	Sodium bicarbonate	
Peripheral nerves	Adrenalin	Magnesium
	Clonidine	Ketorolac
	Sodium bicarbonate	Neostigmine
	Opioids	Ketamine
	Dexamethasone	

- Hadzic A. *Textbook of Regional Anesthesia and Acute Pain Management.* 1st ed. New York, NY: McGraw-Hill Medical; 2006. pp. 139, 153.

A19 D

▶ Opioid receptors have been found to exist in the spinal cord and peripheral nerves as well. Given spinally or epidurally, opioids **reduce the afferent nociception input**, providing analgesia. Thus, they act **synergistically** with local analgesics. Because they help reduce the amount of LA needed, they confer **cardiovascular stability**; however, owing to action on sympathetic ganglia, they may reduce sympathetic outflow, resulting in hypotension.

▶ Intrathecal opioids help reduce the amount of local anaesthetic required, offer added analgesia and may prolong the total duration of analgesia.

However, morphine through this route may increase the risk of **delayed respiratory depression** due to rostral migration through cerebrospinal fluid. Lipophilic opioids like fentanyl and sufentanil hasten the onset but offer limited duration. Sufentanil probably acts systemically rather than spinally, as it is highly lipophilic. Remifentanil is not used via this route as it contains glycine. When used with chlorprocaine, opioids may actually **delay discharge in ambulatory settings**.

▶ Epidural fentanyl reduces volatile requirements when compared with its use intravenously. As a bolus, it acts **spinally**, while as an infusion it is said to exert a **systemic** effect.

▶ Side effects of neuraxial opioids include pruritis, urinary retention, nausea and delayed respiratory depression.

Doses:

Spinal: morphine 100–200 μg, fentanyl 10–25 μg

Epidural: morphine 40 μg/kg, fentanyl 1–2 μg/kg

- Hadzic A. *Textbook of Regional Anesthesia and Acute Pain Management*. 1st ed. New York, NY: McGraw-Hill Medical; 2006. p. 134.

A20 B

▶ Addition of vasoconstrictors helps in reducing total dose, hastens onset and prolongs duration of action of LAs. Although this is mediated postsynaptically (via α1 and α2 receptors), the intrinsic **analgesic effect** is mediated through **presynaptic α2 receptors**. Epidurally administered adrenaline produces **mild vasodilatation** in typical doses. Mean arterial pressure (MAP) is decreased, while the cardiac output (CO) rises. Higher doses result in increased MAP and a fall in CO.

▶ In ambulatory settings, return of bladder function and discharge is delayed, limiting its usefulness. Addition of adrenaline to bupivacaine or ropivacaine does not prolong action to the extent that it prolongs the action of lignocaine. Addition of adrenaline to chloroprocaine causes **flu-like symptoms**. Hence this is not advocated.

Doses:

1 : 200,000 or 5 μg/mL of adrenaline or 0.2 mg phenylephrine

- Hadzic A. *Textbook of Regional Anesthesia and Acute Pain Management*. 1st ed. New York, NY: McGraw-Hill Medical; 2006. p. 135.

A21 A

▸ Alpha-2 adrenergic agonists like clonidine act presynaptically to **reduce the nociceptive input** at **spinal** level. In addition, they **reduce central sympathetic drive** by action on locus ceruleus and nucleus tractus solitarius. Hence they produce sedation, dry mouth, hypotension and bradycardia as main adverse effects.

▸ Though highly lipophilic, they act spinally, acting synergistically with **opioids**. They may reduce anaesthetic requirements when combined with general anaesthesia. Because they lack respiratory depression, pruritis and cause less urinary retention, they may be **better for ambulatory settings**.

Doses:

> Spinal: usual dose 2 µg/kg
> Low dose: 1.5 µg/kg

- Hadzic A. *Textbook of Regional Anesthesia and Acute Pain Management*. 1st ed. New York, NY: McGraw-Hill Medical; 2006. pp. 136–7.

A22. C

▸ Because local anaesthetics are available as solutions of hydrochloride salts, the resultant pH falls to 3.5–4. Addition of bicarbonate to such solutions results in increasing pH toward pKa and increases the fraction of free base present. This **hastens the onset** and may **intensify epidural anaesthesia**. This has not been seen with ropivacaine.

▸ Restoration of pH towards pKa improves adrenaline action, and alkalinisation of adrenaline containing LA solutions may result in **hypotension** (secondary to higher concentration of LA produced by adrenaline).

▸ Excessive carbonation may **precipitate** LAs; hence the following limits are prescribed.

Doses:
> Lignocaine: 1 mL of NaHCO₃ per 10 mL of solution.
> Bupivacaine: 0.1 mL of NaHCO₃ per 10 mL of solution

- Hadzic A. *Textbook of Regional Anesthesia and Acute Pain Management*. 1st ed. New York, NY: McGraw-Hill Medical; 2006. pp. 137–8.

A23 A

- ⟩ **Liposomal morphine** can produce long-lasting analgesia (2 days) when given epidurally. However, it should not be given along with local anaesthetics, as this may cause early and uncontrolled release of morphine, causing loss of advantage and occurrence of adverse effects.
- ⟩ Intrathecal neostigmine produces analgesia by reducing atylcholine breakdown (it is an analgesia at spinal level), but is limited by **hypotension and nausea**. Epidural ketamine and intrathecal ketorolac have not shown neurotoxicity in animal studies. Intrathecal midazolam is effective analgesia, but again, neurotoxicity profile has yet to be evaluated.
  - Hadzic A. *Textbook of Regional Anesthesia and Acute Pain Management*. 1st ed. New York, NY: McGraw-Hill Medical; 2006. pp. 139–40.
  - Viscusi ER, Martin G, Hartrick CT, *et al*. Forty-eight hours of postoperative pain relief after total hip arthroplasty with a novel, extended-release epidural morphine formulation. *Anesthesiology*. 2005; **102**(5): 1014–22.

A24 D

- ⟩ The agents shown to be effective as adjuncts with local anaesthetics in peripheral nerve blocks include **clonidine, dexamethasone, buprenorhine and tramadol**.
- ⟩ **Magnesium, ketorolac and clonidine** are effective in intravenous regional anaesthesia.
- ⟩ **Morphine** reduces donor-site bone pain when infiltrated at the donor bone graft site.
- ⟩ Intra-articluar **morphine, clonidine, neostigmine and ketorolac have produced prolonged analgesia**.
  - Gentili M, Houssel P, Osman M, *et al*. Intra-articular morphine and clonidine produce comparable analgesia but the combination is not more effective. *Br J Anaesth*. 1997; **79**: 660–1.
  - Hadzic A. *Textbook of Regional Anesthesia and Acute Pain Management*. 1st ed. New York, NY: McGraw-Hill Medical; 2006. pp. 139–40.
  - Reuben SS, Connelly NR. Postoperative analgesia for outpatient arthroscopic knee surgery with intraarticular bupivacaine and ketorolac. *Anesth Analg*. 1995; **80**: 1154–7.
  - Yang LC, Chen LM, Wang CJ, *et al*. Postoperative analgesia by intra-articular neostigmine in patients undergoing knee arthroscopy. *Anesthesiology*. 1998; **88**: 334–9.

A25 D

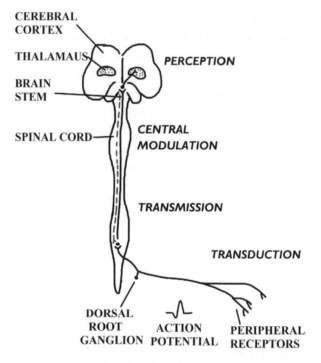

CEREBRAL CORTEX
THALAMAUS
BRAIN STEM
SPINAL CORD

PERCEPTION

CENTRAL MODULATION

TRANSMISSION

TRANSDUCTION

DORSAL ROOT GANGLION **ACTION POTENTIAL** **PERIPHERAL RECEPTORS**

Figure 2.5 Steps involved in pain pathway

Table 2.8 Sites of action of analgesics

Site of action and mechanism	Examples
Transduction: act at the site of injury and prevent action of inflammatory mediators	NSAIDs Antihistaminics Membrane-stabilising agents Opioids Bradykinin and serotonin antagonists Local anaesthetics
Transmission: alter nerve conduction	Local anaesthetics
Modulation: modify spinal and supraspinal modulation	Intrathecal and epidural opioids α2 Agonists NMDA antagonists: ketamine, magnesium, tramadol
Perception: act centrally to reduce perception	Parenteral opioids α2 Agonists General anaesthetics

- Barash PG, Cullen BF, Stoelting RK, *et al. Clinical Anesthesia.* 6th ed. Philadelphia, PA: Lippincott Williams & Wilkins; 2009. p. 1476.

A26 D Opioid receptors are a group of **G protein–coupled receptors** with opioids as ligands. The endogenous opioids are dynorphins, enkephalins, endorphins and nociceptin. Opiate receptors are distributed widely in the brain, spinal cord and peripheral tissues.

Table 2.9 Types of opioid receptors

Receptor type	Endogenous ligand	Desirable actions	Undesirable actions
OP1 (KOP/Ќ)	Dynorphin β-Endorphin	Analgesia	Dysphoria, psychomimetic effects, dieresis
OP2 (DOP/δ)	Enkephalin β-Endorphin	Supraspinal and spinal analgesia, sedation	Constipation, physical dependence
OP3 (MOP/µ)	Enkephalin β-Endorphin	Supraspinal and spinal analgesia, sedation	Respiratory depression, bradycardia, miosis, urinary retention, pruritis, nausea and vomiting, constipation, physical dependence
OP4 (NOP)	Nociception		**Anti-analgesia**

Note:

▶ MOP is present in **para-aqueductal grey (PAG)** of brain and descending inhibitory control pathway, and mediates most of the actions of opioids. It augments descending inhibition (reducing pain or providing analgesia).

▶ KOP inhibits descending inhibitory pathways, hence is **anti-analgesic**.

▶ The effects of **sigma (σ) receptor** are not antagonised by naloxone, and hence this receptor is not classified as an opioid receptor anymore.

  • Smith T, Pinnock C, Lin T, *et al. Fundamentals of Anaesthesia.* 3rd ed. Cambridge: Cambridge University Press; 2009. pp. 587–9.

A27 D

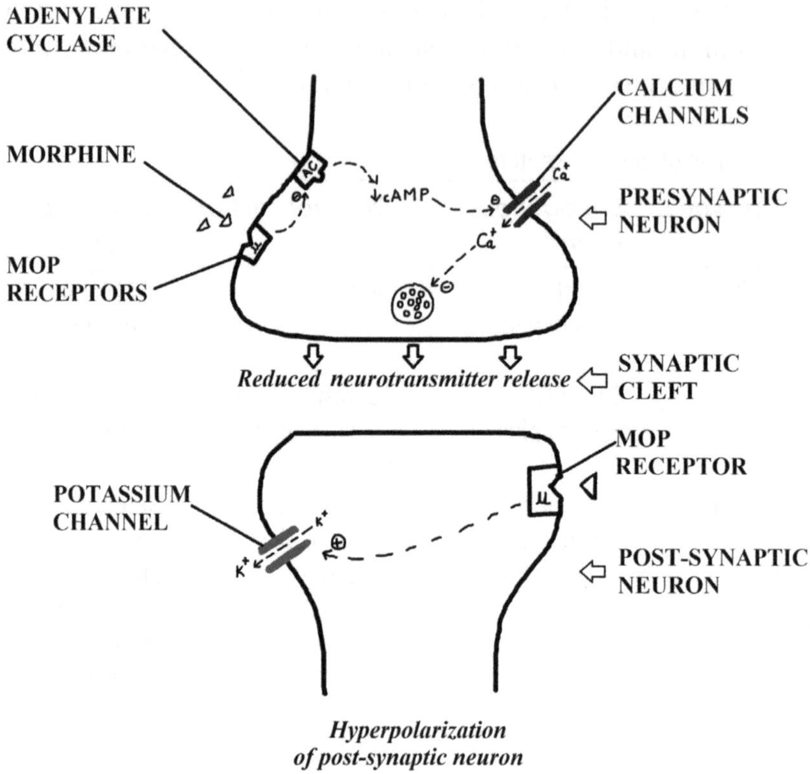

Figure 2.6 Mechanism of action of opioids

Table 2.10 Mechanism of action of opioids

Site and action	Effects	Example
Presynaptic		
Inhibition of adenylate cyclase (needed for Ca+ influx) Inhibition of Ca+ influx Facilitation of K+ efflux (hyperpolarisation)	Failure of excitatory neurotransmitter release (glutamate) at dorsal horn	KOP and NOP: prevent Ca+ influx MOP, DOP: facilitate K efflux
Post-synaptic		
Facilitation of K+ efflux (hyperpolarisation)	Failure of action potential generation	MOP, DOP: facilitate K+ efflux

- McDonald J, Lambert DG. Opioid receptors. *Contin Educ Anaesth Crit Care Pain*. 2005; **5**(1): 22–5.

A28 C **Opiate** refers to only the alkaloids in opium and the natural and semi-synthetic derivatives of opium. The term **'opioid'** includes all naturally occurring or synthetic drugs that have stereospecific actions at opioid receptors, the effects of which can be antagonised by naloxone.

Table 2.11 Classification of opioids by synthesis

Endogenous	Natural	Semi-synthetic	Fully synthetic	Opioid-like drugs
Endorphins	Morphine	Heroin	Pethidine	Tramadol
Enkephalin	Codeine	Hydromorphone	Fentanyl	
Dynorphine	Thebaine	Hydrocodone	Alfentanyl	
Nociception		Oxymorphone	Remifentanyl	
		Oxycodone	Sufentanil	
		Buprenorphine		
		Dextrometharphan		

Table 2.12 Classification of opioids by action

Receptor	Agonist	Partial agonist	Antagonist
MOP (μ)	Morphine, pethidine, methadone, fentanyl, alfentanyl, remifentanyl sufentanil	Buprenorphine	Naloxone Naltrexone **Pentazocine** **Nalorphine**
DOP (δ)	Morphine (μ > δ) **Pentazocine** **Nalorphine**		Naloxone Naltrexone
KOP (Ḱ)			Naloxone

Agonist-antagonists: pentazocine, nalbuphine and butorphanol.

A29 D Tolerance and dependence are induced by chronic exposure to opioids. **Tolerance** means that higher doses of opioids are required to produce the same effect, reducing the maximum response attainable. It is mainly due to **receptor desensitisation**. Tolerance develops to most of the adverse effects as well, like dysphoria, itching, urinary retention and respiratory depression, but occurs more slowly to the analgesia and other physical side effects. **However, tolerance does not develop to constipation or miosis.**

A30 **A** Analgesic efficacy is determined by calculating the '**number needed to treat (NNT)**'. NNT is defined as the average number of patients who need to be treated (with analgesic drug) to prevent one additional bad outcome (pain). It is defined as the **inverse of the absolute risk reduction**.

NNT = 1/(proportion of patients with at least 50% pain relief with analgesic – proportion of patients with at least 50% pain relief with placebo)

Various analgesics have been compared in the Oxford league table of analgesic efficacy. Codeine 60 mg is **least** efficacious, while selective COX-2 inhibitors are **most** efficacious.
*   www.medicine.ox.ac.uk/bandolier/booth/painpag/acutrev/analgesics/lftab. html

A31 **B**

Table 2.13 Opioids and their metabolites

Drug	Enzyme system	Active metabolite	Actions
Morphine	UGT2B7	**Morphine-6-glucuronide** (10% but active) Morphine-3-glucuronide (80% but inactive)	M6G: analgesia M3G: hyperalgesia
Diamorphine	Ester hydrolysis	6-Monoacetylmorphine (MAM) and morphine	Morphine is active component
Pethidine	CYP3A4	Norpethidine	50% analgesic action; neurotoxicity
Codeine	CYP2D6	Morphine, nor codeine	Morphine: analgesia
Tramadol	CYP2D6	O-desmethyltramadol (M1 metabolite)	Analgesia

Note: norfentanyl is an **inactive** metabolite of fentanyl; propacetamol is a prodrug of paracetamol.
*   Nagar S, Raffa RB. Looking beyond the administered drug: metabolites of opioid analgesics. *J Fam Pract.* 2008; **57**(6 Suppl.): S25–32.

A32 D

Table 2.14 Dose equivalence of opioids

Route	Ratio (as compared to oral morphine)	Example
Oral morphine	1 : 1	30 mg
Intravenous morphine	1 : 3	10 mg
Intramuscular morphine	1 : 2	15 mg
Subcutaneous morphine	1 : 2	15 mg
Subcutaneous diamorphine	1 : 4 (as diamorphine has two molecules of morphine)	7.5 mg
Perioperative doses	± 20%	

Epidural dose of morphine is 1 : 10 of oral (up to 5 mg), while intrathecal is 1 : 100 (100–200 mcg).

- Lewis NL, Williams JE. Acute pain management in patients receiving opioids for chronic and cancer pain. *Contin Educ Anaesth Crit Care Pain*. 2005; **5**(4): 127–9.

A33 A **Salient features of morphine** are as follows.

- Particularly effective for **visceral pain**, while less effective for sharp pain.
- Nausea and vomiting: stimulation of **CTZ (5-HT$_3$ and dopamine receptors)**.
- Can cause histamine release if administered rapidly or in large doses, resulting in bronchospasm and hypotension; **take naloxone**.
- Pruritus when given intrathecally or epidurally. It is not histamine-mediated and is treated with **naloxone**. Ondansetron, propofol and antihistaminics have been used. Recent peripherally acting antagonists such as **methylnaltrexone** have been used to reverse peripheral side effects without reversing centrally mediated analgesia.
- Meiosis through stimulation of Edinger–Westphal nucleus; reversed by **atropine**.
- Can induce antidieresis by increasing antidiuretic hormone secretion, resulting in water retention and hyponatremia.
- Chest wall rigidity mediated by interaction with dopaminergic and GABAergic pathways in substantia nigra and striatum. Difficulty in ventilation can result following administration of opioids at induction: **take with muscle relaxants**.
- Morphine is a weak base, hence it is absorbed from the small bowel. This delays absorption and results in slow onset of oral dose. Oral

bioavailability is 30% because of **high first-pass metabolism** in liver. Intravenous and intramuscular bioavailability are higher and onset is faster (10 and 30 minutes, respectively). Neuraxial morphine is associated with rostral spread and **delayed respiratory depression**. Because of low lipid solubility, its absorption from the subcutaneous route is **slow** and so is **usually avoided**.

▶ It is metabolised by **UGT2B7** to **active** morphine-6-glucuronide (M6G) (10%–30%) and an inactive morphine-3-glucuronide (M3G) (70%–90%). M6G is two to four times as potent as morphine, is more hydrophilic, stays in the brain for a longer period and undergoes entero-hepatic circulation. M3G may be associated with **morphine-induced hyperalgesia**.

- Peck TE, Hill S. *Pharmacology for Anaesthesia and Intensive Care*. 3rd ed. Cambridge: Cambridge University Press; 2008. pp. 139–42.

A34 D

Table 2.15 Morphine disposition in susceptible populations

Patient group	Characteristic	Effect and implication
Age < 3 months	Reduced conjugation and renal excretion ability	Prolonged duration, so be cautious; prefer shorter-acting opioids (fentanyl > morphine)
Elderly	Reduced lean mass and hepatic blood flow Increased sensitivity	Reduce doses
High body mass index	Lean body weight < total body weight Higher chances of obstructive sleep apnoea	Calculate doses according to lean body weight Careful use of sedatives and opioids in view of obstructive sleep apnoea
Liver failure	Reduced metabolism and increased elimination half-life Increased sensitivity (along with encephalopathy)	Cautious use in small titrated doses
Renal failure	Accumulation of M6G metabolite (renally excreted) Uraemic encephalopathy may increase sensitivity	Higher chances of toxicity

- Smith T, Pinnock C, Lin T, *et al*. *Fundamentals of Anaesthesia*. 3rd ed. Cambridge: Cambridge University Press; 2009. p. 596.

A35 D **Salient features of diamorphine** are as follows.
- It is diacetylmorphine (having two molecules of morphine). It is a **pro-drug** that is metabolised to **6-monoacetylmorphine (6-MAM)** and then to morphine through **ester hydrolysis**. Its analgesic action is then mediated by morphine.
- Because it has two morphine molecules, it is **twice** as potent.
- It has higher lipid solubility than morphine (but lower than fentanyl/sufentanil). This makes it particularly well suited for subcutaneous administration.
- Orally, it has a high first-pass metabolism.
- Given intrathecally, it has a shorter duration of action than morphine (6 vs 12 hours) because of its higher lipid solubility. This reduces the likelihood of delayed respiratory depression when compared with morphine.
- As it causes high euphoria, it is a drug of abuse (street name is **heroin**).
  - Peck TE, Hill S. *Pharmacology for Anaesthesia and Intensive Care*. 3rd ed. Cambridge: Cambridge University Press; 2008. p. 142.

A36 D **Salient features of methadone** are as follows.
- It is a synthetic opioid agonist used extensively in **opioid de-addiction**.
- It is highly lipid-soluble, has a low first-pass metabolism, high oral bio-availability (80%), high protein binding (90%) and it undergoes rapid *N*-demethylation to inactive metabolites.
- It has a **longer duration of action (30 hours)**, hence prevents withdrawal reactions.
- It is an **NMDA antagonist**, and has been found useful in many opioid-resistant **chronic pain** states.
  - http://pain-topics.org/pdf/OralMethadoneDosing.pdf
  - Peck TE, Hill S. *Pharmacology for Anaesthesia and Intensive Care*. 3rd ed. Cambridge: Cambridge University Press; 2008. p. 143.

A37 D **Salient features of codeine** are as follows.
- It is methylmorphine (prodrug) and has one-tenth the potency of morphine.
- Used orally (bioavailability 50%) or intramuscularly in doses: 30–60 mg (adult) and 0.5–1.0 mg/kg (paediatric). The intravenous route is avoided because of hypotension (histamine release).
- Metabolism is by:
  - glucuronidation (20%) to codeine-glucuronide
  - N-demethylation (10%–20%) to norcodeine

- *O*-demethylation (5%–15%) to morphine by **CYP2D6**: responsible for its analgesic action
- excretion unchanged (15%).

▶ CYP2D6 exhibits **genetic polymorphism**, hence poor metabolisers have poor analgesia. Tramadol undergoes similar *O*-demethylation to *O*-desmethyltramadol (higher affinity than parent compound) via CYP2D6. Poor metabolisers show reduced analgesic activity to tramadol as well.

▶ It is a potent **antitussive**, with **constipation** being its main adverse effect.

▶ Dihydrocodeine is twice as potent.
- Coniam SW, Mendham J. *Principles of Pain Management for Anaesthetists*. 1st ed. London: Hodder Arnold Publication: 2005. p. 44.
- Peck TE, Hill S. *Pharmacology for Anaesthesia and Intensive Care*. 3rd ed. Cambridge: Cambridge University Press; 2008. p. 144.

A38 C **Salient features of tramadol** are as follows.

▶ It is a phenylpiperidine analogue of codeine.

▶ It is an opioid-like drug having a weak agonist effect on MOP (μ) receptors. Its effects are reversed by naloxone.

▶ It is a norepinephrine and serotonin reuptake inhibitor, producing analgesia by enhancing **descending inhibitory pathways** (which need NE and 5-HT for stimulation).

▶ For the same reason, it potentiates 5-HT (serotonin) levels when administered concurrently with MAO inhibitors, producing **serotonin syndrome**.

▶ It may lower seizure threshold and so should be **avoided in epileptics**.

▶ It has high oral bioavailability (70%) and undergoes *O*-demethylation to *O*-desmethyltramadol (higher affinity than parent compound) via **CYP2D6**. Poor metabolisers show reduced analgesic activity to tramadol.

▶ Opioids are used to treat post-operative shivering (pethidine and tramadol in particular).

▶ Nausea is the most limiting side effect (due to 5-HT action on CTZ); take ondansetron.

▶ It has a low abuse potential and hence it is not a controlled drug.
- Coniam SW, Mendham J. *Principles of Pain Management for Anaesthetists*. 1st ed. London: Hodder Arnold Publication: 2005. pp. 44–5.
- Peck TE, Hill S. *Pharmacology for Anaesthesia and Intensive Care*. 3rd ed. Cambridge: Cambridge University Press; 2008. p. 148.

A39 B Pethidine:

- Is an anticholinergic drug that was later found to have analgesic actions.
- Higher lipid solubility hastens the onset, but also offers higher transfer to foetus when given during labour.
- **One-tenth** the potency of morphine.
- Metabolised to **norpethidine** (active metabolite with 50% activity), which can accumulate in renal failure.

Fentanyl:

- **Hundred times** the potency of morphine.
- **Highly lipid-soluble**, hence dissipates to systemic circulation quickly when given intrathecally. This reduces rostral spread potential, reducing the consequent respiratory depression.
- Useful in paediatrics due to its shorter action than morphine.
- Metabolised to **inactive** norfentanyl.

Alfentanil:

- **Ten times** the potency of morphine.
- Lower lipid solubility than fentanyl, but lower pKa (6.5 vs 8.4 at pH 7.4). This results in higher fraction of unionised drug (89% vs 9% with fentanyl) resulting in **faster onset**.

Remifentanil:

- Used as an infusion only. Not used intrathecally (as commercial preparation has glycine).
- Metabolised by ester hydrolysis, having a context-sensitive half-life of **4 minutes**. Hence does not accumulate despite prolonged infusions. However, **analgesia does not continue post-operatively**, and a morphine bolus is required at the end of surgery for postoperative analgesia.
  - Coniam SW, Mendham J. *Principles of Pain Management for Anaesthetists*. 1st ed. London: Hodder Arnold Publication: 2005. pp. 45–6.
  - Peck TE, Hill S. *Pharmacology for Anaesthesia and Intensive Care*. 3rd ed. Cambridge: Cambridge University Press; 2008. pp. 145–7.

A40 C Naloxone:

- It is an opioid receptor antagonist at all three receptors.
- It is an *N*-allyl derivative of **oxymorphone**.
- It is used for opioid overdose rather than dependence (**naltrexone** is used for opioid and alcohol dependence).

▶ It is short-acting, hence is best given as a bolus followed by an infusion.
▶ Opioid reversal can produce withdrawal symptoms, including seizures and pulmonary edema, especially in a neonate.

A41 B Paracetamol:
▶ It is a weak analgesic, antipyretic and and a very weak anti-inflammatory.
▶ It inhibits CNS prostaglandin synthesis.
▶ Metabolised in liver to **N-acetyl-*p*-benzoquinone imine (NAPQI)**, which is very toxic. It is rapidly detoxified by **glutathione**, hence paracetamol overdose results in glutathione depletion and consequent hepatotoxicity. This can be treated with **methionine** (promotes glutathione synthesis) and **N-acetylcysteine** (precursor of glutathione).
▶ Oral/intravenous dose is 20 mg/kg (adult) and 15 mg/kg (paediatric).
▶ Propacetamol is the prodrug form of paracetamol (intravenous formulation). The intravenous formulation is more effective than the oral.
▶ Combined with a weaker opioid (tramadol or codeine), its efficacy may exceed morphine because of synergism.
   • Coniam SW, Mendham J. *Principles of Pain Management for Anaesthetists*. 1st ed. London: Hodder Arnold Publication: 2005. p. 39.
   • www.medicine.ox.ac.uk/bandolier/booth/painpag/acutrev/analgesics/lftab. html

A42 B NSAIDs:
▶ Mechanism: act by **reversible** cyclooxygenase (COX) inhibition. Two isoenzymes are found:
   – **COX-1: constitutively** expressed in kidneys (prostaglandin production for maintenance of renal blood flow) and gastric mucosa (protection against acidity).
   – **COX-2: inducible**. Expressed at the site of injury in response to inflammation.
▶ They have high protein binding and low volume of distribution.
▶ Adverse effects:
   – gastric ulceration (via inhibition of protective prostaglandins)
   – renal damage – via vasoconstriction due to inhibition of prostaglandin synthesis
   – asthma exacerbation – in susceptible individuals (15%) due to unopposed leucotriene synthesis
   – perioperative bleeding – inhibit platelet aggregation
   – affect bone healing (equivocal evidence)
   – hepatotoxicity – transient elevation of transaminases (15%).

▶ Drug interactions: displacement reaction with warfarin (leading to its toxicity).

• Peck TE, Hill S. *Pharmacology for Anaesthesia and Intensive Care*. 3rd ed. Cambridge: Cambridge University Press; 2008. pp. 149–51.

A43 D **Selective COX-2 inhibitors**:

▶ Same risk of gastrointestinal ulcers.

▶ Same risk of renal side effects.

▶ Since they may inhibit vascular prostacyclin synthesis, they may promote platelet aggregation, leading to a higher incidence of **myocardial infarction and stroke** (compared with non-selective COX inhibitors).

▶ Rofecoxib: withdrawn because of higher incidence of **myocardial infarction**.

▶ Celecoxib: contraindicated in **sulphonamide allergy**.

▶ Valdecoxib: withdrawn due to **serious dermatological effects**.

▶ Parecoxib: **parenteral** preparation.

▶ Lumaricoxib: **liver toxicity**.

• Peck TE, Hill S. *Pharmacology for Anaesthesia and Intensive Care. 3rd ed. Cambridge*: Cambridge University Press; 2008. pp. 159–62.

A44 C In the event of a **true allergy** (severe hypotension, skin rash, respiratory difficulty and mucosal oedema), it is advisable to either **avoid opioids** (use non-opioids) or use opioids of a **different chemical class** with close monitoring.

Table 2.16 Chemical classes of opioids

Morphine derivatives	Phenylpiperidines	Diphenylheptanes
Morphine	Fentanyl	Methadone
Hydro/oxycodone	Sufentanil	Propoxyphene
Hydro/oxymorphine	Remifentanil	
Butarphanol	Alfentanil	
Nalbuphine	Pethidine	
Pentazocine		

3

Equipment and physics

Questions

Choose one best answer for each of the following questions.

Q1 Regarding electrical nerve stimulation, which of the following statements is **false**?
a. It is based on the premise that electrical stimulation results in depolarisation of the nerve and hence its identification
b. It is the gold-standard method for nerve blockade
c. It is easier to stimulate motor fibres than sensory fibres
d. It is easier to stimulate a nerve if the needle acts as a cathode rather than an anode

Q2 Which of the following statements regarding rheobase in electrical nerve stimulation is **true**?
a. Rheobase is the minimum duration required to depolarise a nerve
b. Rheobase is the minimum current required to depolarise a nerve
c. Rheobase is the minimum current required to hyperpolarise a nerve
d. Rheobase is the minimum current of indefinite duration required to depolarise a nerve

Q3 The **correct** statement regarding chronaxie in electrical nerve stimulation is which of the following?
a. Chronaxie is the minimum current required to stimulate a nerve
b. Chronaxie is the minimum duration required to stimulate a nerve
c. Chronaxie is the minimum duration of current twice the rheobase required to stimulate a nerve
d. The ease of stimulation is directly proportional to chronaxie

Q4 Regarding properties of electrical nerve stimulation, which of the following statements is **false**?
a. A shorter pulse width is a better discriminator of needle distance from nerve
b. A square-wave pulse is employed
c. Stimulation by cathode is preferred
d. Fixed current is generated

Q5 While performing peripheral nerve stimulation for nerve block, which of the following statements is **false**?
a. The negative pole should be applied to the needle
b. The positive pole should be applied to the patient
c. Applying anode at least 20 cm away from the site of stimulation is critical
d. The motor response is accepted between a current of 0.2 and 0.5 mA

Q6 The most important characteristic of an ideal peripheral nerve stimulator is which of the following?
a. Oscillator
b. Constant current generator
c. Constant voltage generator
d. Display

Q7 While using a peripheral nerve stimulator (PNS), which of the following settings is **not** appropriate?
a. Negative electrode to the needle
b. Starting current of 1–2 mA
c. A pulse width of 0.1 msec
d. A final current of 0.1 mA

Q8 Which of the following statements is **true** about the law that governs the principle of nerve stimulation?

a. The current required is proportional to the distance between the needle and the nerve

b. The current required is inversely proportional to the distance between the needle and the nerve

c. The current required is inversely proportional to the square of the distance between the needle and the nerve

d. The current required is inversely proportional to the square root of the distance between the needle and the nerve

Q9 Which of the following statements regarding use of a PNS for nerve blockade is **false**?

a. Diabetic patients may need a higher current to stimulate their nerves

b. Disappearance of the motor response induced by a low current (0.5 mA) following injection of local anaesthetics or 0.9% saline confirms the proximity of the needle to the nerve

c. The exaggeration of motor response induced by a low current (0.5 mA) following injection of 5% dextrose confirms the needle-to-nerve proximity

d. A current of 1 mA will consistently produce a motor response in more than 90% of cases

Q10 Which of the following statements regarding peripheral nerve stimulators is **correct**?

a. The current range of most PNSs is 5–10 mA

b. Percutaneous nerve stimulation uses a lower current to stimulate a nerve

c. The biomedical department should check PNS machines periodically for current ranges of 1–5 mA

d. None of the above

Q11 Regarding block needles, which of the following statements is **false**?

a. Non-insulated needles have better precision

b. Non-insulated needles may cause local muscle stimulation

c. Insulated needles have a Teflon coating

d. Insulated needles result in less current dispersion than non-insulated needles

Q12 Which of the following statements regarding peripheral nerve block needle-tip design is **true**?

a. Standard bevel needles may cause nerve damage due to blunt injury

b. Nerve injury may be more severe with short bevel needles

c. Short bevel needles result in nerve damage due to sharp cuts

d. The likelihood of nerve trauma is higher with short bevel needles

Q13 Regarding peripheral nerve block needles, which of the following statements is **false**?

a. 18-G Tuohy-tip needle is best suited for continuous catheter technique

b. Blunt-tip 22-G needles are better for single-shot injections

c. Catheters used for continuous peripheral nerve blocks are usually 20-G calibre

d. Superficial and field injections are usually performed using 22-G needles

Q14 Which of the following block approaches is **incorrectly matched** with the recommended needle length?

a. Interscalene block: 25–50 mm

b. Infraclavicular: 50 mm

c. Axillary: 50 mm

d. Sciatic block (posterior): 100 mm

Q15 When using an in-line pressure monitoring device to inject local anaesthetic, which of the following statements is **false**?

a. Its use is based on the premise that high injection pressures are associated with intraneural injections

b. Perineural injections are associated with low injection pressures

c. Injections should be made only when pressures are < 20 psi

d. The device provides a subjective assessment of injection pressures

Q16 Regarding continuous catheter techniques for nerve blocks, which of the following statements is **correct**?

a. Non-stimulating catheters have a higher success rate of secondary block

b. Stimulating catheters involve the bolus dose through the needle and continuous infusion through catheters

c. Leakage is a problem with 'catheter through needle' systems

d. Tunnelling increases the chances of dislodgement

Q17 Regarding ultrasound for regional anaesthesia, which of the following statements is **false**?

a. Ultrasound used for clinical purposes is of the frequency 1–20 KHz
b. B-mode is the most common mode used in regional anaesthesia
c. It is based on the piezoelectric effect
d. The speed of ultrasound waves in tissues is fairly constant at 1540 m/second

Q18 Regarding ultrasound waves, which of the following statements is **false**?

a. Wavelength is inversely related to frequency
b. High-frequency waves have deeper penetration
c. Linear array probes produce higher-frequency ultrasound
d. Curved array probes produce lower-frequency ultrasound

Q19 Regarding ultrasound transducers, which of the following statements is **false**?

a. Linear array probes have best axial resolution
b. Curved array probes produce sectorial images
c. Phased array probes are best for echocardiography
d. J-shaped probes are most suitable for elderly patients

Q20 Which of the following statements is **true**?

a. Axial resolution is the ability of the system to display small structures side by side (same depth) as separate from each other
b. Lateral resolution is the ability of the system to display small structures along the axis of the beam as separate from each other
c. Attenuation is the sum total of reflection, refraction, scattering and absorption
d. Attenuation is inversely proportional to the beam frequency

Q21 Which of the following artefacts is produced during ultrasound scanning?

a. Post-cystic enhancement
b. Reverberation
c. Acoustic shadowing
d. All of the above

Q22 Which of the following structures are **correctly matched** for their echogenicity?
a. Veins – pulsatile hypoechoic
b. Muscle – hyperechoic
c. Central nerve plexus – hypoechoic
d. Peripheral nerves – hypoechoic

Q23 Which of the following aspect of needle technology does **not** enhance needle visualisation under ultrasound?
a. Shallow angle of entry of needle
b. Thicker needles
c. Cornerstone reflectors
d. Compound imaging

Q24 In terms of the advantage of ultrasound-guided regional anaesthesia compared with use of a PNS, which of the following statements is **false**?
a. It provides real-time information of the procedure
b. It prevents nerve damage
c. It shortens the onset times
d. It improves success rate

Q25 Which of the following combinations of ultrasound view and needle approach is most commonly used to perform a single-shot supraclavicular nerve block?
a. Short axis – in plane
b. Short axis – out of plane
c. Long axis – in plane
d. Long axis – out of plane

Q26 Which of the following is **not** a new application of electrical peripheral nerve stimulation?
a. Percutaneous electrode guidance
b. Sequential electrical nerve stimulation
c. Epidural stimulation test
d. Epidural pressure waveform guidance

Q27 Which of the following is **not** an advantage of multi-stimulation technique for nerve blocks?
a. Has a higher success rate
b. Decreases the chances of nerve injury
c. Reduces the total volume required
d. Shorter onset time of the nerve block

Q28 Which of the following blocks is **not** appropriate for multistimulation?
a. Interscalene
b. Supraclavicular
c. Femoral
d. Sciatic nerve

Q29 Regarding the use of peripheral nerve stimulation, which of the following statements is **false**?
a. Initial higher current used has higher sensitivity
b. Subsequent low current has high specificity
c. Clinically used PNS needles with microtip are associated with high specificity of motor response
d. Nerves have low water–lipid ratio, and therefore are most conductive to tissues

Answers

A1 **B**

- Electrical nerve stimulation was first studied by French physiologist **Louis Lapicque** in 1909. It was first used to perform nerve blocks by **Von Perthes** in 1912. Before this, nerves were blocked by direct instillation of local anaesthetics (by dissection and exposure of nerve plexus) or paresthesia techniques.
- The technique of electrical nerve stimulation is based on the premise that a current of sufficient amplitude applied for a sufficient time will depolarise a nerve. In the case of nerve blocks, this means either **motor response or sensory stimulation** (since most nerves are mixed).
- However, it was also noted that stimulating **motor fibres was easier than sensory fibres**, and more importantly, application of a **cathode depolarised** the nerve, while an **anode hyperpolarised** the nerve.
- At present, ultrasound guidance is becoming more popular, but electrical nerve stimulation is still the commonest method employed. **However, no method of nerve blockade is described as gold standard.**
  - Mulroy MF, Bernards CM, McDonald SB, *et al. A Practical Approach to Regional Anesthesia*. 4th ed. Philadelphia, PA: Lippincott Williams & Wilkins; 2008. pp. 93–7.

A2 **D** The total charge (Q) required to depolarise a nerve is the product of the current intensity (I) and the duration (t) for which it is applied.

$$Q = I \times t$$

In turn, the current intensity required to produce depolarisation is given by the following equation (where Ir is the rheobase and **C** is the chronaxie):

$$I = \text{Ir} \times (1 + C/t)$$

By substituting t = infinity, **we get** I = Ir, **and so** Q = Ir. Hence, **rheobase** is the minimum current of **indefinite duration** required to depolarise a nerve.

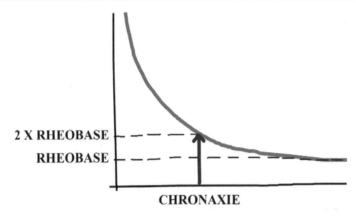

Figure 3.1 Relationship of rheobase and chronaxie

A3   C
- Chronaxie is the **minimum duration** of current **twice the rheobase** required to stimulate a nerve (as shown in the previous answer). It is **inversely proportional** to fibre size and hence ease of stimulation.
- Aα (motor) has a chronaxie of **0.05–0.1 millisecond**, while that of Aδ (sensory) and C (unmyelinated sensory) fibres is **0.15 millisecond** and **0.4 millisecond**, respectively. Hence, stimulating motor nerve requires **shorter pulses** than sensory fibres.

A4   D Desirable properties of electrical nerve stimulation are:
- **Short pulse width**: pulse width refers to the **time duration** for which the current is applied. Shorter pulse width has two advantages:
  - Since the motor fibres have a smaller chronaxie, shorter pulse width stimulates them but not the sensory fibres. This results in **motor responses but not painful paresthesia**, which is undesirable anyway.
  - Shorter pulse width may be superior to longer in **estimating needle-to-nerve distance**.
- **Square-wave current**: a slow rising current allows for **accommodation** (resulting in difficulty in nerve stimulation) of nerve fibres. This can be avoided by the square-wave form of applying current (abrupt rise and abrupt fall).
- **Cathodal stimulation**: it is preferable to stimulate the nerve with needle as cathode, since this then **depolarises** it, whereas needle as anode hyperpolarises the nerve (necessitating application of higher current for stimulation).
- **Constant current generator (not fixed)**: a peripheral nerve stimulator (PNS) should deliver the same current despite changing impedance

applied. This is the **most important** property of the peripheral nervous system (PNS).

▶ **Frequency**: a stimulation frequency of **2 Hz is better than 1 Hz**, since it allows faster manipulation of needle.

- Mulroy MF, Bernards CM, McDonald SB, *et al. A Practical Approach to Regional Anesthesia*. 4th ed. Philadelphia, PA: Lippincott Williams & Wilkins; 2008. pp. 94–9.

A5 C During nerve stimulation, the following things are vital:

▶ **N**egative (cathode) to **n**eedle.

▶ **P**ositive (anode) to **p**atient.

▶ It was considered that the anode site should be at least 20 cm away from the needle site to reduce direct muscle stimulation, but this has been found to be **unnecessary**.

▶ Acceptable current is **between 0.2 and 0.5 mA**. Above 0.5 mA, the needle may be further away from the nerve, and such injections may not be successful. Below 0.2 mA, injection may be intraneural.

- Mulroy MF, Bernards CM, McDonald SB, *et al. A Practical Approach to Regional Anesthesia*. 4th ed. Philadelphia, PA: Lippincott Williams & Wilkins; 2008. pp. 95–8.

A6 B

Table 3.1 The components of a peripheral nerve stimulator

Components	Function
Microcontroller	Brain of the peripheral nervous system: processes variable, like current, pulse width, frequency
Constant current generator (most important)	Generates the same current despite changing impedance
Oscillator	Generates the desired frequency
Clock reference	Synchronises the current with the frequency
LCD display	For current amplitude, frequency and the pulse width selected
Controls	For selecting parameters

- www.nysora.com/regional_anesthesia/equipment/3114-nerve_stimulators.html

A7 A The appropriate settings of a PNS for performing a nerve block include:
- negative lead to needle
- positive lead to patient
- a **square-wave** impulse (to prevent accommodation)
- pulse duration **0.1 millisecond** (for stimulating motor nerve fibres preferably)
- frequency of **2 Hz** (better than 1 Hz)
- an initial current of **1–2 mA**
- a final current of **0.2–0.5 mA** (> 0.5 mA, the needle may be further away from the nerve, and such injections may not be successful; < 0.2 mA, the injection may be intraneural).
  - *Nerve Location: The Art and Science of Finding Peripheral Nerves.* B. Braun Satellite Symposium XXII. ESRA Congress Malta, September 2003.

A8 C The **inverse-square law (Coulomb's Law)** dictates that the current required (I) to stimulate a nerve, is proportional to the minimal current (i), and inversely to the square of the distance (r) from the nerve (k is a constant).

$$I = k(i/r^2)$$

Hence as the needle approaches the nerve, less current is needed to stimulate it and vice versa. The motor response amplitude will increase if the current is not reduced. Practically, the current is decreased till final amplitude of **0.2–0.5 mA**. At currents less than 0.2 mA, the nerve tip may lie within the nerve, and hence such injections may lead to nerve injury.
  - www.nysora.com/regional_anesthesia/equipment/3114-nerve_stimulators. html

A9 D
- Usually, a motor response between 0.2 and 0.5 mA is sought and considered appropriate. However, in **elderly, diabetics or those with neurological diseases**, higher currents may be needed due to slower nerve velocities and lower motor amplitudes.
- The disappearance of the motor response induced by a low current (0.5 mA) following injection of local anaesthetics or normal saline (**conducting solutions**), confirms the proximity of needle to the nerve and constitutes the **Raj test**. This does not result due to the physical displacement of the nerve but due to the **dissipation of current density** near the nerve.

- The exaggeration of motor response induced by a low current (0.5 mA) following injection of 5% dextrose (**non-conducting solutions**), confirms the needle-to-nerve proximity as well and constitutes the **Tsui test**.

- In a study performed by Urmey and Stanton in 2002, the authors concluded that a sensory response (paraesthesia), presumably due to nerve contact, was not associated with ability to elicit a motor response in 70% of patients. This lack of motor response occurred in the majority of patients despite increasing amperage to 1.0 mA, which exceeds the minimal value accepted by most anaesthesiologists. **Results of this study provided evidence that a lack of motor response does not rule out the possibility of sensory nerve contact by the injection needle.**

  - Cousins MJ, Bridenbaugh PO, Carr DB, *et al. Cousins and Bridenbaugh's Neural Blockade in Clinical Anesthesia and Pain Medicine*. 4th ed. Philadelphia, PA: Lippincott Williams & Wilkins; 2008. p. 172.

  - Mulroy MF, Bernards CM, McDonald SB, *et al. A Practical Approach to Regional Anesthesia*. 4th ed. Philadelphia, PA: Lippincott Williams & Wilkins; 2008. pp. 98–103.

  - Urmey WF, Stanton J. Inability to consistently elicit a motor response following sensory paresthesia during interscalene block administration. *Anesthesiology*. 2002; **96**(3): 552–4.

A10 D

- The optimal range for a PNS is **0–5 mA**. This is because some patients may need higher current for stimulation (diabetics, elderly, neurologic disease). Newer devices may have higher ranges (**0–10 mA**) used for epidural stimulation. Higher ranges (**0–80 mA**) are used in neuromuscular monitors.

- Percutaneous nerve stimulation is a new technique involving the stimulation of nerves non-invasively. The current needed for this is **higher than invasive stimulation**, but offers the identification of insertion points in especially difficult cases (obese).

- Biomedical engineering departments have measured the accuracy of PNS in the higher current ranges (**> 1 mA**) in the past. It was subsequently argued that since the current used for performing nerve blocks is in the range of **0.2–0.5 mA**, it is prudent to check the accuracy in this range. This has been adopted by some manufacturers.

  - Hadzic A, Vloka J, Hadzic N, *et al*. Nerve stimulators used for peripheral nerve blocks vary in their electrical characteristics. *Anesthesiology*. 2003; **98**(4): 969–74.

- Hadzic A. *Textbook of Regional Anesthesia and Acute Pain Management*. 1st ed. New York, NY: McGraw-Hill Medical; 2006. p. 314.
- Urmey WF, Grossi P. Percutaneous electrode guidance: a noninvasive technique for prelocation of peripheral nerves to facilitate peripheral plexus or nerve block. *Reg Anesth Pain Med.* 2002; **27**(3): 261–7.

A11 A

▶ **Non-insulated needles** were the first to be used. Both the tip and the shaft were conductive, causing current dispersion and lower accuracy. They also caused local muscle stimulation through the shaft of the needle.

▶ The development of **Teflon-coated insulated needles** resulted in better precision. This is because only the tip is conductive, and hence the current is not dispersed.

- Hadzic A. *Textbook of Regional Anesthesia and Acute Pain Management*. 1st ed. New York, NY: McGraw-Hill Medical; 2006. p. 310.
- www.aagbi.org/sites/default/files/149-Nerve-stimulation-for-peripheral-nerve-blockade.pdf

A12 B Various needle-tip designs are prevalent. Among the sharp needles, the tip may have a **long (standard, 15°) bevel** or **short (30° or 45°) bevel**.

▶ The long-bevel needles may cause **sharp cuts** on nerves, while the short bevel leads to **blunt** nerve damage.

▶ Although nerve injury is **more frequent** with long-bevel needles, it may be **more severe** if it occurs using a short-bevel needle.

▶ Blunt-bevel needles offer more resistance as they pass through tissue planes and thus give a **better feel**. Hence they are most commonly used nowadays.

- Hadzic A. *Textbook of Regional Anesthesia and Acute Pain Management*. 1st ed. New York, NY: McGraw-Hill Medical; 2006. p. 310.
- Neal JM, Rathmell JP. *Complications in Regional Anesthesia and Pain Medicine.* 1st ed. Philadelphia, PA: Saunders; 2006. pp. 130–1.

A13 D Needle gauge is an important consideration while performing blocks. Superficial injections are best given using **25/26-G needles**. The **21/22-G** needles are best for single-shot injections, whereas the **18/19-G** Tuohy-tip needles are best suited for continuous catheter techniques. In such cases, **20-G** catheters are used.

- Hadzic A. *Textbook of Regional Anesthesia and Acute Pain Management.* 1st ed. New York, NY: McGraw-Hill Medical; 2006. pp. 310–11.

A14 B Needle length is an important consideration when doing nerve blocks. Shorter needle may not be sufficient, while longer needles may have potential for tissue damage if introduced further than needed.

Table 3.2 Appropriate needle lengths for nerve blocks

25 mm	50 mm	100 mm	150 mm
Interscalene	Cervical plexus	Infraclavicular	Sciatic (anterior)
	Supraclavicular	Popliteal (lateral)	
	Axillary	Paravertebral	
	Femoral	Lumbar plexus	
	Popliteal (posterior)	Sciatic (posterior)	

- Hadzic A. *Textbook of Regional Anesthesia and Acute Pain Management.* 1st ed. New York, NY: McGraw-Hill Medical; 2006. p. 311.

A15 D An in-line pressure-monitoring device measures pressure while injecting local anaesthetic. It provides an **objective assessment** of pressures rather than subjective feel. The latter can vary between individuals and devices. Intraneural injection pressures are **> 20 psi** while those made perineurally have lower pressures of **5–20 psi**. Therefore, the device guides placement of the tip according to injection pressures.
- www.macostamedicalusa.com

A16 C
- The continuous catheter technique involves the use of larger needles (Tuohy-, Sprotte- or facet-tipped 18/19 G) and fine stimulating catheters (20 G). Once a nerve is stimulated using the needle, the catheter is threaded through the needle.
- In the case of non-stimulating catheters, the perineural space is dilated by injecting saline and threading the catheter **3–5 cm** beyond the needle tip. Although the use of catheters helped to prolong post-operative pain relief, they were limited by **secondary block failures** (primary block refers to the block following initial injection, while secondary block is one following continuous infusion).
- This was improved by **stimulating catheters**. They are threaded along the nerve, and their position confirmed using electrostimulation in real

time. This is followed by initial bolus and continuous infusion, both through the catheter. This has reduced secondary failures.

▶ Systems with 'catheter over needle' and 'catheter through needle' are available. Though the latter are more prevalent, their use is often plagued by **leakage** through the injection site (because the hole made by the needle is larger than the catheter size). Tunnelling the catheter **reduces the chances of dislodgement** and helps maintain the catheter for a **longer time**.

- Hadzic A. *Textbook of Regional Anesthesia and Acute Pain Management*. 1st ed. New York, NY: McGraw-Hill Medical; 2006. pp. 649–53.

A17 **A** **Ultrasound waves (> 20 KHz)** are waves beyond the audible frequency range of **audible sound (20–20 000 Hz)**. Clinically used ultrasound is in the **1–20-MHz** frequency range. Ultrasound waves are generated by applying an electric field to piezoelectric crystals to produce a series of **pressure waves**. The pressure waves are transmitted from the probe head and reflected back dependent upon the tissue type. The returning pressure waves are detected and generate an electric current that is converted into a **two-dimensional image**. This interpretation assumes the speed of sound in soft tissues to be **1540 m/second**.

The various modes of ultrasound in use are:

▶ **A-mode**: the **simplest type** of ultrasound. A **single transducer** scans a line through the body with the echoes plotted on screen as a **function of depth**.

▶ **B-mode: the commonest mode**. A **linear array of transducers** simultaneously scans a plane through the body that can be viewed as a **two-dimensional image** on screen.

▶ **M-mode**: M stands for **'motion'**. Ultrasound pulses are emitted in quick succession, recording a video in ultrasound. This can be used to determine the **velocity** of specific organ structures such as cardiac valves and jets.

▶ **Doppler mode**: This mode makes use of the **Doppler effect** (change in frequency of a wave for an observer moving relative to the source of the wave) in measuring and visualising blood flow.

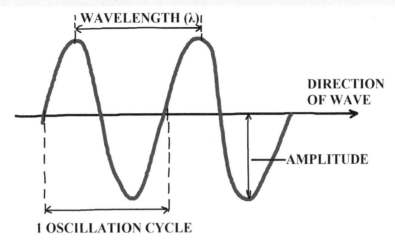

Figure 3.2 Characteristics of a sound wave

A18 B

Ultrasound waves are sound waves.

- ❱ Wavelength (λ): distance between two consecutive corresponding points of the same phase.
- ❱ Amplitude (A): maximum height of the wave.
- ❱ Frequency (f): number of complete cycles per second.
- ❱ Period (τ): time taken for one complete wave cycle to occur.
- ❱ Velocity (c): speed at which sound waves pass through a medium. It may be calculated using the equation: $c = \lambda \times f$

Since the velocity within a medium is constant, this implies that wavelength and frequency bear an **inverse relationship**.

- ❱ **Higher-frequency beams experience more attenuation** (directly proportional) and hence have lesser penetration. They are used for performing superficial blocks (interscalene and supraclavicular).
- ❱ **Low-frequency beams have better** penetration and allow visualisation of deep structures (infraclavicular and sciatic nerve blocks).

Linear transducers generate high-frequency ultrasound, while curved array probes low-frequency ultrasound.

- • www.aagbi.org/sites/default/files/199-The-physics-of-ultrasound-part-1.pdf

A19 D

Table 3.3 Characteristics of various ultrasound transducer array

Linear array	Curved array	Phased array
High frequency **(6–13 MHz)**	Low frequency **(2–5 MHz)**	Consists of many small
Greatest axial resolution	Decreased axial resolution	ultrasonic elements
More attenuation	Less attenuation	High-resolution beam
Limited depth of penetration	Deeper penetration	Characteristic image is sector-shaped
Rectangular images	**Sector-shaped** image	Used for
Best for superficial structures (e.g. brachial plexus)	Best for large or deep structures (e.g. sciatic nerve)	**echocardiography**

J-shaped (hockey-stick footprint) probes are linear array probes which are small in size and hence ideally suited for **paediatric** usage.

- www.aagbi.org/sites/default/files/218-The-Physics-of-Ultrasound-part-2.pdf

A20 C

- **Axial resolution** is the ability of the system to display small structures along the axis of the beam as separate from each other. It is **directly proportional to the frequency** of the beam.
- **Lateral resolution** is the ability of the system to display small structures side by side (same depth) as separate from each other.
- **Attenuation** is the sum total of reflection, refraction, scattering and absorption. It leads to loss of clarity of the image. It can be corrected by time-gain compensation (also called depth-gain compensation). Attenuation is **directly proportional** to the frequency. So higher frequency ultrasound beams undergo higher attenuation and allow the best visualisation of superficial structures.

A21 A An artefact is an image, or part of it, that does not correspond to the anatomy of the structure being examined. The most important artefacts are as follows.

- **Shadowing**: when the ultrasound beam cannot pass through a structure (e.g. bone), the beam is reflected back and the tissues immediately behind the structure appear dark.
- **Post-cystic enhancement**: when the ultrasound beam passes through a **fluid-filled structure** such as the urinary bladder, cysts or blood vessels, very little is reflected, and therefore the tissues behind the fluid appear bright.

▶ **Reverberation**: occurs when ultrasound is repeatedly reflected between two highly reflective surfaces.
▶ **Anisotropy**: is the property of tendons, nerves and muscles to vary in their ultrasound appearance depending on the **angle of insonation** of the incident ultrasound beam.
  • www.usra.ca/imageartifacts.php
  • www.aagbi.org/sites/default/files/218-The-Physics-of-Ultrasound-part-2. pdf

A22 C On returning to the transducer, the amplitude of an echo is represented by **the degree of brightness (i.e. echogenicity)** of a dot on the display. Each tissue displays a different echogenicity, allowing identification of structures.
▶ **Anechoic**: veins/arteries offer no reflection and appear **black**.
▶ **Hypoechoic**: muscle and central nerve plexus offer weak reflections and appear **dark**.
▶ **Hyperechoic**: bone and peripheral nerves offer strong reflections and appear **bright**.
  • www.usra.ca/tissueecho.php

A23 D

Table 3.4 Factors determining needle visualisation under ultrasound

Factor	Deteriorates	Improves
Technique	Out of plane	In plane
Size of needle	Smaller (22 G)	Larger (17-G Tuohy)
Angle of insertion	Steep	Shallow
Depth of insertion	Deep	Shallow
Echogenicity	Non-echogenic	Echogenic (cornerstone reflectors)

▶ **Cornerstone reflectors**: introduced by some companies (Pajunk), these are intended to improve needle visibility under ultrasound, even at steep angles. They do so by reflecting all ultrasound waves without losses.
▶ In **real-time spatial compound imaging**, a transducer array is used to rapidly acquire several overlapping scans of an object from different angles. These scans are averaged to form a compound image that shows improved image quality because of reduction of artefacts.
▶ Other technologies involve either one of the following:
  – **Needle-guidance systems**: Sonic GPS (Ultrasonics) and eTrAX needle systems (CiVCO).

  – **Newer imaging modalities**: Multibeam (Sonosite), Cross XBeam (GE) and Flexi Focus (BK Medical).
  * www.bkmed.com/Ultrasound_scanners_Flex_Focus_Family_en.htm
  * www.civco-etrax.com/etrax/
  * www.sonosite.com
  * www.ultrasonix.com/products/sonixgps
  * www.gehealthcare.com/promo/venue40/us_development/
  * www.pajunk.com/

A24 B

▶ Ultrasound provides **real-time** visualisation of the nerve and surrounding structures during regional anaesthesia.

▶ It allows detection of **anatomical variations** and demonstrates spread of local anaesthetic during injection.

▶ **Intraneural or intravascular** injection can be detected by ultrasound.

▶ Evidence shows ultrasound-guided peripheral nerve blocks can be **more successful** than peripheral nerve stimulator techniques and have a **faster onset** time.

▶ However, evidence to clearly demonstrate that ultrasound-guided regional anaesthesia is safer (in terms of neural injury) than using a peripheral nerve stimulator is still **not available**.
  * Marhofer P, Schrögendorfer K, Koinig H, *et al*. Ultrasonographic guidance improves sensory block and onset time of three-in-one blocks. *Anesth Analg*. 1997; **85**: 854–7.
  * Williams SR, Chouinard P, Arcand G, *et al*. Ultrasound guidance speeds the execution and improves the quality of supraclavicular block. *Anesth Analg*. 2003; **97**: 1518–23.
  * www.usra.ca/general.php

A25 A Structures may be visualised under ultrasound in either the **short axis or long axis**.

▶ In the short-axis view, tubular structures such as nerves and blood vessels appear as though they have been **sliced across their diameter**, like discs of salami.

▶ In the long-axis view, tubular structures are **sliced longitudinally along the length** of the tube.

The needle approach is described as in-plane if the needle remains parallel to the ultrasound beam, allowing visualisation of the tip and shaft.

- In the **out-of-plane approach**, the needle is inserted more perpendicular to the ultrasound beam and can only be visualised as a dot when the needle crosses the beam.
- An **in-plane needle approach** with a short-axis view of the brachial plexus is most commonly used to perform a supraclavicular nerve block.

Note: for insertion of catheters at this level, an out-of-plane approach is preferred by many.

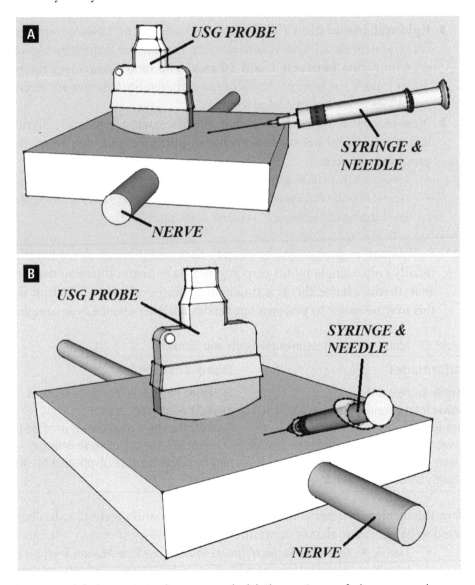

Figure 3.3 (A) Short-axis in-plane approach; (B) Short-axis out-of-plane approach

A26 D The newer applications of electrical nerve stimulation include the following.

▶ **Percutaneous electrode guidance**: involves percutaneous stimulation of peripheral nerves to identify a nerve before skin puncture. This reduces the number of unsuccessful painful insertion and helps identify the best insertion point.

▶ **Sequential electrical nerve stimulation (SENS)**: delivers current at 3 Hz with sequential pulses of 0.1, 0.3 and 1 msecond to improve motor response.

▶ **Epidural stimulation (Tsui test)**: the placement of wired epidural catheters threaded into epidural space can be confirmed by electrical stimulation **between 1 and 10 mA**. The motor responses elicited direct toward the level of the tip of the catheter. Stimulation at currents < 1 mA indicate intrathecal placement.

▶ **Non-electrical methods** to confirm the placement of epidural catheters include **epidural pressure waveform guidance and electrocardiographic guidance**.

- Cousins MJ, Bridenbaugh PO, Carr DB, *et al. Cousins and Bridenbaugh's Neural Blockade in Clinical Anesthesia and Pain Medicine*. 4th ed. Philadelphia, PA: Lippincott Williams & Wilkins; 2008. pp. 172–3.

A27 B Although a given nerve block may have components nerve bundles, usually only a single motor response is sought before injecting the local anaesthetic. Hence this is a single-stimulation technique. Technically, this may be easier to perform but carries a higher chance of incomplete

Table 3.5 Multistimulation techniques: merits and demerits

Advantages	Disadvantages
Higher success rate	Increased patient discomfort because of multiple needle redirections
Lower total volume of local anaesthetic needed	Time for the entire procedure is increased
Shortening of onset times of nerve blocks	Theoretically, the risk of nerve damage may be higher because of repeated needle passage
Lower potential of local-anaesthetic toxicity because of lower doses	

Note: the incidence of nerve injury with multistimulation technique has been found to be similar to that of conventional techniques.

- Hadzic A. *Textbook of Regional Anesthesia and Acute Pain Management*. 1st ed. New York, NY: McGraw-Hill Medical; 2006. p. 618.

block of other bundles (in a given plexus), lowering the success rate and necessitating the use of higher volume to ensure spread to all components. **Multistimulation technique** involves seeking specific component bundle motor responses separately and then blocking the component nerves individually. For example, for the axillary block, the radial, ulnar, median and musculocutaneous responses are sought individually.

A28 B

▶ Multistimulation technique has been found to be useful for interscalene, axillary, infraclavicular, mid-humeral, femoral and sciatic nerve blocks.
▶ However, frequent redirections in the **supraclavicular area** may increase the risk of arterial puncture and pneumothorax, and **are not advised**.
  • Hadzic A. *Textbook of Regional Anesthesia and Acute Pain Management*. 1st ed. New York, NY: McGraw-Hill Medical; 2006. p. 618.

A29 D

▶ While performing a peripheral nerve block, all efforts are directed toward improving the sensitivity and specificity of nerve stimulation and consequent motor response. As the current needed to stimulate a nerve is **inversely proportional to the square of the distance from the needle**, high currents help in finding the nerve initially. Hence they **increase the likelihood** of finding the nerve. Subsequently, lowering the current as the needle approaches the nerve helps to **improve the specificity** of the response.
▶ The resistance encountered by a stimulating electrode depends directly on the tissue resistance and inversely on the conductive area of the electrode. Stimulating a nerve using a **microtip** electrode (i.e. despite high resistance) **improves the specificity** of the stimulation.
▶ Water–lipid ratio of tissues is proportional to conductance, and since **nerves have a high water–lipid ratio, they have higher conductance** than skin, muscle, fat or bone; hence they are stimulated in preference upon application of a current.

4
Central neuraxial blocks

Questions

Distribution

Questions 1–20:   Spinal anaesthesia

Questions 21–33:   Epidural anaesthesia

Questions 34–40:   Combined spinal–epidural anaesthesia

Questions 41–46:   Caudal anaesthesia

Choose one best answer for each of the following questions.

Q1   Absolute contraindication for spinal anaesthesia is:
   a. Aortic stenosis
   b. Multiple sclerosis
   c. Severe hypovolaemia
   d. Systemic sepsis

Q2   The **false** statement regarding anatomy of spinal cord is:
   a. Supraspinous ligament extends from foramen magnum to sacrum
   b. Dura mater extends from foramen magnum to S2 level
   c. Pia mater ends at filum terminale
   d. Arachnoid mater ends at S2 level

Q3 Of the following, which is the **incorrect** statement about spinal nerves?
a. There are 31 pairs of spinal nerves, each composed of anterior motor root and posterior sensory root
b. The spinal nerves are named according to upper vertebral body from which they exit
c. The spinal nerve roots and the spinal cord are sites of action of local anaesthetic in spinal anaesthesia
d. Most ventral nerve roots of the spinal nerve exit as a single bundle

Q4 Which is not an important factor in determining the distribution of local anaesthetic?
a. Baricity
b. Dose
c. Position of patient
d. Concentration of drug

Q5 Regarding additive drugs (along with local anaesthetic) for spinal anaesthesia, the **false** statement is:
a. Epinephrine may cause anterior spinal artery ischemia
b. Phenylephrine may increase the risk of transient neurological symptoms
c. Neostigmine causes nausea, vomiting, agitation and lower-limb weakness
d. Clonidine only prolongs sensory blockade

Q6 All of the following are risk factors for hypotension during subarachnoid block **except:**
a. Emergency surgery
b. Low BMI
c. History of hypertension
d. Combined general and spinal anaesthetic

Q7 The **False** statement concerning hypotension during spinal anaesthesia is:
a. Pure alpha agonists are superior to combined alpha and beta agonists in treating hypotension
b. Phenylephrine mainly causes systemic vasoconstriction
c. Epinephrine causes systemic vasoconstriction and increases cardiac output
d. Hypotension is avoided by fluid infusion at the time of induction

Q8 Which of the following do not represent adequate sensory blockade level for the given surgery?
a. Urological surgeries – T6
b. Caesarean section – T4
c. Transurethral resection of prostate – T12
d. Perineal surgery – S2–S5

Q9 Risk factors for bradycardia during subarachnoid block are all of the following **except**:
a. ASA class 1
b. Age > 60 years
c. Male sex
d. Preoperative beta blockade

Q10 The **true** statement about high spinal block is:
a. Usually it does not affect cervical area
b. Arterial blood gas measurements are affected in spontaneously breathing patients
c. It affects inspiratory and expiratory muscles of respiration
d. If the patient is having dyspnoea, they should be intubated

Q11 The **false** statement regarding spinal needles is:
a. Whitacre and Sprotte needles are pencil-point needles with a non-cutting bevel
b. Quincke–Babcock needles have a medium cutting bevel
c. Greene needles have a sharp cutting bevel
d. Pitkin needles have a short cutting bevel

Q12 Which of the following statement regarding the Taylor approach to subarachnoid block is **false**?
a. The Taylor approach is a paramedian approach at L4–L5 interspace
b. The needle is inserted 1 cm medial and inferior to the posterior superior iliac spine
c. The needle is angled cephalad at 45°–55°
d. The Taylor approach to subarachnoid block can be performed with the patient in the sitting position

Q13 The **False** statement about intrathecal additives is:
  a. Opioids and local anaesthetics have synergistic analgesic properties in intrathecal space
  b. Small doses of fentanyl intensify subarachnoid block without prolonging it
  c. Clonidine intensifies and prolongs only sensory blockade
  d. Intrathecal neostigmine provides analgesia by increasing the levels of acetylcholine

Q14 The **true** statement regarding the sensitivity of different nerve fibres to local anaesthetics is:
  a. The preganglionic sympathetic fibres (B fibres) are less sensitive to local anaesthetic as compared to C fibres
  b. Among the sensory fibres, the sequence of blockade is C > Aδ > Aβ
  c. The Aα motor fibres are more sensitive to local anaesthetics than sensory fibres
  d. The recovery of the nerve fibres occurs in the same sequence as their blockade

Q15 All of the following statements are true **except**:
  a. Baricity is the ratio of density of a local anaesthetic to the density of cerebrospinal fluid
  b. Specific gravity is the ratio of density of a substance to the density of water
  c. Hyperbaric solutions have prolonged duration of action
  d. Cerebrospinal fluid density changes with temperature

Q16 Regarding the occurrence of post-dural puncture headache (PDPH), the **correct** statement is:
  a. The incidence of PDPH with experts using non-cutting needles is < 1%
  b. The incidence is slightly higher in the obstetric population
  c. Should a dural puncture occur with a Tuohy needle, 50%–80% of such patients experience PDPH
  d. All of the above

Q17 A proposed mechanism for the development of PDPH includes:
  a. Loss of cerebrospinal fluid
  b. Cerebral vasodilatation
  c. Raised intracranial pressure
  d. All of the above

Q18 Which of the following characteristics goes against the diagnosis of PDPH?
a. Typically bilateral headache
b. Delayed onset (within 48 hours)
c. No change in severity with position
d. History of a possible dural puncture

Q19 Which of the following is **not** a risk factor for the development of PDPH?
a. Old age
b. Female sex
c. Using a cutting-tip needle
d. Previous history of PDPH

Q20 Which of the following is considered gold standard for the treatment of PDPH?
a. Non-steroidal anti-inflammatory drugs
b. Epidural saline
c. Epidural blood patch
d. Sumatriptans

Q21 Which of the following is a **true** statement about epidural space?
a. Epidural space is a potential space between dura mater and arachnoid mater
b. Epidural space extends into the skull
c. Batson's venous plexus is a valveless system
d. Ligamentum flavum forms its anterior boundary

Q22 Which of the following statements is **false**?
a. The spinous processes of lower thoracic and lumbar vertebrae are horizontal
b. The spinous processes of cervical vertebraes are caudally inclined
c. The greatest degree of angulation of spinous processes is at the T3–T7 level
d. Insertion of an epidural needle in the mid-thoracic region is easier by paramedian approach

Q23 Which of the following vertebral levels and corresponding anatomical landmarks is **incorrectly** matched?
a. C7 – most prominent spinal process in the neck
b. T3 – spine of scapula
c. T7 – inferior angle of scapula
d. S1 – line connecting the posterior inferior iliac spine

Q24 All of the following are absolute contraindications of epidural anaesthesia **except**:
a. Patient refusal
b. Platelet count < 100 000 per mL
c. Raised intracranial pressure
d. Allergy to local anaesthetic

Q25 All of the following are physiological effects of epidural anaesthesia **except**:
a. Lung volumes like tidal volume and vital capacity are unchanged with high thoracic epidural
b. Thoracic epidural maintains stable visceral perfusion
c. Neuroendocrine stress response is more effectively reduced in upper-abdominal surgery than with lower-abdominal surgery
d. Renal function is minimally altered with epidural anaesthesia

Q26 Which of the following statements about drugs used in epidural space is **incorrect**?
a. Addition of epinephrine to local anaesthetic solution increases the incidence of hypotension due to its beta-blocking properties
b. Addition of bicarbonate 1 mEq/10 mL to bupivacaine fastens the onset of action
c. Combining long- and short-acting anaesthetics has not proven better
d. Clonidine has possible antibacterial activity against *Staphylococcus*

Q27 Which of the following is a **true** statement about factors affecting height of epidural blockade?
a. Concentration of drug affects the height of the block
b. Volume affects the height of the block
c. Weight affects the height of the block
d. Height of the patient affects the height of the block

Q28 Which of the following is a **false** statement about loss-of-resistance (LOR) technique to identify epidural space?
a. The LOR-to-air technique was described by Dogliotti
b. With LOR to saline, the incidence of dural puncture is low
c. In LOR-to-air technique, timing with respiratory cycle is not needed
d. With LOR to saline, entry into epidural space is more dependent on the visual sign than feel

Q29 Which of the following statements about intravascular placement of an epidural catheter is **false**?
a. The test dose for epidural anaesthesia includes 3 mL of 1.5% lignocaine with epinephrine 15 mcg
b. Change in heart rate of 10 bpm is an indication of intravascular placement
c. Change in systolic blood pressure of > 20 mmHg is an indication of intravascular placement in patients on beta blockers
d. Vascular injection is detected in children by ECG changes

Q30 Concerning epidurals in elderly patients, which of the following is **correct**?
a. Require the same dose as adults for the same level of block
b. There is limited cephalad spread
c. The size of interverterbral foramina decreases with age
d. All of the above

Q31 Which of the following does **not** represent the pharmacokinetic differences of epidurally administered local anaesthetic in children when compared with adults?
a. Reduced duration of action
b. Higher doses according to weight
c. Higher rate of continuous infusions
d. Higher potential for toxicity

Q32 Which of the following statements about paediatric epidurals is **incorrect**?
  a. Single-isomer local anaesthetics are preferred
  b. Additives are preferred in infants to reduce doses of local anaesthetics needed
  c. Monitoring ECG changes is considered to be a more specific and more reliable marker of epidural placement than heart-rate changes
  d. It is easier to insert catheters to higher levels from lower approaches

Q33 When comparing lumbar epidural and thoracic epidural for abdominal surgery, the disadvantage of lumbar epidural is:
  a. Hypotension and bradycardia is more common
  b. Rescue analgesia is required more often
  c. Motor block is extensive
  d. All of the above

Q34 The **incorrect** statement about combined spinal epidural (CSE) is:
  a. CSE provides surgical anaesthesia as rapidly as single-shot subarachnoid block
  b. Surgical anaesthesia with epidural anaesthesia is slower as compared with CSE
  c. CSE reduces the incidence of patchy blockade and poor sacral spread
  d. CSE prolongs the duration of the first stage of labour in primiparous patients

Q35 Which of the following is a **false** statement about CSE?
  a. Posterior epidural space distance is important with CSE needle-through-needle technique (NTN)
  b. Spinal block failure with CSE NTN technique is the same as with median or paramedian approach
  c. The spinal needle protrudes 10–15 mm beyond the epidural needle in NTN technique
  d. Posterior epidural space distance is widest at the lumbar region

Q36 Which of the following is an **incorrect** statement about CSE?
a. NTN technique is associated with less discomfort for the patient than separate needle technique
b. Confirmation of epidural placement of catheter is done with test dose (3 mL of 1.5% lignocaine with epinephrine 1 : 200 000)
c. Nerve stimulation may be used as a technique for confirmation of epidural placement of catheter
d. All of the above

Q37 All of the following statements about confirmation of epidural space are true **except**:
a. Tsui test can be used for confirmation of epidural placement of catheter
b. With the use of nerve stimulator to confirm proper placement of epidural catheter, presence of a motor response with > 10 mA indicates inappropriate catheter location
c. With the use of nerve stimulator to confirm proper placement of epidural catheter, presence of a motor response with < 1 mA indicates appropriate catheter location
d. Both sensitivity and specificity of Tsui test is 100%

Q38 Which of the following statements about CSE is **false**?
a. With CSE, there is a possibility of migration of epidural catheter into subarachnoid space
b. With CSE, epidural administration of local anaesthetic may lead to higher block levels as compared with the same dose used in epidural block alone
c. Subarachnoid placement of local anaesthetic with CSE may lead to higher block levels as compared to single-shot spinal block
d. With CSE, use of long spinal needles decreases the incidence of failed spinal block

Q39 Which of the following statements about CSE is **correct**?
a. There is increased risk of foetal bradycardia when CSE is used for labour analgesia
b. There is a high risk of PDPH with CSE
c. There is increased risk of metal deposition with CSE
d. The risk of neurologic injury is same with single-shot spinal and CSE

Q40 Concerning 'epidural volume extension' technique, which of the following statements is **correct**?
   a. It helps in reducing the intrathecal dose by half
   b. It extends the dermatomal spread by at least two segments
   c. It shortens the motor block duration
   d. It produces significantly fewer haemodynamic changes

Q41 Which of the following statements about anatomy of the sacral canal is **false**?
   a. The sacrococcygeal ligament forms the roof of the sacral canal and is a continuation of ligamentum flavum
   b. The superior articular process of S5 forms the sacral cornua
   c. The sacral canal is triangular in shape
   d. The sacral canal contains spinal meninges, epidural venous plexus and cauda equina

Q42 Which of the following statements about the technique of administering caudal anaesthetic is **correct**?
   a. Caudal in children is best performed in prone position
   b. A long-bevel needle is best used to penetrate the tough sacrococcygeal ligament
   c. A 22-G intravenous cannula is best used for the procedure
   d. The needle is inserted in horizontal plane followed by tilting it at an angle of 45° to the sacrum

Q43 Which of the following statements about caudal block is **false**?
   a. Less peripheral vasodilatation is seen with caudal block than with lumbar epidural
   b. There is limited autonomic block with caudal block
   c. The local anaesthetic dose required is more with caudal block than lumbar epidural for the same level of block
   d. The sacral contribution to the sympathetic system to bladder and the bowel are blocked

Q44 Regarding methods of confirmation of caudal placement of the Tuohy needle, which of the following is **incorrect**?
a. Caudal placement of the needle can be identified with the 'whoosh' test
b. Caudal placement of the needle can be identified with nerve stimulation with gluteus muscle contraction as the appropriate end response
c. Thoracic placement of epidural catheters via the caudal approach is confirmed with epidural electrocardiography
d. Loss of resistance to air or saline

Q45 Which of the following statements about caudal block is **false**?
a. Caudal block is used for surgical procedures only below the diaphragm in children
b. Caudal epidural block may be used for lower gynaecological surgeries
c. Caudal block is mainly used for chronic pain management in adults
d. None of the above

Q46 Which of the following statements about caudal block is **true**?
a. Epidural adhesions in caudal space are identified by the 'Christmas tree' appearance after injection of caudal contrast
b. The incidence of local anaesthesia toxicity is more common with caudal block than brachial plexus block
c. In paediatric patients, P-wave changes on ECG are suggestive of intravascular injection of local anaesthesia during caudal bock
d. There is no difference in incidence of local anaesthesia toxicity with lumbar and caudal epidural

Answers

A1   C
- **Absolute contraindications** for spinal anaesthesia include patient refusal, raised intracranial hypertension, neurological disease of indeterminate origin, coagulopathy, severe hypovolaemia and local infection.
- **Relative contraindications** include systemic sepsis, surgery of indeterminate duration, arthritis, kyphoscoliosis and previous lumbar surgery.
- Central neuraxial block in patients with multiple sclerosis is controversial. There is no clinical study which has shown that spinal anesthesia worsens pre-existing neurological disease. Perioperative surgical stress may exacerbate the condition, and hence a central neuraxial block may be preferred.
  - Hadzic A. *Textbook of Regional Anesthesia and Acute Pain Management*. 1st ed. New York, NY: McGraw-Hill Medical; 2006. p. 195.

A2   A Spinal cord has three coverings:
- **Dura mater** (outermost) extends from foramen magnum to S2.
- **Arachnoid mater** (middle) extends to S2.
- **Pia mater** (innermost) ends in the filum terminale.

  Supraspinous ligaments extend from C7 to sacrum connecting the tips of the spinous processes. Above C7, they are called the **ligamentum nuchae**. The spinous processes are interconnected by the interspinous ligaments. The laminae are connected by the ligamentum **flavum**. The vertebral bodies are held together by the **anterior and the posterior longitudinal ligaments**.
- Structures pierced while performing a spinal anaesthetic via **midline approach** are skin, subcutaneous tissues, supraspinous ligaments, interspinous ligaments, ligamentum flavum, dura mater, subdural space, arachnoid mater and subarachnoid space.
- However, via the **paramedian approach** all the above structures are encountered except the supraspinous and interspinous ligaments.
  - Hadzic A. *Textbook of Regional Anesthesia and Acute Pain Management*. 1st ed. New York, NY: McGraw-Hill Medical; 2006. p. 196.

A3 B

▶ **Thirty-one** pairs of spinal nerves arise from the spinal cord with anterior motor and posterior sensory roots. The spinal nerves are named as per the intervertebral foramen from which they exit.

▶ In the **cervical region**, they are named according to the lower cervical vertebral body (C3 emerges from intervertebral foramen formed by C2 and C3), but in the **thoracic and lumbar region** they are named according to the upper vertebral body (L3 emerges from intervertebral foramen formed by L3 and L4).

▶ The dorsal nerve roots divide into two or three bundles during their exit and redivide further before forming dorsal root ganglia.

▶ Most ventral nerve roots exit as a single bundle, explaining the slower onset of motor blockade because of smaller surface area for local anaesthetic action.

- Barash PG, Cullen BF, Stoelting RK, *et al. Clinical Anesthesia*. 6th ed. Philadelphia, PA: Lippincott Williams & Wilkins; 2009. p. 911.
- Hadzic A. *Textbook of Regional Anesthesia and Acute Pain Management*. 1st ed. New York, NY: McGraw-Hill Medical; 2006. p. 197.
- Mulroy MF, Bernards CM, McDonald SB, *et al. A Practical Approach to Regional Anesthesia*. 4th ed. Philadelphia, PA: Lippincott Williams & Wilkins; 2008. pp. 65–6.

A4 D The factors affecting the spread of local anaesthetic in subarachnoid space include the following.

▶ **Drug factors**: baricity, volume, specific gravity and dose of local anaesthetic.

▶ **Patient factors**: raised intra-abdominal pressure (pregnancy, obesity, ascites), spinal column anatomy, patient position and patient height.

▶ **Technique**: direction of the needle bevel and site of injection.

Concentration has no effect on the spread of local anaesthetic, as a new concentration is formed after mixing with the cerebrospinal fluid (CSF).

- Hadzic A. *Textbook of Regional Anesthesia and Acute Pain Management*. 1st ed. New York, NY: McGraw-Hill Medical; 2006. p. 202.

A5 D

▶ Epinephrine and phenylephrine are both vasoconstrictors. They **prolong** the duration of action of local anaesthetic by decreasing their systemic absorption. Because of its vasoconstrictive properties, epinephrine may cause **anterior spinal artery ischaemia**.

▶ The risk of transient neurological symptoms (TNSs) has been shown to increase with the use of phenylephrine.
▶ Clonidine prolongs **both sensory and motor blockade**.
▶ Acetylcholinesterase inhibitors like neostigmine exert their effect by increasing acetylcholine and nitric oxide. However, their use is limited by side effects such as **nausea, vomiting, agitation, bradycardia, restlessness and lower-limb weakness**.
  • Hadzic A. *Textbook of Regional Anesthesia and Acute Pain Management*. 1st ed. New York, NY: McGraw-Hill Medical; 2006. pp. 203–4.

A6   **B** The risk factors for **hypotension** following spinal anaesthetic include:
▶ obesity (high body mass index)
▶ pre-existing hypertension
▶ hypovolaemia
▶ age > 40 years
▶ combined general and spinal anaesthetic
▶ chronic alcohol consumption
▶ emergency surgery
▶ high sensory blockade
▶ addition of vasoconstrictor to local anaesthetic solution.
  • Hadzic A. *Textbook of Regional Anesthesia and Acute Pain Management*. 1st ed. New York, NY: McGraw-Hill Medical; 2006. p. 204.

A7   **A**
▶ Combined alpha and beta agonists are superior to pure alpha agonist in treating hypotension, and **ephedrine is currently the drug of choice**. Phenylephrine can be used, especially if tachycardia is present.
▶ **Coloading** of fluids at the time of induction has been shown to be superior to the prior infusion of fluids.
▶ **Reverse Trendelenburg position** may stop the cephalad anaesthetic spread, but may lead to marked hypotension because of venous pooling in lower limbs.
▶ **Flexion of the operation table** may be helpful by elevating the legs but preventing cephalad spread of local anaesthetic.
  • Mulroy MF, Bernards CM, McDonald SB, *et al. A Practical Approach to Regional Anesthesia*. 4th ed. Philadelphia, PA: Lippincott Williams & Wilkins; 2008. pp. 94–5.

A8 C Appropriate sensory levels of blockade for common surgeries are as follows:

- Caesarean section/upper abdominal surgery – T4
- gynaecological and urological surgeries – T6
- vaginal delivery of foetus – T10
- transurethral resection of prostate – T10
- lower extremity surgery with tourniquet – T10
- perineal surgery – S2–S5.
  - Hadzic A. *Textbook of Regional Anesthesia and Acute Pain Management.* 1st ed. New York, NY: McGraw-Hill Medical; 2006. p. 200.
  - Mulroy MF, Bernards CM, McDonald SB, *et al. A Practical Approach to Regional Anesthesia.* 4th ed. Philadelphia, PA: Lippincott Williams & Wilkins; 2008. p. 71.

A9 B The following are the risk factors for **bradycardia** with spinal anaesthetic:

- ASA class 1
- prolonged PR interval (heart blocks)
- preoperative beta-blocker therapy
- male gender
- baseline heart rate < 60 bpm
- sensory block above T5
- younger age groups (age < 40 years).
  - Mulroy MF, Bernards CM, McDonald SB, *et al. A Practical Approach to Regional Anesthesia.* 4th ed. Philadelphia, PA: Lippincott Williams & Wilkins; 2008. p. 94.

A10 A

- A high spinal block **does not** affect the cervical segments usually.
- High spinal block paralyses the abdominal and intercostal muscles **affecting forced expiration**. Therefore, there is a decrease in expiratory reserve volume, peak expiratory flow and maximum minute ventilation (all forced expiratory volumes).
- There is **relative sparing** of phrenic nerve and cervical area. Hence, inspiration is minimally affected.
- Arterial blood gas measurements **do not change** in a spontaneously breathing patient.
- Inability to feel the chest wall may result in **dyspnoea**. This is addressed by reassurance (not intubation).

- Hadzic A. *Textbook of Regional Anesthesia and Acute Pain Management*. 1st ed. New York, NY: McGraw-Hill Medical; 2006. p. 206.

A11 C

Table 4.1 Various types of spinal needles

Type	Example
Pencil-point needles	Sprotte and Whitacre
Needles with cutting bevels	Pitkin (short cutting bevel)
	Quincke (medium cutting bevel)
Needle with non-cutting bevel	Greene needle

Although the pencil-point needles require **more force** to insert than bevel-tip needles, they provide **better tactile sensation** of the layers of the ligaments encountered. The incidence of **post-dural puncture headache** (PDPH) can be reduced by directing the bevel of the needle longitudinally. Spinal needles with introducers help by preventing contamination of CSF with epidermis, which may lead to formation of dermal spinal tumors. The introducer is placed in the interspinous ligament.

- Hadzic A. *Textbook of Regional Anesthesia and Acute Pain Management*. 1st ed. New York, NY: McGraw-Hill Medical; 2006. pp. 211–12.

A12 A The Taylor approach is a paramedian approach at **L5–S1** interface, which is the largest interspace. It can be done in the **sitting, prone or lateral positions**. The needle is inserted **1 cm inferior and 1 cm medial to the posterior superior iliac spine** and directed at an angle of **45°–55° cephalad**.

- Hadzic A. *Textbook of Regional Anesthesia and Acute Pain Management*. 1st ed. New York, NY: McGraw-Hill Medical; 2006. p. 215.

A13 C

▶ Opioids act **synergistically** along with local anaesthetics in intrathecal space by binding to μ-opioid receptors.

▶ Morphine may cause **delayed respiratory depression** (24 hours), whereas lipophilic opioids like fentanyl and sufentanil cause **immediate respiratory depression** (20–30 minutes).

▶ Small doses of fentanyl **intensify** the blockade without prolonging it.

▶ Clonidine intensifies and prolongs **both sensory and motor blockade**. This effect is seen with intrathecal, oral (premedication) or intravenous route of clonidine.

▶ Neostigmine, an acetylcholinesterase inhibitor, increases the availability of endogenous acetylcholine. Activation of acetylcholine receptors is thought to contribute to an endogenous form of analgesia. However, it is not used because the incidence of nausea and vomiting is high.

- Cousins MJ, Bridenbaugh PO, Carr DB, *et al. Cousins and Bridenbaugh's Neural Blockade in Clinical Anesthesia and Pain Medicine*. 4th ed. Philadelphia, PA: Lippincott Williams & Wilkins; 2008. p. 217.

A14 B The sequence of blockade of nerve fibres is as follows:

B fibres (preganglionic sympathetic) > C fibres (cold sensation) > Aδ (pinprick) > Aβ (touch) > Aα (motor)

The recovery is in the reverse order. This explains one of the reasons for the zone of **differential blockade** in spinal anaesthesia: sympathetic block is two segments higher than sensory block, which is two segments higher than motor blockade. These zones of differential blockade remain constant during emergence from spinal anaesthetic.

- Cousins MJ, Bridenbaugh PO, Carr DB, *et al. Cousins and Bridenbaugh's Neural Blockade in Clinical Anesthesia and Pain Medicine*. 4th ed. Philadelphia, PA: Lippincott Williams & Wilkins; 2008. p. 219.

A15 C The density of CSF varies from 1.00033 g/mL to 1.00067 g/mL. It decreases with increase in temperature.

Baricity is ratio of density of local anaesthetic to CSF.
- ▶ Hyperbaric solutions have greater density to CSF. Local anaesthetics are made hyperbaric by adding **glucose 50–80 mg/mL**.
- ▶ Isobaric solutions have the same density as CSF whereas hypobaric are less dense than CSF.
- ▶ Local anaesthetics are made hypobaric by adding **distilled water**. Hypobaric anaesthetic solution may be used for rectal and perineal surgery in lateral decubitus or prone jackknife position.

Specific gravity is the ratio of density of a substance to the density of water.

Local anaesthetics behave as isobaric solution if the density of the solution is within the mean of plus or minus the standard deviation of density of CSF.

Note:
- ▶ Hyperbaric and hypobaric solutions can be made to **spread by altering patient position**.

▶ Hyperbaric solutions allow for providing a **saddle block**.

▶ In a **supine patient**, spread of a hyperbaric solution is the maximum, followed by isobaric solutions, while it is the **least with hypobaric solutions**.

▶ Hypobaric solutions are **not available commercially** and must be prepared at bedside.

▶ Hyperbaric solutions have **a shorter duration** of action than plain solutions.

  • Cousins MJ, Bridenbaugh PO, Carr DB, *et al. Cousins and Bridenbaugh's Neural Blockade in Clinical Anesthesia and Pain Medicine*. 4th ed. Philadelphia, PA: Lippincott Williams & Wilkins; 2008. p. 222.

A16 D Regarding the occurrence of PDPH:

▶ Incidence is **< 1%** if procedure is performed by an expert using non-cutting needles (**Whitacre or Sprotte**).

▶ Incidence is **higher in the obstetric population (1.7%)**, since the procedure is technically difficult (exaggerated lordosis) and pregnant patients may not be able to sit very still for the procedure.

▶ Should a dural tear happen using a **Tuohy needle** (**16 G** is usually used for adults), then **50%–80%** of those patients go on to develop PDPH.

▶ **Higher with cutting needles** (Quincke) than with non-cutting needles (Whitacre or Sprotte).

  • Hadzic A. *Textbook of Regional Anesthesia and Acute Pain Management*. 1st ed. New York, NY: McGraw-Hill Medical; 2006. p. 1041.

A17 D The proposed mechanism in the development of PDPH includes:

▶ The **loss of CSF** from the intrathecal space: this leads to intracranial hypotension to start with, causing the **sagging** of cranial structures in **upright** position, resulting in headache.

▶ Compensatory **cerebral venodilatation** (in keeping with the **Monro–Kelly doctrine**, which states that the sum of volumes of the brain, CSF and intracranial blood is constant).

▶ **Raised intracranial pressure**: secondary to cerebral venodilatation.

  • Hadzic A. *Textbook of Regional Anesthesia and Acute Pain Management*. 1st ed. New York, NY: McGraw-Hill Medical; 2006. p. 1041.

  • Turnbull DK, Shepherd DB. Post-dural puncture headache: pathogenesis, prevention and treatment. *Br J Anaesth*. 2003; **91**(5): 718–29.

A18 C Typical features of PDPH are as follows.

> **History** of a dural puncture (following spinal) or a possible dural tap (following epidural).
> Onset is usually delayed (**12–48 hours**) but can be seen up to 5 days after a procedure.
> Headache is typically **positional** in character (most severe in upright position, while decreases with patient recumbent).
> Is almost always **bilateral** in distribution.
> **Associated symptoms** of nausea, vomiting, neck stiffness, visual/auditory disturbances or cranial nerve involvement.

Note: an increase in severity of the headache on standing is the sine qua non of PDPH.

- Turnbull DK, Shepherd DB. Post-dural puncture headache: pathogenesis, prevention and treatment. *Br J Anaesth*. 2003; **91**(5): 718–29.

A19 A

Table 4.2 Risk factors for the development of post-dural puncture headache

Patient-related	Procedure-related
Young adults (vs elderly)	Larger-gauge needles (vs finer needles)
Female sex (vs males)	Cutting needles (vs non-cutting)
Obstetric patients (vs non-obstetric patients)	Higher number of dural punctures
History of previous headaches	Insertion of needle bevel perpendicular to the direction of fibres of ligamentum flavum (cutting rather than splitting)
	Non-expert operator
	Dural puncture following epidural than a spinal (bigger defect)

Note: paramedian approaches may allow better sealing of defects, lowering the incidence of PDPH. Recent evidence suggests that threading a catheter into the subarachnoid space may reduce the incidence of PDPH.

- Hadzic A. *Textbook of Regional Anesthesia and Acute Pain Management*. 1st ed. New York, NY: McGraw-Hill Medical; 2006. p. 1043.
- Sharpe P. Accidental dural puncture in obstetrics. *Contin Educ Anaesth Crit Care Pain*. 2001; **1**(3): 81–4.

A20 C

Table 4.3 Management of post-dural puncture headache

Conservative
bed rest, hydration, abdominal binders
Pharmacological
paracetamol, non-steroidal anti-inflammatory drugs, codeine
strong opioids (as temporary measure)
cerebral vasoconstrictors: caffeine, methylxanthine, theophylline
5-HT$_1$ agonist: sumatriptan
adrenocorticotropic hormone
Interventional
intrathecal opioids
epidural saline
epidural blood patch (considered 'gold standard'): success rate is **70%–90%**

Note: prophylactic blood patch in asymptomatic patients who have had a dural puncture is not advised.

- Sharpe P. Accidental dural puncture in obstetrics. *Contin Educ Anaesth Crit Care Pain.* 2001; **1**(3): 81–4.

A21 C

▸ Epidural space (extradural) lies between spinal dura mater and walls of vertebral canal.

▸ It extends from the base of the skull to the sacral hiatus.

▸ It contains fat, lymphatics, areolar tissue, nerves and venous plexus. There is no free fluid present.

▸ **Batson's venous plexus**, present in the epidural space, is a valveless system in continuity with the pelvic veins and venous system of the abdominal and thoracic body wall.

▸ This explains the more common blood vessel puncture in **pregnant patients**, as epidural veins are engorged due to caval compression (especially in **paramedian insertions**).

▸ The anterior dura is heavily innervated by nerves, but the posterior dura is poorly supplied. The periosteum is pain-sensitive but the **ligamentum flavum is not**. This allows spinal anaesthetic with little pain.

▸ The ligamentum flavum forms the posterior boundary of epidural space.

Note: epidural fat increases with obesity and decreases with age. This explains why epidural local anaesthetic requirement is **lower in the elderly**.

- Hadzic A. *Textbook of Regional Anesthesia and Acute Pain Management*. 1st ed. New York, NY: McGraw-Hill Medical; 2006. p. 235.
- Richardson J, Groen GJ. Applied epidural anatomy. *Contin Educ Anaesth Crit Care Pain*. 2005; **5**(3): 98–100.

A22 B

▶ The spinous processes of cervical, thoracic and lumbar vertebrae have different angulation.

▶ They are **relatively straight**, posteriorly directed **at cervical, lower thoracic and lumbar levels**.

▶ But they are **caudally inclined at thoracic levels**.

▶ The greatest degree of angulation is at **T3–T7**, making **medial approach** to epidural space technically **difficult**. Hence a **paramedian approach is easier** at this level.

- Hadzic A. *Textbook of Regional Anesthesia and Acute Pain Management*. 1st ed. New York, NY: McGraw-Hill Medical; 2006. p. 232.

A23 D

▶ C7: vertebrae prominens

▶ T3: spine of scapula

▶ T7: inferior angle of scapula

▶ L4: line connecting iliac crest

▶ S2: line connecting posterior inferior iliac spine.

- Hadzic A. *Textbook of Regional Anesthesia and Acute Pain Management*. 1st ed. New York, NY: McGraw-Hill Medical; 2006. p. 240.

A24 B Absolute contraindications for epidural blockade include patient refusal, infection at injection site, allergy to local anaesthetic, raised intracranial pressure and hypovolemia. **Relative contraindications** include a platelet count < 100 000 per mL, hypertension, sepsis, anatomical abnormality of spine, previous spinal surgery and an uncooperative patient.

- Hadzic A. *Textbook of Regional Anesthesia and Acute Pain Management*. 1st ed. New York, NY: McGraw-Hill Medical; 2006. p. 232.

A25 C

Table 4.4 The physiological effects of epidural anaesthesia

System	Effects
Cardiovascular	*Block below T4:* venodilation and arterial dilation, decrease in venous return and systemic vascular resistance compensatory reflex vasoconstriction above the blockade *Block above T4:* blocks the cardio-acceleratory fibres, resulting in bradycardia and hypotension
Respiratory	Minimal effects on pulmonary function Vital capacity, tidal volume, minute ventilation and dead space are maintained Forced expiratory volumes reduced
Renal	Urinary retention may occur from blockade of S2–S4 fibres Due to renal autoregulation, renal blood flow is maintained.
Gastrointestinal	Increase in secretions, peristalsis and a contracted gut occur because of unopposed parasympathetic action The visceral perfusion is well maintained Nausea from increased gastric peristalsis
Neuroendocrine	Epidural blockade abolishes the stress response to surgery by blocking the afferent sensory fibres Thoracic epidural prevents an increase in post-operative nor-epinephrine release, which causes vasospasm, thus offering cardioprotective benefits

Epidural anaesthesia more effectively decreases stress response with lower-abdominal and lower-limb surgeries than upper-abdominal and thoracic surgeries. This is because not all the nociceptive afferent fibres in upper-abdominal and thoracic surgeries may be blocked.

- Hadzic A. *Textbook of Regional Anesthesia and Acute Pain Management.* 1st ed. New York, NY: McGraw-Hill Medical; 2006. p. 241.

A26 B

▶ Epinephrine added to local anaesthetic solution (short- and medium-acting) **prolongs the duration** of action both by pharmacodynamic and pharmacokinetic effect. Pharmacokinetic effect – slower drug clearance from epidural space, resulting in decrease in peak plasma concentration, mainly by decreasing blood flow in the dura mater. Pharmacodynamic effect – acts on α2 receptors, decreasing pain transmission.

- Epinephrine may **increase the incidence of hypotension**, because of its β2 (vasodilatation) effect.
- Adding bicarbonate to local anaesthetic increases the unionised form, hence more drug can penetrate the lipid membrane, thereby **increasing the speed of onset**.
- Combining long and short anaesthetic solutions **has not been proven to be better**. Additionally, it may potentiate toxicity (as this is additive).
- Clonidine **prolongs and intensifies epidural** blockade. It modulates the stress response to surgery and has possible antibacterial activity against *Staphylococcus*.

Note: recommended solutions of sodium bicarbonate to be added to local anaesthetic are 1 mEq/mL for lignocaine and other shorter-acting agents, and 0.1 mEq/mL for bupivacaine and ropivacaine.

- Hadzic A. *Textbook of Regional Anesthesia and Acute Pain Management*. 1st ed. New York, NY: McGraw-Hill Medical; 2006. p. 243.
- Mulroy MF, Bernards CM, McDonald SB, *et al. A Practical Approach to Regional Anesthesia*. 4th ed. Philadelphia, PA: Lippincott Williams & Wilkins; 2008. pp. 108–9.

A27 B

- Site of epidural injection is important (should correlate with the dermatome of surgical incision for maximal effect).
- Concentration of local anaesthetic mainly affects the **density of the block**.
- Volume affects the **height of the block**. Usually 1–2 mL per segment is used for epidural blockade.
- Weight and height have **no correlation with the spread** of epidural drug, except in extreme scenarios.
  - Hadzic A. *Textbook of Regional Anesthesia and Acute Pain Management*. 1st ed. New York, NY: McGraw-Hill Medical; 2006. p. 245.

A28 A

- The loss or resistance (LOR) to fluid to identify the epidural space was first decribed by **Dogliotti**. It mainly gives a **visual sign** of entry into epidural space and is not dependent on the feel. If a large volume of saline is used it may produce inadequate blockade due to dilution of local anaesthetic. Fluid obtained later after catheter placement can be differentiated from CSF by **urine reagent strip**.

▶ LOR using air might result in false LOR, as air is **compressible**. Use of air may cause venous air embolism, headache, pneumocephalus and patchy block.

  • Hadzic A. *Textbook of Regional Anesthesia and Acute Pain Management.* 1st ed. New York, NY: McGraw-Hill Medical; 2006. pp. 250–2.

A29 **B**

▶ The test dose for epidural anaesthesia **includes 3 mL of 1.5% lidocaine with epinephrine 15 mcg**.

▶ An increase in heart rate by 20% is indicative of intravascular placement, except in patients on beta blockers, pregnant patients in active labour and patients under general anaesthetic.

▶ Systolic blood pressure changes of about 20 mmHg are used as an indicator of intravascular placement in patients on beta blockers.

▶ Peaked P waves and T-wave changes on ECG indicate intravascular placement in paediatrics.

▶ Dense motor block within 5 minutes of test dose indicates intrathecal placement.

▶ In patients in active labour, the test dose must be given **after a contraction**.

  • Hadzic A. *Textbook of Regional Anesthesia and Acute Pain Management.* 1st ed. New York, NY: McGraw-Hill Medical; 2006. pp. 250–2.

A30 **C** In elderly patients, there is a **reduction in size of the intervertebral foramina**, limiting the spread of local anaesthetics out of the epidural space. Additionally, reduction in the fat content allows a **more cephalad spread**. Hence, the same dose as in adults will lead to a higher block. Consequently, dosing for the elderly should be **reduced**.

  • Hadzic A. *Textbook of Regional Anesthesia and Acute Pain Management.* 1st ed. New York, NY: McGraw-Hill Medical; 2006. pp. 245.

A31 **C** Pharmacokinetic considerations of epidural in children:

▶ **Higher CNS toxicity**: blood–brain barrier is more permeable.

▶ Lower α1-acid glycoprotein levels: **higher free fraction** and higher potential for toxicity.

▶ **Higher initial plasma concentrations** due to high cardiac output increasing the uptake of local anaesthetic agents from neuraxial spaces.

▶ **Decreased duration of action** due to high cardiac output and increased uptake away from neuraxis.

▶ **Drug accumulation** after a continuous infusion.

▶ **Reduced drug metabolism and clearance**: immature liver and kidneys. Due to this, decrease infusion rate after 24 hours.

- Patel D. Epidural analgesia for children. *Contin Educ Anaesth Crit Care Pain*. 2006; **6**(2): 63–6.

A32 B Regarding paediatric epidurals:

▶ The **single isomers** like ropivacaine and levobupivacaine are preferred. The reduced toxicity and less motor blockade offer immense benefits particularly in infants and neonates. Prolonged infusion of ropivacaine (72 hours) has not shown increased toxicity. The vasoconstrictive properties of ropivacaine may delay its systemic absorption, reducing systemic toxicity.

▶ **Test doses**: convulsions, arrhythmias and respiratory or cardiac arrest may be the first signs of toxicity in children, as procedures are mostly performed under general anaesthetic. Monitoring ECG changes is a specific and more reliable method of detecting intravascular spread.

▶ **Additives**: because of concerns regarding spinal cord toxicity and the risk of apnoea, additives are not commonly used below 6 months of age.

▶ **Anatomy**: because the spinal cord extends till L3 and subarachnoid space till S3–S4 in infants, caudal epidural is preferred over lumbar epidurals. Also, due to less fat and fibrous tissue, it is easier to insert catheters to higher levels from lower approaches.

- Patel D. Epidural analgesia for children. *Contin Educ Anaesth Crit Care Pain*. 2006; **6**(2): 63–6.

A33 D Difficulties in needle insertion, uncertain placement of catheters and the potential of neurological problems with thoracic epidural are the reasons for **hesitancy** in its use for abdominal surgery. On the other hand, extension of lumbar block may be accepted as a compromise. But this may not be ideal for several reasons, as follows.

▶ Higher chances of bradycardia, vasodilatation and hypotension (Bezold–Jarisch reflex) with lumbar epidural.

▶ Lumbar blocks are difficult to maintain (frequent regression seen) and need frequent rescue doses.

▶ Lumbar block cause more hypotension, and reflex vasoconstriction above the block may lead to myocardial ischaemia.

▶ Evidence suggests that lumbar epidurals should be avoided in patients undergoing abdominal or thoracic procedures.

- McLeod GA, Cumming C. Thoracic epidural anaesthesia and analgesia. *Contin Educ Anaesth Crit Care Pain*. 2004; **4**(1): 16–19.

A34 D Combined spinal epidural (CSE) offers benefits of both spinal and epidural.

▶ The **onset** of surgical anaesthesia is comparable with a single-shot spinal and is faster than epidural anaesthesia.

▶ CSE allows the use of **lower dose of anaesthetic** for spinal and later prolongation of block if required with epidural administration of local anaesthetic.

▶ There is significant **reduction in the duration of first-stage labour** in primiparous patients.

There are a few disadvantages of CSE:

▶ Inability to test the epidural catheter after spinal injection.

▶ Possibility of failed epidural catheter.

▶ The risk of greater spread of spinal drug after epidural injection.

• Hadzic A. *Textbook of Regional Anesthesia and Acute Pain Management.* 1st ed. New York, NY: McGraw-Hill Medical; 2006. p. 286.

A35 B CSE can be done with two techniques: needle-through-needle technique (NTN) and two separate injections at different levels.

▶ The knowledge of posterior epidural space distance (PED) is very important with NTN technique.

▶ **Underestimation** of PED may result in spinal block failure and **overestimation** may cause damage to neural structures.

▶ PED is widest in the lumbar region and narrowest in the cervical region.

▶ The dural sac is **triangular in shape**, and thus paramedian approach increases the risk of failed spinal block with NTN technique.

• Hadzic A. *Textbook of Regional Anesthesia and Acute Pain Management.* 1st ed. New York, NY: McGraw-Hill Medical; 2006. p. 288.

A36 B The two techniques of performing CSE are NTN and separate needle technique (SNT).

▶ **NTN**: This involves use of two separate needles for epidural and spinal, but use of same intervertebral space. This is associated with **single skin puncture** and hence less discomfort to the patient. However, as **spinal block is given prior** to epidural catheterisation, confirmation of epidural placement of catheter is **not possible**.

▶ Separate spinal and epidural block (SNT) at two different intervertebral spaces. This is slightly **more uncomfortable** to the patient because of two skin punctures. It also **takes more time** than the NTN technique.

▶ The test dose (3 mL of 1.5% lignocaine and epinephrine 1:200 000) is used to rule out intravascular placement or intrathecal placement. If the catheter is intravascular, there would be tachycardia due to epinephrine, whereas a dense block with test dose will confirm intrathecal placement. **The test dose does not confirm proper epidural placement.**

▶ Nerve stimulation may be used as a technique for confirmation of epidural placement of catheter.

- Hadzic A. *Textbook of Regional Anesthesia and Acute Pain Management.* 1st ed. New York, NY: McGraw-Hill Medical; 2006. pp. 290–2.

A37 **C** Various tests are used to confirm epidural placement of catheter, the use of nerve stimulators (Tsui test) being one of them. Epidural placement of catheter is confirmed if a motor response is obtained with a current strength of **1–10 mA**. A motor response with **> 10 mA** indicates that the catheter is **outside** the epidural space, whereas a motor response with **< 1 mA** indicates **subarachnoid location** of catheter. Its sensitivity and specificity is 100%.

- Hadzic A. *Textbook of Regional Anesthesia and Acute Pain Management.* 1st ed. New York, NY: McGraw-Hill Medical; 2006. p. 293.

A38 **D** Failure of spinal block with CSE is mainly because:

▶ spinal needle too short – not able to reach dura

▶ spinal needle too long – deviation from the midline

▶ with NTN technique as spinal needle enters via the epidural needle, it is not stabilised by the surrounding ligaments. Therefore, the hand must be very stable during injection of drug. Slight movement of hand may result in inappropriate drug delivery.

There is a possibility of depositing **metallic debris** in the intrathecal space with NTN technique due to friction between the needles. There may be subarachnoid flux of epidurally administered local anaesthetic with CSE, leading to **higher block** than the same dose administered solely epidurally. Similarly intrathecally administered local anaesthetic may lead to higher block with CSE than single-shot spinal, as epidurally administered air or saline **decreases the lumbar CSF volume.**

- Hadzic A. *Textbook of Regional Anesthesia and Acute Pain Management.* 1st ed. New York, NY: McGraw-Hill Medical; 2006. pp. 294–6.

A39 A

▶ There is increased risk of **foetal bradycardia** with CSE as compared with single-shot spinal. The rapid onset of analgesia with CSE causes a fall in catecholamine levels, leading to foetal bradycardia. However, this effect is transient, lasting only few minutes.

▶ The incidence of PDPH is **rare** with CSE because of the use of **small-gauge atraumatic spinal needles**.

▶ There is a higher risk of neurological injury with CSE when compared with a single-shot spinal.

▶ There is **no increased risk** of metal deposition with NTN combined spinal epidural.

  • Hadzic A. *Textbook of Regional Anesthesia and Acute Pain Management*. 1st ed. New York, NY: McGraw-Hill Medical; 2006. pp. 296–98.

A40 C 'Epidural volume extension' (EVE) via a combined spinal–epidural (CSE) technique is the enhancement of a small-dose intrathecal block by epidural saline boluses. The **advantages** are as follows.

▶ Theoretically, it may help reduce the total intrathecal local anaesthetic dose required. However, a recent study did not find the technique dose-sparing.

▶ It allows a faster motor recovery.

▶ It does not alter the pain scores (VAS), peak sensory block height, time for sensory regression (to T10) and lowest systolic blood pressures.

  • Beale N, Evans B, Plaat F, *et al*. Effect of epidural volume extension on dose requirement of intrathecal hyperbaric bupivacaine at caesarean section. *Br J Anaesth*. 2005; **95**(4): 500–3.

  • Lew E, Yeo SW, Thomas E. Combined spinal-epidural anesthesia using epidural volume extension leads to faster motor recovery after elective cesarean delivery: a prospective, randomised, double-blind study. *Anesth Analg*. 2004; **98**(3): 810–14.

A41 B

▶ The sacral vertebral foramina form a triangular canal called the **sacral canal**, which is a continuation of the lumbar spinal canal.

▶ **Sacral hiatus** is formed by failure of the laminae of S5 to meet, thus exposing its dorsal surface.

▶ **Sacral cornuae** are formed by inferior articular process of S5 of each side.

▶ Practically, the sacral hiatus is identified by drawing an equilateral triangle, the base of which is formed by the posterior superior iliac spine.

  • Hadzic A. *Textbook of Regional Anesthesia and Acute Pain Management*. 1st ed. New York, NY: McGraw-Hill Medical; 2006. pp. 270–2.

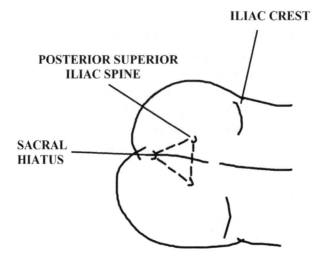

Figure 4.1 Landmarks for caudal anaesthesia

A42 **C** Regarding the technique for caudal block:

▶ Best position for children is **lateral decubitus** with hips and knees flexed at 90°. Adults are best positioned **prone** for this block.

▶ A **22-G intravenous canula** or a **needle with a stellate** is best used to avoid tissue coring into a hollow needle.

▶ The needle should be **short-bevel** to appreciate penetration of sacro-coccygeal membrane.

▶ **Strict asepsis** is stressed because of frequent soiling from the anal area.

▶ The needle is first placed at an **angle of 45°** to the plane of the sacrum, and placed at the sacral hiatus to pierce the sacrococcygeal ligament. Then it is placed **horizontally** and advanced by **2–3 mm**.

Table 4.5 Doses of local anaesthetic for caudal block (as described by Armitage)

Level needed	Agent	Dose
Sacro-lumbar	0.25% bupivacaine	0.5 mL/kg
Upper abdominal	0.25% bupivacaine	1 mL/kg
Mid-thoracic	0.25% bupivacaine	1.25 mL/kg

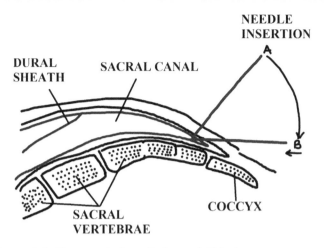

Figure 4.2 Placement of needle in caudal block

- Armitage EN. Local anaesthetic techniques for prevention of postoperative pain. *Br J Anaesth*. 1986; **58**: 790–800.
- O Raux, C Dadure, J Carr, *et al. Paediatric Caudal Anaesthesia. Updates in Anaesthesia*. Available at: http://update.anaesthesiologists.org/2010/12/01/paediatric-caudal-anaesthesia

A43 D

- ▶ Caudal block results in less peripheral vasodilatation than lumbar epidural, as **sympathetic outflow** from the spinal cord **ends at L2**.
- ▶ Caudal block results in blockage of **S2–S4** contribution to **parasympathetic system**, affecting the bladder and the bowel distal to the colonic splenic flexure.
- ▶ The sacral canal varies widely anatomically, requiring almost **double the dose** of local anaesthetic as compared with lumbar epidural in order to achieve the same level of blockade.
    - Hadzic A. *Textbook of Regional Anesthesia and Acute Pain Management*. 1st ed. New York, NY: McGraw-Hill Medical; 2006. pp. 270–2.

A44 B

- ▶ **Whoosh test**: injection of 2–3 mL of air in the caudal epidural space and auscultation over the thoracolumbar area produces the characteristic sound. It may cause patchy block and air embolism.
- ▶ **Swoosh test**: in paediatric patients, local anaesthetic or saline is used instead of air.
- ▶ Correct needle placement in the epidural space can be identified with a

nerve stimulator (current 1–10 mA) and **anal sphincter contraction** as the end response.

▶ Ultrasound may be useful in children < 6 months old, as after this age there is **ossification** of vertebral bodies preventing good visualisation.

- Hadzic A. *Textbook of Regional Anesthesia and Acute Pain Management*. 1st ed. New York, NY: McGraw-Hill Medical; 2006. pp. 274–9.

A45 A Uses of caudal epidural block:

▶ Caudal block is used for surgical procedures both **above and below the diaphragm** in paediatrics.

▶ It may be used for labour analgesia, gynaecological, lower-limb and anal surgeries.

▶ It is mainly used for chronic pain management in adults.

- Hadzic A. *Textbook of Regional Anesthesia and Acute Pain Management*. 1st ed. New York, NY: McGraw-Hill Medical; 2006. p. 272.

A46 B

▶ **'Christmas tree'** appearance is normally seen on injection of contrast in the caudal space. It is due to spread of the dye in the caudal canal and along the nerve roots as they exit the vertebral column. **Epidural adhesions** are diagnosed with its characteristic **absence**.

▶ The risk of local anaesthetic toxicity is as follows: **caudal > brachial plexus block > lumbar or thoracic epidural**.

▶ **T-wave changes** on the ECG are the **earliest changes** in paediatric patients following intravascular placement of local anaesthetic following caudal block. These are then followed by heart rate and blood pressure changes.

- Hadzic A. *Textbook of Regional Anesthesia and Acute Pain Management*. 1st ed. New York, NY: McGraw-Hill Medical; 2006. p. 281.

5
Peripheral nerve blocks

Questions

Choose one best answer for each of the following questions.

Q1   Regarding brachial plexus anatomy, which of the following statements is **true**?
   a. The brachial plexus is derived from the dorsal rami of C5–T1 spinal nerves
   b. The plexus divides into horizontally arranged trunks immediately before forming three cords
   c. The brachial plexus unites into three cords immediately forming three trunks before dividing into five nerves
   d. Passes over the first rib and under the clavicle

Q2   Which of the following statements regarding the anatomy of brachial plexus is **correct**?
a. The brachial plexus anatomy is quite variable
b. The divisions lie above the clavicle and are blocked in a supraclavicular approach
c. The cords are arranged around the first part of the axillary artery
d. The median nerve is the terminal branch of posterior cord

Q3   Which of the following nerves does **not** originate from the brachial plexus in the supraclavicular region?
a. Dorsal scapular nerve
b. Long thoracic nerve
c. Nerve to subclavius
d. Phrenic nerve

Q4   Which of the following nerves is **correctly matched** with the cord of the brachial plexus?
a. Lateral cord – ulnar nerve
b. Posterior cord – musculocutaneous nerve
c. Medial cord – median nerve
d. Posterior cord – axillary nerve

Q5   Which of the following nerves are **correctly** derived from the corresponding nerve roots?
a. Musculocutaneous – C8, T1
b. Axillary nerve – C6, C7
c. Radial nerve – C5–T1
d. Median nerve – C8, T1

Q6   Regarding the brachial plexus, which of the following statements is **incorrect**?
a. The musculocutaneous nerve continues as the lateral cutaneous nerve of the forearm
b. The axillary nerve continues as the lateral cutaneous nerve of the arm
c. The radial nerve continues as the posterior cutaneous nerve of the forearm
d. The median nerve continues as the medial cutaneous nerve of the forearm

Q7 The following pairs are correctly matched for the dermatomal supply **except**:
a. Shoulder tip – C4
b. Thumb – C6
c. Little finger – C7
d. Medial epicondyle – T1

Q8 Which of the following reflexes are **correctly matched** for their root value?
a. Biceps – C5, C6
b. Triceps – C6, C7
c. Patella – L2, L3
d. Ankle – L5, S1, S2

Q9 Regarding the nerve supply to the hand, which of the following is **correct**?
a. All thenar muscles are supplied by the median nerve
b. Radial nerve supplies flexor carpi radialis
c. Median nerve supplies palmar surface of lateral three and a half fingers
d. Ulnar nerve supplies dorsal surface of lateral one and a half fingers

Q10 Which of the following peripheral nerve block sites are **incorrectly matched** with the level of the brachial plexus?
a. Interscalene block – roots
b. Supraclavicular block – trunks
c. Infraclavicular block – divisions
d. Axillary – terminal nerves

Q11 Which of the following blocks are **correctly matched** for the surgery?
a. Interscalene – clavicle
b. Supraclavicular – hand
c. Infraclavicular – elbow
d. Axillary – upper arm

Q12 Regarding the brachial plexus 'sheath' concept, which of the following statements is **true**?
a. The 'sheath' is derived from prevertebral fascia
b. Winnie popularised this concept, postulating the sheath allowed single injections to produce effective blocks
c. Below the clavicle, the sheath is less robust
d. All of the above

Q13 Which of the following landmarks is **not** needed to perform an interscalene block?
a. Sternal head of sternocleidomastoid
b. Clavicular head of sternocleidomastoid
c. Clavicle
d. First rib

Q14 Which of the following statements is **not** an absolute contraindication to performing an interscalene block?
a. Contralateral phrenic nerve paresis
b. Patient refusal
c. Active bleeding in an anticoagulated patient
d. Local anaesthetic allergy

Q15 Regarding the interscalene block, which of the following statements is **false**?
a. Bicep or tricep stimulation can be accepted
b. Ulnar distribution is often spared
c. Posterior arthroscopic port insertion can be accomplished without pain
d. Phrenic nerve is almost always blocked

Q16 Regarding approaches for a peripheral nerve stimulator (PNS)-guided interscalene block, which of the following statements is **correct**?
a. Modified lateral approach of Borgeat is at the level of C6
b. Pippa's posterior approach involves 5°–10° anterolateral angulation
c. Winnie's classic approach angulates the needle in the horizontal plane
d. Meire's approach is not suitable for catheter placement

Q17 Which of the muscle responses is **not** correctly matched with the trouble-shooting actions listed while performing a PNS-guided interscalene block?
a. Diaphragmatic twitches – redirect needle posterolaterally
b. Scapular twitches – redirect needle anteriorly
c. Trapezius twitches – redirect needle anteriorly
d. Pectoral twitches – redirect needle medially

Q18 Which of the following is **not** a complication of interscalene block?
a. Oculosympathetic palsy
b. Pourfour duPetit's syndrome
c. Hemidiaphragmatic paresis
d. Pneumothorax

Q19 Regarding ultrasound-guided interscalene block, which of the following statements is **false**?
a. A high-frequency probe is used
b. The upper roots have a 'traffic signal light' appearance
c. It may prevent intraneural injection
d. The most commonly applied approach is 'in-plane'

Q20 Regarding phrenic nerve paresis due to interscalene block, which of the following statements is **correct**?
a. Classic PNS-guided interscalene block results in 50% incidence of hemidiaphragmatic paresis
b. Ultrasound-guided block eliminates the occurrence of this complication
c. Reducing the volume of injectate reduces the chances of phrenic nerve paresis
d. Interscalene block at C7 increases the risk of phrenic nerve paresis

Q21 Which of the following statements about the brachial plexus anatomy at the supraclavicular area is **false**?
a. The brachial plexus is organised into a 'bunch of grapes' within a common sheath
b. It passes under the clavicle but over the first rib
c. The subclavian vessels lie lateral to the plexus
d. The pleural dome is medial to the plexus

Q22 Regarding different supraclavicular block approaches, which of the following statements is **false**?
   a. Kulenkampff's original technique had a high risk of pneumothorax
   b. Winnie's approach has a high risk of vascular puncture
   c. Brown's plumb-bob technique advocates anteroposterior plane of needle insertion in parasagittal plane
   d. Dupré and Danel's approach uses the internal jugular as a landmark for needle insertion

Q23 Which of the following muscle responses are **not** correctly matched with the troubleshooting actions listed while performing a PNS-guided supraclavicular block?
   a. Diaphragmatic twitches – redirect needle posterolaterally
   b. Deltoid twitches – inject, since this is an appropriate response
   c. Scapular twitches – redirect needle anteriorly
   d. Little-finger twitches – redirect needle laterally

Q24 Regarding supraclavicular block, which of the following statements is **false**?
   a. It provides anaesthesia for almost the entire upper limb with a single injection
   b. The plexus is located medial to the subclavian artery
   c. It causes less hemidiaphragmatic paresis than interscalene block
   d. The most feared complication is pneumothorax

Q25 Which of the following statements regarding the anatomy of infraclavicular brachial plexus is **correct**?
   a. The brachial plexus in this area is covered by pectoralis major superiorly and pectoralis minor inferiorly
   b. The block involves injection at the level of terminal nerves
   c. The plexus is arranged around the second part of the axillary artery
   d. The medial cord is rarely present medial to the axillary artery

Q26 Regarding the different infraclavicular block approaches, which of the following statements is **false**?

a. Modified Raj's approach entails lateral insertion of needle towards axilla

b. In vertical infraclavicular approach, needle is directed vertically downwards

c. Coracoid approach involves medial needle direction

d. Klaastad's approach is commonly employed while doing ultrasound-guided blocks

Q27 Which of the following muscle responses is **not** an acceptable end point for performing PNS-guided infraclavicular block?

a. Biceps twitch

b. Wrist extension

c. Thumb opposition

d. Finger flexion

Q28 Regarding infraclavicular block, which of the following statements is **false**?

a. It is the best site for catheter insertion

b. It is ideally performed using a high-frequency ultrasound probe

c. Bilateral blocks may be performed

d. It is the best block for elbow surgery

Q29 Which of the following statements about the anatomy of nerves in the axillary area is **false**?

a. The radial nerve lies posterior to the axillary artery

b. The ulnar nerve lies medial and below the artery

c. The musculocutaneous nerve lies above the biceps muscle, innervating as it continues to forearm

d. The arm is abducted at 90° to facilitate block

Q30 Regarding different axillary block approaches, which of the following statements is **false**?

a. De Jong introduced the concept of the neurovascular sheath, enabling single-injection technique

b. Multistimulation technique involves blocking all four nerves separately

c. In the transarterial technique, injectate is deposited deep to the artery

d. Ultrasound-guided blocks are commonly performed using high-frequency probes, in a short-axis view with in-plane needle insertion

Q31 Which of the following statements regarding the axillary block is **incorrect**?
   a. It is well suited for catheter placement
   b. Multistimulation technique has higher success rate
   c. Musculocutaneous sparing is the most common inadequacy of single- injection technique
   d. Tourniquet use needs blocking intercostobrachially by subcutaneous infiltration at axillary floor

Q32 Assessment of the adequacy of brachial plexus block can be made by which of the following methods?
   a. Pull-pull-pinch-pinch
   b. Push-pull-pinch-pinch
   c. Pull-pull-punch-punch
   d. Push-push-pinch-punch

Q33 Regarding tourniquet pain, which of the following statements is **false**?
   a. It is mediated by sympathetic fibres
   b. It is due to accumulation of metabolites
   c. The hypertensive response associated with tourniquet pain can be reduced with ketamine
   d. Epidural clonidine can reduce tourniquet pain

Q34 Regarding nerve block at the level of the elbow, which of the following statements is **correct**?
   a. The median nerve can be blocked lateral to brachial artery
   b. The radial nerve can be blocked lateral to biceps tendon
   c. The ulnar nerve should be blocked between medial epicondyle and olecrenon
   d. Insufficient anaesthesia resulting from block of nerves at the elbow may be supplemented by blocks at the axilla

Q35 Regarding blocks at the wrist, which of the following statements is **false**?
   a. Radial nerve block at the wrist needs a single injection above the radial styloid
   b. Median nerve is blocked between the tendons of palmaris longus and flexor carpi radialis
   c. Ulnar nerve should be blocked medial to flexor carpi ulnaris
   d. Wrist block is adequate for AV fistula surgery

Q36   Regarding suprascapular nerve block, which of the following statements is **correct**?

    a. The suprascapular nerve provides most of the nerve supply to the glenohumeral joint

    b. Its root value is C6–C7

    c. It is blocked superficially, medial to the midpoint of the spine of the scapula

    d. Ultrasound cannot identify this nerve, as it is deeply situated

Q37   Regarding cervical plexus blockade, which of the following statements is **false**?

    a. Cervical plexus is derived from C1–C4

    b. Its cutaneous branches are greater occipital, lesser auricular (largest), transverse cervical and supraclavicular nerves

    c. The phrenic nerve is derived from it

    d. It supplies motor branches to sternocleidomastoid

Q38   Regarding superficial cervical plexus block, which of the following statements is **false**?

    a. Superficial plexus is derived from C1–C4

    b. Superficial cervical plexus may be blocked at midpoint of lateral margin of sternocleidomastoid

    c. Carotid surgery may be performed under a superficial plexus block

    d. Surgery involving the clavicle may be performed using this block

Q39   Regarding deep cervical plexus and its block, which of the following statements is **true**?

    a. Injection is made at the C6 tubercle

    b. The needle is directed medially

    c. The main advantage is it does not produce phrenic nerve paresis

    d. It is essentially a paraverterbral block

Q40   Which of the following statements regarding lumbosacral plexus is **false**?

    a. It comprises two distinct and separate plexus

    b. Lumbar plexus block anaesthetises both the lumbar and sacral components by a single injection

    c. It originates from the anterior rami of the T12–S3 spinal nerves

    d. Continuous lumbosacral plexus block is as effective as an epidural for postoperative analgesia

Q41 Regarding lumbar plexus anatomy, which of the following statements is **true**?
a. It is derived from the anterior primary rami of L1–L4
b. It lies within the body of the quadratus lumborum
c. The lateral cutaneous nerve of thigh (LCN), femoral nerve (FN) and obturator nerve (ON) are its most important branches
d. The LCN, FN and ON are arranged vertically within the quadratus lumborum

Q42 Which of the following branches of lumbar plexus is **correctly matched** with the muscles it supplies?
a. ON supplies pectinius
b. LCN supplies vastus lateralis
c. Ilioinguinal nerve supplies cremaster
d. FN supplies gracilis

Q43 Which of the following statements regarding innervation to joints by the lumbar plexus is **correct**?
a. LCN of thigh innervates the hip joint
b. Posterior division of the femoral nerve innervates the knee joint
c. Anterior division of the obturator innervates the knee joint
d. Posterior division of the obturator innervates the hip joint

Q44 Regarding lower-limb block, which of the following statements is **correct**?
a. Lumbar plexus block consistently blocks the sciatic nerve
b. Femoral nerve block is best performed at the level of the inguinal ligament
c. Surgery over medial malleolus can be done by blocking the femoral nerve
d. Sciatic nerve block is an essential component of postoperative analgesia for total knee arthroplasty

Q45 Regarding the dermatomal supply of the lower limb, which of the following statements is **false**?
a. Pocket area of the trouser is L3
b. Kneecap is L4
c. Medial malleolus is S2
d. Perianal area is S4–S5

Q46 Which of the following landmarks is **not** needed to perform lumbar plexus block?
a. Anterior superior iliac spine
b. Posterior superior iliac spine
c. Iliac crest
d. Spinous processes of lumbar vertebrae

Q47 Regarding the lumbar plexus block, the following statement is **false**:
a. The needle is inserted perpendicular to skin
b. A 100-mm needle is needed
c. Transverse process is usually contacted at 6–8 cm depth
d. Transverse process to lumbar plexus distance is dependent on patient size

Q48 Which of the following troubleshooting manoeuvres for lumbar plexus block is **correctly matched**?
a. Stimulation of erector spinae – withdraw needle
b. Hip flexion – withdraw needle
c. Hamstring twitch – redirect caudally
d. Contact with bone – redirect medially

Q49 While performing the lumbar plexus block, which of the following precaution(s) is/are important?
a. The patient should not be anticoagulated
b. The needle should not be inserted 2–3 cm beyond the transverse process
c. Medial angulation of the needle should be avoided
d. All of the above

Q50 Which of the following is/are complication(s) of lumbar plexus block?
a. Epidural anaesthesia
b. Sympathetic block
c. Spinal anaesthesia
d. All of the above

Q51 Which of the following statements regarding femoral nerve anatomy is **correct**?

a. It is derived from the anterior divisions of the anterior rami of the L2–L4 spinal nerves

b. Passes under the inguinal ligament medial to femoral artery

c. Lies under fascia lata and fascia iliaca

d. Saphenous nerve originates from anterior branch of FN and lies within adductor canal

Q52 Regarding the various techniques of femoral nerve block, which of the following statements is **correct**?

a. Femoral nerve block using PNS is ideally performed at the level of the inguinal ligament

b. The anterior superior iliac spine and pubic tubercle form the landmarks needed for a fascia iliaca block

c. Femoral three-in-one block consistently blocks all three main branches of lumbar plexus

d. Use of ultrasound guidance reduces chances of neural damage

Q53 Regarding PNS-guided femoral block, which of the following statements is **true**?

a. Femoral nerve is at its widest at the level of the inguinal ligament

b. Continuous femoral nerve block provides analgesia for femoral neck fractures

c. End point of needling technique is the stimulation of anterior branch of femoral nerve

d. The catheter should be threaded beyond 10 cm to reach the lumbar plexus for better-quality block

Q54 Which of the following statements regarding femoral nerve block is **correct**?

a. Fascia iliaca block is difficult to perform as the fascial layers cannot be relied upon

b. Femoral three-in-one block is inadequate for popliteal surgeries

c. Continuous femoral nerve block leaves catheter below fascia lata

d. Stimulating catheters have shown enormous benefits when compared with non-stimulating catheters for femoral nerve block

Q55 Which of the following statements regarding saphenous nerve block is **false**?
a. It does not cause any motor block
b. Trans-sartorial approach has the highest success rate
c. It provides cutaneous anaesthesia over the lateral malleolus
d. An ultrasound-guided approach uses the descending genicular artery as a landmark, as the saphenous nerve lies next to it

Q56 Which of the following statements regarding the obturator nerve is **true**?
a. It has a root value of L1–L4
b. It is derived from posterior division of dorsal primary rami
c. The posterior division passes deep to the adductor brevis but superficial to adductor magnus
d. The anterior division passes superficial to the adductor longus and adductor magnus

Q57 Regarding obturator nerve block, which of the following statements is **false**?
a. Classic Winnie's approach is painful
b. The classic approach advocates needle positioning towards obturator foramen
c. Ultrasound guidance helps to block both branches of ON
d. Successful obturator block is established by anaesthesia over medial thigh

Q58 Which of the following statements regarding the lateral cutaneous nerve of the thigh is **false**?
a. It has no motor innervation
b. It is derived from the dorsal division of anterior rami of L2–L3
c. Lies on the iliacus, and courses towards the anterior superior iliac spine (ASIS)
d. Can be blocked 2 cm medial and 2 cm cranial to the ASIS

Q59 Which of the following statements regarding the sacral plexus is **false**?
a. It is derived from the anterior primary rami of L4–S3 spinal nerves
b. Most nerves exit through the greater sciatic foramen
c. Sciatic nerve is the main nerve of this plexus
d. It lies anterior to the iliac vessels

Q60 Regarding sciatic nerve and its branches, which of the following statements is **correct**?
a. Sciatic nerve enters the thigh at the midpoint of greater trochanter and sacral hiatus
b. Tibial and common peroneal nerves are two distinct nerves from the very start contained within the same common sheath
c. Sciatic nerve divides into its two main branches at mid-thigh level
d. At the level of the lower thigh, it courses lateral to the tendon of biceps femoris

Q61 Which of the following nerves does **not** innervate the hip joint?
a. Posterior cutaneous femoral nerve
b. Femoral nerve
c. Obturator nerve
d. Sciatic nerve

Q62 Regarding the performance of a parasacral block, which of the following statements is **false**?
a. Posterior superior iliac spine (PSIS) and ischial tuberosity form important landmarks
b. It consistently blocks both the terminal nerves of sacral plexus
c. It is more advantageous than popliteal block for below-knee procedures
d. Tibial nerve motor response is associated with higher success rate

Q63 Which of the following statements regarding the parasacral plexus block is **correct**?
a. It usually leads to a drop in blood pressure
b. Obturator nerve can be reliably blocked by proximal sacral block approaches
c. It has been shown that posterior cutaneous femoral nerve (PCFN) block provides better tolerance of a thigh tourniquet during below-knee surgery
d. In combination with femoral nerve block, it can be used for operations on the entire lower limb

Q64 Which of the following statements regarding proximal sciatic nerve blockade is **false**?
   a. The posterior transgluteal approach to the sciatic nerve block uses
      PSIS, greater trochanter and sacral hiatus as landmarks
   b. The subgluteal approach uses greater trochanter and ischial
      tuberosity as landmarks
   c. The infragluteal approach uses the lateral margin of biceps femoris
      tendon as a landmark
   d. The anterior approach uses the lesser trochanter as landmark

Q65 Which of the following statements regarding the advantages or disadvantages of proximal sciatic nerve block is **correct**?
   a. Labat's approach is simple to follow and perform
   b. Subgluteal approach is difficult, as the sciatic nerve lies under the
      gluteus muscle
   c. Raj's approach is ideal for supine positioning
   d. In infragluteal approach, BF twitch are reliable end points for
      injection

Q66 Which of the following statement regarding the EMR obtained while
performing sciatic nerve block is **false**?
   a. Eversion of the foot produces the best success rate, as it indicates
      that the tip of the needle is centrally located
   b. Inversion of the foot produces the best success rate, as it indicates
      that the tip of the needle is centrally located
   c. Plantar flexion is due to stimulation of tibial nerve component
   d. Dorsiflexion is due to stimulation of common peroneal nerve
      component

Q67 Regarding the block of sciatic nerve in the popliteal fossa, which of the
following statements is **false**?
   a. It is the most common block employed to block sciatic nerve
   b. It is performed at the apex of the triangle formed by the biceps
      femoris and semimembranosus
   c. Multistimulation technique reduces total volume of local
      anaesthetic needed, and onset times for block
   d. Lateral approach to this block uses the groove between biceps
      femoris and vastus lateralis as a landmark

Q68 Regarding ultrasound-guided popliteal block technique, which of the following statements is **correct**?
a. A low-frequency array probe is used
b. The sciatic nerve is situated deep to popliteal vessels
c. The ultrasound probe needs to be tilted cranially to eliminate anisotropy
d. The local anaesthetic needs to be deposited circumferentially around the nerves

Q69 Which of the following structures is **correctly matched** with its cutaneous nerve supply?
a. Lateral malleolus – saphenous nerve
b. Web space between the first and second toes – deep peroneal nerve
c. Medial malleolus – sural nerve
d. Heel – superficial peroneal nerve

Q70 Regarding the nerve supply to the ankle, which of the following nerves is blocked deep?
a. Sural nerve
b. Superficial peroneal nerve
c. Saphenous nerve
d. Posterior tibial nerve

Q71 Regarding landmarks for ankle block, which of the following statements is **false**?
a. Deep peroneal nerve is blocked medial to dorsalis pedis artery
b. Saphenous nerve is blocked at medial malleolus
c. Posterior tibial nerve is blocked deep to posterior tibial artery
d. Sural nerve is blocked at lateral malleolus

Q72 Regarding regional blocks for foot surgery, which of the following statements is **false**?
a. Ankle blocks are superior to subcutaneous infiltration
b. Popliteal block is superior to both ankle block and subcutaneous infiltration
c. Mayo block is an alternative to ankle blocks for foot surgery
d. Adrenaline is best avoided in ankle blocks

Q73 Regarding pain relief for thoracic surgery, which of the following is **false**?
   a. Uncontrolled acute pain is related to development of chronic pain syndromes
   b. Intercostal blocks help in preserving lung function
   c. Thoracic paravertebral block provides comparable analgesia to epidural, but fewer side effects
   d. None of the above

Q74 Which of the following statements is **correct** regarding the anatomy of intercostal nerves (ICNs)?
   a. They arise from posterior primary rami of T1–T12
   b. At the angle of the rib, ICNs lie between the internal intercostals and the innermost intercostals
   c. Lateral cutaneous branches form the ICNs
   d. ICNs lie in the intercostal grooves above the superior edge of the rib

Q75 Which of the following is the **correct** statement regarding performance of intercostal block?
   a. It is usually performed anterior to mid-axillary line
   b. It is best performed with patient in supine position
   c. After contacting the rib, the needle should be walked off the inferior edge by directing it caudally
   d. None of the above

Q76 Regarding intercostal nerve blocks, which of the following statements is **false**?
   a. ICN block also blocks the visceral pain component
   b. Multiple injections are usually needed due to overlap of nerve supply
   c. Injection at a single level may spread to multiple segments because of medial spread
   d. They may spread to subarachnoid space

Q77 Regarding interpleural anaesthesia, which one of the following statements is **correct**?
  a. Anaesthesia is attained by diffusion to epidural and subarachnoid spaces
  b. The technique may be performed under general anaesthesia and positive pressure ventilation
  c. Keeping the operative side up may lead to sympathetic blockade
  d. None of the above

Q78 Which of the following is **not** a good indication for interpleural block?
  a. Open cholecystectomy
  b. Renal surgery
  c. Unilateral breast procedures
  d. Thoracotomy

Q79 Which of the following is **true** regarding rectal sheath blocks?
  a. It's easy to perform in obese individuals
  b. A single injection on either side suffices for a midline incision
  c. Local anaesthetic is injected above the posterior rectus sheath
  d. Injections above the umbilicus cover the infra-umbilical area as well

Q80 Regarding inguinal block, which of the following statements is **correct**?
  a. Iliohypogastric and ilioinguinal nerves arise from L1 spinal nerve root
  b. Iliohypogastric nerve lies between internal and external oblique at the anterior superior iliac spine
  c. Ilioinguinal nerve lies between transversus abdominis and internal oblique initially, and between internal and external oblique medial to the anterior superior iliac spine
  d. All of the above

Q81 Regarding inguinal hernia block, which of the following is **false**?
  a. It is performed medial to anterior superior iliac spine
  b. Genitofemoral nerve is best blocked medial to anterior superior iliac spine
  c. Does not provide visceral anaesthesia
  d. Femoral block may result if injection is made too deep

Q82 Which of the following statement concerning transversus abdominis plane (TAP) block is **false**?
a. Local anaesthetic is deposited between the external oblique and the internal oblique
b. Reliably provides anaesthesia to lower abdominal wall
c. Triangle of Petit is bounded anteriorly by the external oblique and posteriorly by latissimus dorsi
d. Injections are made posterior to mid-axillary line in the landmark-based technique

Q83 All of the following blocks are correctly matched for the critical bony landmark needed for performing them, **except** which option?
a. Intercostal nerve block and inferior edge of the rib
b. Inguinal block and anterior superior iliac spine
c. TAP block and iliac crest
d. Paravertebral block and spinous process

Q84 Which of the following constitutes the boundaries of the thoracic paravertebral space?
a. Superior costotransverse ligament superiorly
b. Vertebral body medially
c. Posterior intercostals membrane posteriorly
d. Parietal pleura medially

Q85 The following are all differences between thoracic and lumbar paravertebral blocks **except**:
a. Loss-of-resistance technique is particularly suited to lumbar levels and not the thoracic levels
b. The needle is walked off cephalad at thoracic levels and caudad at lumbar levels to block the corresponding spinal nerves
c. A single large-volume injection may spread cephalad or caudad in the thoracic region, rather than the lumbar spaces
d. In both thoracic and lumbar regions, the spinal nerves leave the intervertebral foramen inferior to the transverse process of its corresponding vertebra

Q86 Which of the following is **incorrect** regarding the paravertebral blocks?
a. They provide good analgesia for fractured ribs
b. Easy threading of catheter is most vital for reliable placement of paravertebral catheter
c. Excessive medial angulation of needle while performing a paravertebral block increases the chances of epidural spread
d. Excessive lateral angulation of needle may increase chances of pneumothorax

Q87 Regarding intravenous regional anaesthesia (IVRA), which of the following is **false**?
a. It was first introduced by August Bier
b. It is easier to perform in the arm than in the leg
c. Lignocaine is most commonly used
d. The only absolute contraindication is an anticoagulated patient

Q88 What is the correct sequence of employing IVRA?
a. Intravenous cannulation, exsanguination, distal cuff inflation, local anaesthetic (LA) injection, proximal cuff inflation, distal cuff deflation
b. Exsanguination, intravenous cannulation, proximal cuff inflation, LA injection, distal cuff inflation, proximal cuff deflation
c. Intravenous cannulation, exsanguination, proximal cuff inflation, LA injection, distal cuff inflation, proximal cuff deflation
d. Exsanguination, intravenous cannulation, distal cuff inflation, LA injection, proximal cuff inflation, distal cuff deflation

Q89 Regarding IVRA, the **false** statement is:
a. Bupivacaine is best avoided
b. Rapid injections (over 10 seconds) result in faster onset of block
c. Antecubital veins are best avoided
d. Cuff should not be deflated before 20 minutes

Q90 Which of the following is considered to be the most useful adjunct to LA for IVRA?
a. Non-steroidal anti-inflammatory drugs
b. Opioids
c. Clonidine
d. Neostigmine

Q91 Which of the following does **not** pass through the superior orbital fissure?
a. Oculomotor nerve
b. Trochlear nerve
c. Abducens nerve
d. Zygomatic branch of maxillary

Q92 What is the eye movement possible even after a correctly performed retrobulbar block?
a. Medial movement of the eye
b. Opening of the eye
c. Upward movement of the eye
d. Closing of the eye

Q93 Regarding the use of cocaine for topical ophthalmic anaesthesia, which of the following statements is **correct**?
a. Cocaine is the safest agent available
b. Cocaine-induced hypertension is best treated by propranolol
c. Koller was the first to use cocaine for ophthalmic anaesthesia
d. The maximum dose of cocaine used in adults is 500 mg

Q94 Which of the following statements is **correct** regarding retrobulbar block?
a. The traditional Atkinson position of superonasal gaze during inferotemporal needle placement is recommended
b. Chances of globe perforation are higher in myopic eyes
c. Non-cutting-edge blunt needles have lower scleral perforation pressures than those with cutting edge
d. Globe perforation presents with pain, increasing proptosis and frequently subconjunctival or eyelid ecchymosis

Q95 Regarding complications of retrobulbar block, which of the following statements is **true**?
a. ECG needs to be monitored for several hours after a retrobulbar haemorrhage
b. Globe perforation is the most common complication
c. Retrobulbar haemorrhage presents as intense immediate pain with sudden loss of vision
d. In oculocardiac reflex, vagus nerve is the afferent

Q96 Which of the following statements regarding alternatives to retrobulbar block for ophthalmic anaesthesia is **incorrect**?

a. Peribulbar block does not enter the cone of extraocular muscles

b. In sub-Tenon's block use of longer rigid metallic cannulae is preferable to shorter plastic cannulae

c. The onset of block in peribulbar block is slow, while in sub-Tenon's block it is rapid

d. Peribulbar block is associated with the same incidence of postcataract ptosis as retrobulbar block

Q97 Regarding the landmarks for performing facial nerve block for ophthalmic anaesthesia, which of the following is **correctly matched**?

a. Classical Van Lint approach and zygomatic arch

b. Classical Atkinson approach and lateral orbital rim

c. O'Brien approach and mandibular condyle

d. Nadbath–Rehman approach and infraorbital foramen

Q98 Which of the following nerves **does not** innervate the scalp?

a. Greater auricular nerve

b. Auriculotemporal nerve

c. Greater occipital nerve

d. Lesser occipital nerve

Q99 Which of the following is a **correct** landmark for a scalp block?

a. Auriculotemporal nerve – behind the auricle

b. Zygomaticotemporal nerve – against the zygoma

c. Greater occipital – medial to occipital protuberance

d. Supratrochlear – between the eyebrows

Q100 Regarding the nerve supply of the face, which of the following statements is **false**?

a. The tip of the nose is supplied by ophthalmic division of the trigeminal nerve

b. The upper lip is supplied by the maxillary division of the trigeminal nerve

c. The lower lip is supplied by the mandibular division of the trigeminal nerve

d. The angle of the jaw is supplied by the facial nerve

Q101 Which of the following statements concerning trigeminal nerve anatomy is **correct**?

a. It is the longest cranial nerve
b. It forms the Gasserian ganglion in Meckel's cave
c. It is associated with four small intracranial sympathetic ganglia
d. Maxillary branch carries motor fibres apart from sensory

Q102 Which of the following nerves is **correctly matched** with the foramen it exits?

a. Ophthalmic nerve – inferior orbital fissure
b. Maxillary nerve – foramen rotundum
c. Mandibular nerve – foramen spinosum
d. Infraorbital nerve – infraorbital notch

Q103 Which of the following statements regarding the ophthalmic branch (V_1) of the trigeminal nerve is **true**?

a. It is the biggest branch of the trigeminal nerve
b. It exits the cranium through the inferior orbital fissure
c. The supraorbital nerve can be blocked at the medial margin of the orbit
d. Only its extracranial components can be blocked

Q104 Which of the following statements regarding the maxillary branch (V_2) of the trigeminal nerve is **incorrect**?

a. It is a purely sensory nerve
b. It exits the cranium through the foramen rotundum
c. Infraorbital block can be used for analgesia in cleft palate surgery
d. One of its branches supplies the scalp and hence it needs to be anaesthetised for scalp block

Q105 Regarding the mandibular nerve (V_3) and its branches, which of the following statements is **false**?

a. It has a small motor root
b. It emerges from the foramen ovale
c. The inferior alveolar nerve emerges from the mental foramen
d. Auriculotemporal nerve supplies the temporomandibular joint

Q106 All of the following terminal branches of the trigeminal nerve (CNV) can be blocked in a vertical line **except**:
a. Supraorbital nerve
b. Supratrochlear nerve
c. Infraorbital nerve
d. Mental nerve

Q107 Regarding maxillary nerve block, which of the following is **incorrect**?
a. It is performed using a lateral approach through the pterygopalatine fossa
b. The needle is redirected anteriorly off the lateral pterygoid plate
c. Refractory headaches can be effectively treated by blocking the sphenopalatine ganglion by this approach
d. It can lead to transient blindness

Q108 Regarding mandibular nerve block, which of the following is **incorrect**?
a. It is blocked at the level of foramen ovale
b. The needle is redirected posteriorly off the lateral pterygoid plate
c. It may lead to xerophthalmia
d. It can provide analgesia for hemimandibulectomy

Q109 Which of the following reflex is **not** blunted as a result of airway anaesthesia for awake intubation?
a. Gag reflex
b. Glottis closure reflex
c. Cough reflex
d. Stapedial reflex

Q110 Regarding airway anaesthesia, which of the following nerves is **not blocked**?
a. Cranial nerve V
b. Cranial nerve VII
c. Cranial nerve IX
d. Cranial nerve X

Q111 Which of the following statements regarding airway blocks is **false**?
a. No single nerve block can anaesthetise the entire airway
b. No single manoeuvre can anaesthetise the entire airway
c. Mandibular branches of trigeminal need not be blocked
d. Facial nerve need not be blocked

Q112 Regarding anaesthesia of nasal cavity, which of the following statements is **correct**?
  a. The anterior ethmoidal nerve and sphenopalatine nerves are derived from V_2
  b. The maximum dose of cocaine is 300 mg
  c. The instillation technique is most comforting for the patient
  d. Applicator at the middle turbinate is most important

Q113 Regarding anaesthesia of oropharynx for fibreoptic intubation, which of the following is **false**?
  a. Simplest method for this is atomisation of local anaesthetic
  b. Atomisation provides uniform and reliable anaesthesia for this procedure
  c. Glossopharyngeal nerve can be blocked intraorally at the base of the anterior tonsillar pillar
  d. Maximum safe plasma level of lignocaine is 5 mg/L

Q114 Concerning anaesthesia of the larynx and trachea for airway block, which of the following statements is **correct**?
  a. The external branch of the superior laryngeal nerve needs to be blocked
  b. Sensory innervation above the vocal cords is from the external branch of the superior laryngeal nerve
  c. Recurrent laryngeal nerve is blocked by transtracheal injection through the thyrohyoid membrane
  d. Transtracheal injection blocks both superior and recurrent laryngeal nerve

Answers

A1   D

- The brachial plexus originates from the **anterior primary rami of C5–T1 spinal nerves** and supplies the upper limb. There may be a contribution from **C4 or T2** occasionally, resulting in a pre-fixed (C4–C8) or post-fixed (C6–T2) brachial plexus.
- The brachial plexus supplies the entire upper limb except the trapezius muscle (**spinal accessory** nerve) and the skin of axilla (**intercostobrachial** nerves).
- It is comprised of **roots (five), trunks (three), divisions (six) and cords (three)**. There are **five terminal branches** and **numerous collateral branches** that leave the plexus at various points. The roots first **converge** to form three vertical trunks (upper, middle and lower), which each **divide** into anterior and posterior divisions (totalling six); the divisions **merge** variously to form the three cords (lateral, posterior and medial) that finally give the five terminal branches. The cords are described in terms of their relation to the axillary artery.
- The plexus travels between the anterior and middle scalene muscles (interscalene groove or the apex of scalene triangle) in the neck, over the first rib, under the midpoint of the clavicle, medial to the coracoid process to the axillary artery. This **line of Grossi** presents an anatomical perspective to guide the localisation of the brachial plexus.
  - Mulroy MF, Bernards CM, McDonald SB, *et al. A Practical Approach to Regional Anesthesia.* 4th ed. Philadelphia, PA: Lippincott Williams & Wilkins; 2008. pp. 172–5.

A2   A The brachial plexus displays marked anatomical variations, and **29 different variations** have been described, mainly below the level of the clavicle. Over 60% of individuals have different brachial plexus anatomy in each arm. However, the high success rate of upper-limb blocks is because of the superficial and reliable landmarks for accessing blockade of nerves.

- The five **roots** are the five anterior rami of the spinal nerves.
- These roots **merge** to form three **vertically arranged trunks**:
  - 'superior' or 'upper' (C5–C6)
  - 'middle' (C7)
  - 'inferior' or 'lower' (C8–T1).
- Each trunk then splits into two, to form six **divisions**:
  - anterior divisions of the upper, middle and lower trunks
  - posterior divisions of the upper, middle and lower trunks.
- These six divisions will **regroup** to become the three **cords**. The cords are named by their position with respect to the **second part of the axillary artery**.
  - The posterior cord is formed from the three posterior divisions of the trunks (C5–T1)
  - The **lateral cord** is the anterior divisions from the upper and middle trunks (C5–C7)

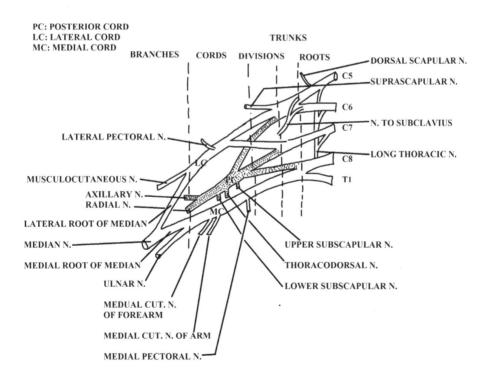

Figure 5.1 Brachial plexus anatomy

    – The **medial cord** is simply a continuation of the anterior division of the lower trunk (C8–T1).
- The five **terminal branches** are as follows:
  - the **musculocutaneous** nerve is derived from the lateral cord
  - the **ulnar** nerve is derived from the medial cord
  - the **median** nerve is derived from both the lateral and medial cords
  - the **axillary** and **radial** nerves are derived from the posterior cord.
  - Cousins MJ, Bridenbaugh PO, Carr DB, *et al. Cousins and Bridenbaugh's Neural Blockade in Clinical Anesthesia and Pain Medicine*. 4th ed. Philadelphia, PA: Lippincott Williams & Wilkins; 2008. p. 316.

A3 D

Table 5.1 Supraclavicular branches of brachial plexus

Level	Nerve	Root value	Innervations
Roots	Dorsal scapular nerve	C5	Rhomboid muscles and levator scapulae
Roots	Long thoracic nerve	C5, C6, C7	Serratus anterior
Upper trunk	Nerve to the subclavius	C5, C6	Subclavius muscle
Upper trunk	Suprascapular nerve	C4, C5, C6	Supraspinatus and infraspinatus

Phrenic nerve is a branch of the **cervical plexus** (C3–C5) and not brachial plexus, although it receives a contribution from C5.

A4 D The branches of the cords are:
- **Posterior cord branches (ULTRA)**: upper subscapular, lower subscapular, thoracodorsal, radial and axillary nerves
- **Lateral cord branches (LML)**: lateral pectoral, musculocutaneous and lateral root of the median nerve
- **Medial cord branches (M4U)**: medial pectoral, medial cutaneous nerve of arm, medial cutaneous nerve of forearm, medial root of the median nerve and ulnar nerve.

A5 C Root value of terminal nerves:
- Musculocutaneous: C5, C6, C7
- Median: medial root, C5, C6, C7; lateral root: C8, T1
- Axillary: C5, C6.
- Radial: C5–T1.
- Ulnar: C8, T1.

A6 D The **axillary nerve** continues as the lateral cutaneous nerve of the arm, while the **musculocutaneous nerve** continues as the lateral cutaneous nerve of the forearm. The **radial nerve** continues as the posterior cutaneous nerve of the forearm. The medial cutaneous nerve of the arm and the medial cutaneous nerve of the forearm originate from the medial cord. The **median, ulnar and radial nerves** provide cutaneous supply to the hand.

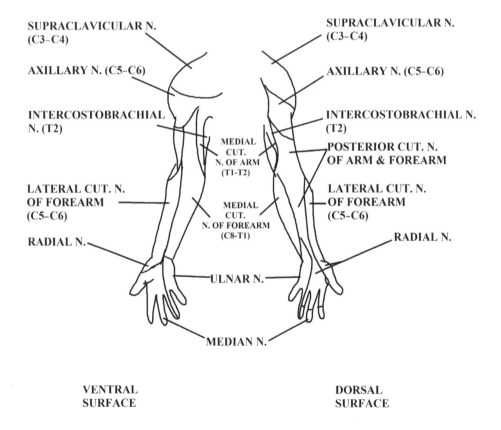

Figure 5.2 Cutaneous supply of the upper limb

A7 C

Dermatomal supply of the upper limb can be summarised as:

- ◗ C4 – shoulder tip
- ◗ C5 – radial side of upper arm, lateral epicondyle
- ◗ C6 – radial side of forearm, thumb
- ◗ C7 – middle three fingers
- ◗ C8 – little finger, ulnar side of forearm
- ◗ T1 – medial epicondyle, ulnar side of upper arm
- ◗ T2 – skin of axilla.

A8 A **Root values of common reflexes:**

- ◗ Biceps reflex (C5, C6)
- ◗ Brachioradialis reflex (C5, C6)
- ◗ Triceps reflex (C7, C8)
- ◗ Finger reflex (C8, T1)
- ◗ Patellar reflex or knee-jerk reflex (L3, L4)
- ◗ Ankle-jerk reflex (Achilles reflex) (S1, S2)
- ◗ Plantar reflex or Babinski reflex (L5, S1, S2).

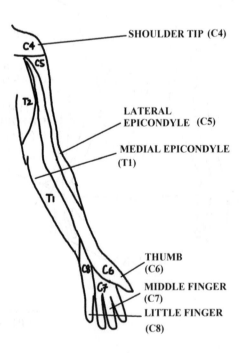

Figure 5.3 Dermatomes of the upper limb

A9   C

Table 5.2 Structures supplied by nerves of the upper extremity

Nerve	Muscular innervation	Cutaneous innervation
Axillary – C5, C6	Deltoid Teres minor	Lateral shoulder
Musculocutaneous – C5, C6, C7	Biceps brachii Brachioradialis Coracobrachialis	Lateral forearm
Radial – C5–T1	**BEAST** **B**rachioradialis **B**rachialis **E**xtensors of forearm and hand (abductor pollicis longus) **A**nconeus **S**upinator **T**riceps	Posterior lower arm and forearm Dorsum of hand (lateral three and a half fingers except terminal phalynx)
Ulnar – C8, T1	Forearm: flexor carpi ulnaris flexor digitorum profundus (medial part) Hand: hypothenar muscles interossei lumbricals (third and fourth) adductor pollicis	Both surfaces of medial one and a half finger
Median – C5–T1	Forearm: pronator teres flexor carpi radialis flexor digitorum sperficialis flexor digitorum profundus (lateral part) **Hand: LOAF** **L**umbricals (first and second) **O**pponens pollicis **A**bductor pollicis brevis **F**lexor pollicis brevis	Palm of hand (lateral three and a half fingers)

Note: the median and ulnar nerves do not innervate any structure above the elbow joint.

A10 C

Table 5.3 Levels of brachial plexus block

Level	Block	Nearby bony structures	Nearby artery
Root	Interscalene	Verterbral transverse processes	Vertebral artery
Trunks	Supraclavicular	Above first rib	Subclavian artery
Divisions	None	Under clavicle	N/A
Cords	Infraclavicular	Medial to coracoid process	Second part of axillary artery
Terminal nerves	Axillary	N/A	Third part of axillary artery

Note: no block is possible under the clavicle, and hence none involves the divisions. Occasionally, divisions may be present above clavicle, hence supraclavicular block may be at the level of trunks (mostly) or divisions (infrequently).

- Mulroy MF, Bernards CM, McDonald SB, *et al. A Practical Approach to Regional Anesthesia.* 4th ed. Philadelphia, PA: Lippincott Williams & Wilkins; 2008. pp. 172–3.

A11 C Appropriate blocks for surgeries are:
- Clavicle: superficial and deep cervical plexus block
- Shoulder: interscalene
- Upper humerus: interscalene + supraclavicular
- Elbow: infraclavicular
- Hand: axillary.

A12 D
- The brachial plexus sheath is said to be derived from the invagination of **prevertebral fascia**. The concept of the brachial plexus sheath was put forth by **Winnie**. He supported the concept of **single-injection blocks** for brachial plexus anaesthesia resulting from widespread distribution of local anaesthetic solution.
- However, this concept has been challenged by others, and recent cryo-microtome evidence suggests that below the clavicle, this sheath is less robust, actually being a **multicompartment space**. This is supported clinically, since infraclavicular and axillary blocks have a higher success rate when a **multistimulation** technique is used rather than a single injection.

- Cousins MJ, Bridenbaugh PO, Carr DB, *et al. Cousins and Bridenbaugh's Neural Blockade in Clinical Anesthesia and Pain Medicine.* 4th ed. Philadelphia, PA: Lippincott Williams & Wilkins; 2008. p. 318.
- Mulroy MF, Bernards CM, McDonald SB, *et al. A Practical Approach to Regional Anesthesia.* 4th ed. Philadelphia, PA: Lippincott Williams & Wilkins; 2008. pp. 174–5.

A13 D The landmarks needed to identify the interscalene groove and perform the interscalene block are:
- sternal head of sternocleidomastoid
- clavicular head of sternocleidomastoid
- upper border of cricoids cartilage (**C6 – Chassaignac's tubercle**)
- clavicle.

These landmarks can be accentuated by asking the patient to **lift their head** or take a **deep sniff**. The first rib cannot be palpated in all but the thinnest of individuals. The brachial plexus passes over the first rib, hence walking over the first rib helps with doing the supraclavicular block.
- Hadzic A. *Textbook of Regional Anesthesia and Acute Pain Management.* 1st ed. New York, NY: McGraw-Hill Medical; 2006. p. 407.

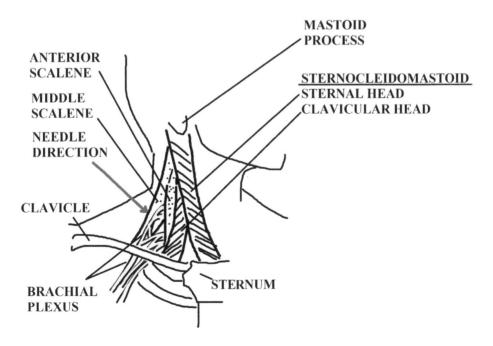

Figure 5.4 Landmarks for interscalene block

A14 A

Table 5.4 Contraindications to upper-limb blocks

Absolute	Relative
Patient refusal	Pre-existing neurological deficit
Local infection at the site of block	Chronic obstructive pulmonary disease
Allergy to local anaesthetics	Pre-existing contralateral lung disease
Active bleeding in anticoagulated patient	Contralateral phrenic or recurrent laryngeal nerve paresis
A vital capacity < 1 L	Incapacity to endure a decrease of 25% of vital capacity

Note: in the case of pre-existing lung disease, or phrenic/recurrent laryngeal nerve paresis, an axillary block is a suitable option. No block should be performed in the absence of a competent practitioner and resuscitation facilities.

- Hadzic A. *Textbook of Regional Anesthesia and Acute Pain Management.* 1st ed. New York, NY: McGraw-Hill Medical; 2006. p. 404.

A15 C

▶ Interscalene block is most suitable for shoulder surgery, as it blocks the **upper trunk (C5–C6); however, ulnar sparing** makes it unsuitable for forearm or hand surgery.

▶ Although **deltoid twitch** is the preferred response to neurostimulation, bicep, pectoral or triceps muscle response offers a similar success rate.

▶ Because of the proximity of the **phrenic nerve** to the interscalene groove, blocks at this level (especially if performed at a high level in the neck) **nearly always** lead to its paresis.

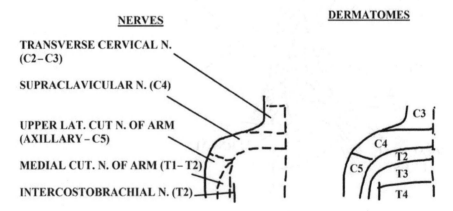

Figure 5.5 Dermatomal and cutaneous supply of the shoulder area

Shoulder innervation is through both cervical and brachial plexus.

Cutaneous innervation:
Clavicle and shoulder tip: supraclavicular nerve (C2–C4)
Anterior and lateral deltoid: upper lateral cutaneous branch of the axillary nerve (C5, C6)
Posterior deltoid: axillary nerve
Medial side of the arm: medial cutaneous nerve of the arm (C8–T1)
Axilla: intercostobrachial nerve (T2).

Joint innervation:
Acromioclavicular joint: suprascapular nerve
Glenohumeral joint: suprascapular nerve (superior), axillary nerve (inferior), subscaplular nerve and musculocuatneous nerve (minor).

▶ The anterior and lateral port insertion is usually painless, as these areas are well anaesthetised by an interscalene block.

▶ However, an axillary port placement requires the blockade of the intercostobrachial nerves.

▶ Posterior arthroscopic port insertion is often **painful** in an awake patient, as this area is supplied by the **suprascapular nerve** (which leaves the plexus early at the level of trunk and is spared by an interscalene block). Infiltrating the posterior port insertion site with local anaesthetic anaesthetises the posterior part of joint capsule.

- Beecroft CL, Coventry DM. Anaesthesia for shoulder surgery. *Contin Educ Anaesth Crit Care Pain*. 2008; **8**: 193–8.
- Hadzic A. *Textbook of Regional Anesthesia and Acute Pain Management*. 1st ed. New York, NY: McGraw-Hill Medical; 2006. p. 405.

A16 B

Table 5.5 Various approaches to interscalene block

Approach	Level	Direction of needle	Advantages	Disadvantages
Anterior approach				
Winnie's (classic)	*Cricoid cartilage* (CC) at C6	Perpendicular in all planes (**50°** caudal and posterior)	Reliable with both paraesthesia and peripheral nervous system	High risk of complications from medial direction (vertebral artery/spinal cord injections); difficult catheter insertion
Meire's (modified lateral)	**2–3 cm above** CC or *superior thyroid notch*	**30°** caudal and posterior towards middle or lateral third of clavicle	Reduced complications and **allows catheter placement**	Needs peripheral nervous system to guide placement
Borgeat's (modified lateral)	**0.5 cm below** CC	**30°** caudal and posterior towards middle or lateral third of clavicle	Reduced complications and allows catheter placement	N/A
Posterior approach				
Pippa's (cervical paravertebral approach)	Between C6 and C7	**3 cm lateral to midline,** directed **5°–10° anterolaterally** towards posterior edge of the sternocleidomastoid muscle at the level of CC	**Lateral angulation** is intended to reduce some neurological adverse effects	Painful, therefore needs local anaesthetic infiltration

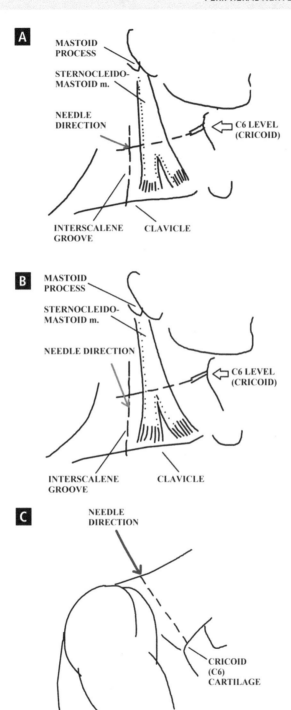

Figure 5.6 (A) Winnie's classic approach; (B) Borgeat's modified lateral approach; (C) Pippa's posterior approach

Boezaart cervical paravertebral approach is a modification of Pippa's posterior approach, and involves the insertion of a stimulating Tuohy needle at C6 level at the apex of 'V' formed by levator scapulae and trapezius, **directed antero-medially** (instead of anterolateral) and 30° caudad (aiming for the suprasternal notch). The needle is advanced until a deltoid twitch is stimulated, and then a catheter may be inserted.

- Hadzic A. *Textbook of Regional Anesthesia and Acute Pain Management*. 1st ed. New York, NY: McGraw-Hill Medical; 2006. pp. 408–9.

A17 D

Table 5.6 Troubleshooting for interscalene block muscle responses

Twitch	Interpretation	Action (redirect needle)
Diaphragm	Phrenic nerve stimulation (anterior to anterior scalene)	Posterolateral redirection
Trapezius	Accessory spinal nerve stimulation (posterior to interscalene groove)	Redirect anteriorly
Scapular	Dorsal scapular nerve (posterior) Thoracodorsal nerve (posterior) Long thoracic nerve (posterior)	Redirect anteriorly
Biceps, deltoid, triceps, pectoral	All part of brachial plexus	Alright to inject at this point

- Hadzic A. *Textbook of Regional Anesthesia and Acute Pain Management*. 1st ed. New York, NY: McGraw-Hill Medical; 2006. p. 411.

A18 D Complications of interscalene block are:

▶ **Vascular**:
  - intravascular injection into **vertebral or carotid artery** can result in rapid-onset **seizures (local anaesthetic toxicity)** hence the doses should always be fractionated and only injected after gentle negative aspiration
  - **Bezold–Jarisch reflex** – sudden bradycardia and hypotension (15%–30%) favoured by sitting position, awake patient and hypovolaemia; it is treated by atropine and ephedrine.

▶ **Neurologic**:
  - phrenic nerve – paresis results almost always causing hemidiaphragmatic paresis
  - recurrent laryngeal nerve palsy – hoarseness of voice (20%)

- sympathetic chain block – **Claude Bernard-Horner's syndrome or oculosympathetic palsy** (40%–60%); it is characterised by ptosis, enophthalmos, miosis and anhidrosis
- sympathetic chain irritation – **Pourfour du Petit's syndrome**: exophthalmia, mydriasis and inability to close the ipsilateral eye rarely occurs
- epidural injection
- intrathecal injection (**rachianaesthesia**)
- spinal cord injection
- nerve damage: temporary or permanent.

❱ Other: haematoma, bruising, infection, bronchospasm (due to sympathetic blockade) and rare pneumothorax.

- Cousins MJ, Bridenbaugh PO, Carr DB, *et al*. *Cousins and Bridenbaugh's Neural Blockade in Clinical Anesthesia and Pain Medicine*. 4th ed. Philadelphia, PA: Lippincott Williams & Wilkins; 2008. pp. 321–5.
- Hadzic A. *Textbook of Regional Anesthesia and Acute Pain Management*. 1st ed. New York, NY: McGraw-Hill Medical; 2006. pp. 414–16.

A19 C

Ultrasound-guided interscalene block:

❱ **High frequency (6–13 MHz)** probe is preferred (poor penetration), as brachial plexus at interscalene groove is at 1–2 cm depth.

❱ At this level, the C5–C7 nerve roots are seen as 'traffic signal lights' appearance, sandwiched between the anterior scalene muscle medially and the middle scalene laterally.

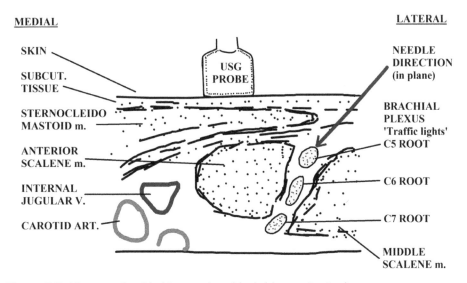

Figure 5.7 Ultrasound-guided interscalene block (short-axis view)

- ▶ **Below C6**, the vertebral artery is not protected by the vertebral transverse process and is exposed to being punctured or injected into if a low approach is used.
- ▶ The plexus may be identified in two ways:
  - **Medial-to-lateral search**: the probe is initially placed in the midline of the neck and moved laterally, identifying trachea, carotid artery, internal jugular vein, tail of sternocleidomastoid and eventually the nerve roots lying between the two scalene muscles.
  - **Inferior-to-superior search**: the probe is placed first in the supraclavicular area to identify the subclavian artery, with the brachial plexus anterolateral to it. As the plexus is traced proximally, the interscalene groove is seen and the roots are identified.
- ▶ Ultrasound can help improve success rate, reduce time to onset of block and reduce the volume of local anaesthetic needed; however, it cannot eliminate intraneural injections completely, since this is limited by operator skill and image resolution.
  - • Mulroy MF, Bernards CM, McDonald SB, *et al. A Practical Approach to Regional Anesthesia*. 4th ed. Philadelphia, PA: Lippincott Williams & Wilkins; 2008. pp. 177–9.

A20 C

- ▶ The phrenic nerve is derived from the **cervical plexus** (C3–C5) and passes over the anterior surface of anterior scalene muscle. An interscalene block is performed in the groove between the anterior and middle scalene muscles.
- ▶ The classic peripheral nervous system (PNS)-guided interscalene block results in **100%** incidence of hemidiaphragmatic paresis. This is said to occur by **spread upwards to C3–C4 level** or by **spilling over anterior scalene** to involve the phrenic nerve. The risk of phrenic nerve paresis is increased by medially directed injections, high-volume injections (30–40 mL), injections at C6 (vs C7) level or PNS-guided blocks.
- ▶ At C6, the phrenic nerve and brachial plexus are close together (at the apex of interscalene groove); however, subsequently (i.e. at C7 and C8) the phrenic nerve moves **medially** while the brachial plexus moves **laterally** toward midpoint of the clavicle. As this distance increases, the risk of injectate spilling over the belly of anterior scalene and affecting the phrenic nerve reduces. Hence low-volume injections (5–10 mL), injections at C7 (vs C6) and ultrasound-guided blocks may have a phrenic sparing effect.
  - • Kessler J, Schafhalter-Zoppoth I, Gray AT. An ultrasound study of the phrenic nerve in the posterior cervical triangle: implications for the interscalene brachial plexus block. *Reg Anesth Pain Med*. 2008; **33**: 545–55.

- Renes SH, Rettig HC, Gielen MJ, *et al*. Ultrasound-guided low-dose inter-scalene brachial plexus block reduces the incidence of hemidiaphragmatic paresis. *Reg Anesth Pain Med*. 2009; **34**(5): 498–502.
- Riazi S, Carmichael N, Awad I, *et al*. Effect of local anaesthetic volume (20 vs 5 mL) on the efficacy and respiratory consequences of ultrasound-guided interscalene brachial plexus block. *Br J Anaesth*. 2008; **101**: 549–56.
- Urmey WF, Talts KH, Sharrock NE. One hundred percent incidence of hemidiaphragmatic paresis associated with interscalene brachial plexus anesthesia as diagnosed by ultrasonography. *Anesth Analg*. 1991; **72**(4): 498–503.

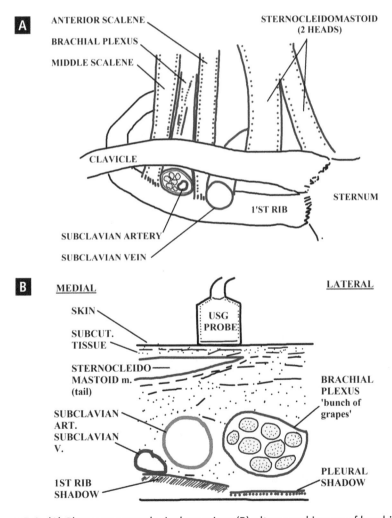

Figure 5.8 (A) Plexus at supraclavicular region; (B) ultrasound image of brachial plexus in supraclavicular area

A21 C The brachial plexus forms **trunks** in the supraclavicular area in a **compact bundle** within a sheath, resulting in high success if injection is made at this site. Under ultrasound, the plexus is seen as a '**cluster of grapes**', with the subclavian vessels lying medial to the plexus, the first rib inferiorly and the clavicle lies superiorly. The pleural dome lies far medially. See Figure 5.8 on p. 143.

- Mulroy MF, Bernards CM, McDonald SB, *et al. A Practical Approach to Regional Anesthesia.* 4th ed. Philadelphia, PA: Lippincott Williams & Wilkins; 2008. p. 174.
- www.usra.ca/supanatomy.php

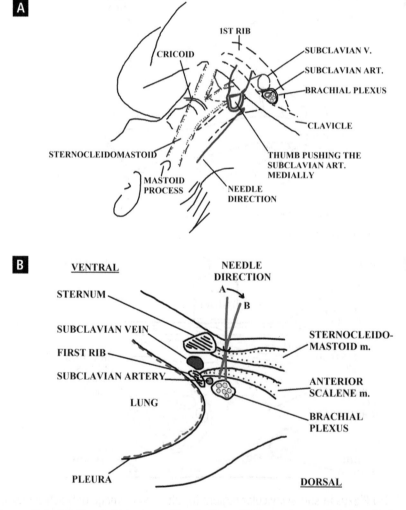

Figure 5.9 (A) Classic Kulenkampff technique; (B) Brown's plumb-bob technique

A22 **D** Various techniques have been advocated for performing supraclavicular block. Traditionally, lower and medial approach (**Kulenkampff**, 1911) has resulted in a higher risk of pneumothorax (up to **6%**) and the modifications advocated have attempted to reduce this complication. Various methods are presented in Figure 5.9 and Table 5.7.

Table 5.7 Various approaches at supraclavicular level

Approach and description	Advantage	Disadvantage
Classic Kulenkampff technique: at the midpoint of clavicle, the subclavian artery is held medially and the needle inserted 1 cm above the clavicle in the parasagittal plane to induce paraesthesia of the brachial plexus	Simple landmarks	Pneumothorax + + + Cannot insert catheter – – –
Winnie and Collins' subclavian perivascular: needle is inserted at the base of the interscalene groove, posterior to the subclavian artery, in the horizontal plane	Easy and simple landmarks	Haematoma + + +
Brown's plumb-bob technique: needle inserted just above the clavicle, at the lateral edge of the clavicular head of the sternocleidomastoid, in the parasagittal plane perpendicular to the brachial plexus; the needle is directed only anteroposteriorly	Pneumothorax + non-experts can do block	
Dupré and Danel's technique: uses the external jugular vein as a landmark (approximately 2 cm above the midclavicular point)	Catheter + + +	Complex landmarks

A23 B

Table 5.8 Troubleshooting for supraclavicular block muscle responses

Twitch	Interpretation	Action (redirect needle)
Diaphragm	Phrenic nerve stimulation (anterior to anterior scalene)	Posterolateral redirection
Scapular	Suprascapular nerve (posterior)	Redirect anteriorly
Deltoid	Stimulating upper trunk	Redirect inferiorly toward middle trunk
Ulnar	Medial cord is far medially near pleura	Danger of pleural puncture, hence redirect laterally
Hit the rib	First rib is anterior to the plexus in the parasagittal plane	Walk off the rib **posteriorly**
Biceps, triceps or forearm/ hand twitch	All part of the brachial plexus	Alright to inject at this point

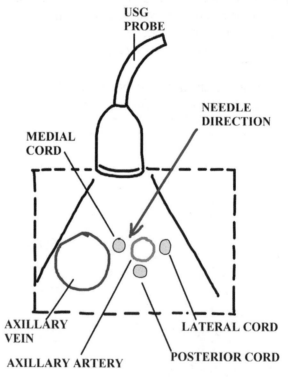

Figure 5.10 Ultrasound image of cords around axillary artery

A24 **B** Salient features of supraclavicular block are as follows.

▶ Consistently provides anaesthesia to the upper limb (except shoulder) with a **single injection**.

▶ The needle should **not be directed medially**, for fear of puncturing the pleura.

▶ **Ulnar sparing** is most common since the inferior trunk is situated far medially. This can be overcome using ultrasound, as it allows medial injections under vision.

▶ The plexus is situated **posterolateral** to the subclavian artery.

▶ The most feared complication is **pneumothorax**; however, the risk is reduced with a modified technique and use of ultrasound. Pneumothorax presents as a **pleuritic chest pain** and dyspnoea. Some anaesthetists avoid this block for outpatient surgery.

▶ Phrenic nerve paresis is **less common** than interscalene blocks.

• Cousins MJ, Bridenbaugh PO, Carr DB, *et al. Cousins and Bridenbaugh's Neural Blockade in Clinical Anesthesia and Pain Medicine.* 4th ed. Philadelphia, PA: Lippincott Williams & Wilkins; 2008. pp. 330–1.

A25 **C** Infraclavicular block involves blocking the brachial plexus at the level of **cords** that lie around the **second part of the axillary artery**. At this level, the plexus is bounded by the clavicle above, the ribcage medially and the coracoid process laterally. It is covered by both pectoralis major and pectoral minor. Medial to the coracoid process, the lateral cord of the plexus lies **superolaterally**, the posterior cord lies **posteriorly** and the medial cord lies **posteromedially** with respect to the axillary artery. See Figure 5.10.

• Sandhu NS, Capan LM. Ultrasound-guided infraclavicular brachial plexus block. *Br J Anaesth*. 2002; **89**: 254–9.

A26   C

Table 5.9 The various approaches to infraclavicular block

Approach	Landmarks	Needle direction	Advantages	Disadvantages
Modified Raj's (modification of classic Raj's approach)	**3 cm below** the midpoint of line joining jugular notch and acromio-clavicular joint (mid-clavicular point)	100-mm needle, directed 45°–60° **laterally** toward axillary artery	As needle is directed laterally, no danger of pneumothorax	Long intramuscular trajectory is painful
Kilka's vertical infraclavicular	**Immediately below** the midpoint of line joining jugular notch and acromioclavicular joint (mid-clavicular point)	50-mm needle directed **90° vertically** and is kept in the parasagittal plane (cranio-caudal adjustments)	Less depth needed to reach plexus	Higher risk of pneumothorax
Whiffler's coracoid approach	**2 cm medial and 2 cm inferior** to tip of coracoid process	80-mm needle directed **90° vertically** and is kept in the parasagittal plane (cranio-caudal adjustments)	Less risk of pneumothorax	N/A
Klaastad ultrasound guidance approach	Intersection between clavicle and coracoid process	80-mm needle inserted at a **30° angle** in the sagittal plane	Appropriate for ultrasound guidance	N/A

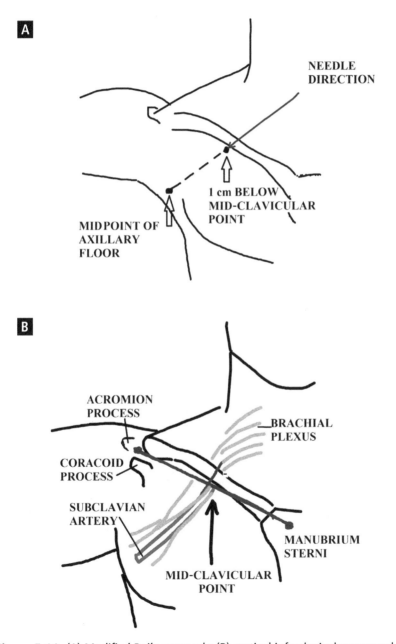

Figure 5.11 (A) Modified Raj's approach; (B) vertical infraclavicular approach

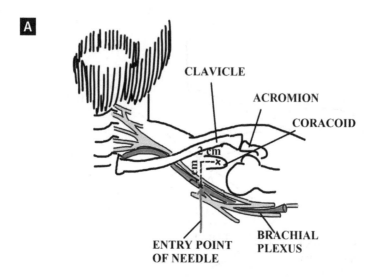

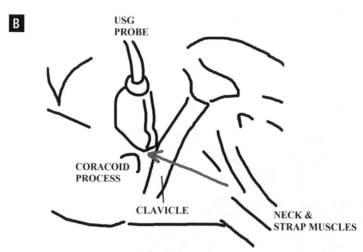

Figure 5.12 (A) Coracoid approach; (B) Klaastad's approach

- Hadzic A. *Textbook of Regional Anesthesia and Acute Pain Management*. 1st ed. New York, NY: McGraw-Hill Medical; 2006. pp. 434–8.

A27 **A** Infraclavicular block is made at the level of cords. Hence, the appropriate responses are given by the mnemonic '**at the cords, pinkie (fifth digit) towards**'.

Table 5.10 Neurostimulation of cords of brachial plexus

Cord	Nerve	Muscle responses	Pinkie movement
Lateral cord	Median (lateral root)	Pronation, elbow flexion, finger flexion, thumb opposition	Laterally (due to pronation)
Posterior cord	Radial and axillary	Finger and wrist extension, abduction of thumb	Posteriorly (due to wrist extension)
Medial cord	Ulnar	Medial finger flexion, ulnar deviation of wrist	Medial (due to ulnar deviation of wrist)

Table 5.11 Inappropriate muscle responses during neurostimulation of cords of brachial plexus

Twitch	Interpretation	Action (redirect needle)
Biceps twitch	Due to musculocutaneous nerve stimulation; needle too superior, as the musculocutaneous nerve leaves the plexus superiorly	Redirect inferiorly
Deltoid	Due to axillary nerve stimulation; needle is inferior, as the axillary nerve originates lower down	Redirect superiorly
Pectoral	Direct muscle stimulation	Redirect deeper

- Cousins MJ, Bridenbaugh PO, Carr DB, *et al. Cousins and Bridenbaugh's Neural Blockade in Clinical Anesthesia and Pain Medicine*. 4th ed. Philadelphia, PA: Lippincott Williams & Wilkins; 2008. p. 332.
- Hadzic A. *Textbook of Regional Anesthesia and Acute Pain Management*. 1st ed. New York, NY: McGraw-Hill Medical; 2006. pp. 382–3.

A28 B Salient features of infraclavicular block are as follows.

- The lateral cord is the **first** to be stimulated.
- The medial cord is usually situated **between the axillary artery and the axillary vein**.
- Posterior cord stimulation is met with the **best success rate** and most widespread block.
- The musculocutaneous nerve leaves the lateral cord more proximally, hence biceps twitch is **not an appropriate response**.
- Classic infraclavicular block can be made with the **arm by the side**. However, recent analysis has revealed that arm abduction to 90° will stretch the brachial plexus and make it taut. This will bring the three cords closer together and will enhance nerve visualisation under ultrasound.
- It is the best block for **catheter placement** (since muscle bulk holds catheter well).
- It is the best block for **elbow surgery**.
- It can be performed **bilaterally**, since it does not cause hemidiaphragmatic paresis.
- A **low-frequency** (higher penetration) probe is best suited for an ultrasound approach. Usually a **short-axis view** of the anechoic pulsatile axillary artery is used with in-plane needle advancement in a **postero-caudal** direction.
- A multistimulation technique takes longer, but offers a higher success rate.
- Infraclavicular blocks are **large-volume blocks** (40 mL) and a lower success rate is reported with lower volumes.
  - Cousins MJ, Bridenbaugh PO, Carr DB, *et al. Cousins and Bridenbaugh's Neural Blockade in Clinical Anesthesia and Pain Medicine*. 4th ed. Philadelphia, PA: Lippincott Williams & Wilkins; 2008. pp. 332–3.
  - Hadzic A. *Textbook of Regional Anesthesia and Acute Pain Management*. 1st ed. New York, NY: McGraw-Hill Medical; 2006. pp. 427–9.
  - Mulroy MF, Bernards CM, McDonald SB, *et al. A Practical Approach to Regional Anesthesia*. 4th ed. Philadelphia, PA: Lippincott Williams & Wilkins; 2008. pp. 189–90.

A29 C Median and musculocutaneous nerves lie **above** the axillary artery, while the ulnar and radial nerves lie **below** it. The musculocutaneous nerve actually lies away from the artery **under the coracobrachialis muscle**. Each of these **four terminal nerves** must be blocked for effective anaesthesia. Abduction of the arm at 90° facilitates access to the axilla. See Figure 5.13 and Table 5.12 on p. 153.

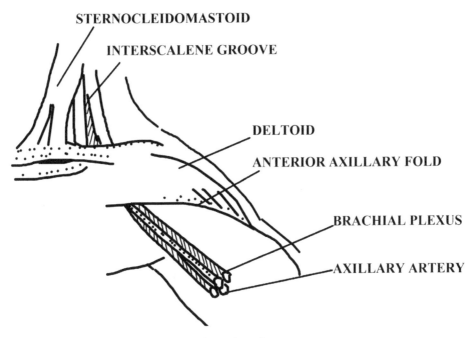

STERNOCLEIDOMASTOID

INTERSCALENE GROOVE

DELTOID

ANTERIOR AXILLARY FOLD

BRACHIAL PLEXUS

AXILLARY ARTERY

Figure 5.13 Brachial plexus passing through axillary area

Table 5.12 Appropriate muscle responses during neurostimulation of branches of brachial plexus in the axillary area

Nerves	Muscle responses
Musculocutaneous	Elbow flexion
Median	Pronation, finger flexion, thumb opposition
Radial	Finger and wrist extension, abduction of thumb
Ulnar	Medial finger flexion, ulnar deviation of wrist

- Hadzic A. *Textbook of Regional Anesthesia and Acute Pain Management*. 1st ed. New York, NY: McGraw-Hill Medical; 2006. pp. 442–4.

A30 C Various techniques used for axillary block are as follows.

▶ **Single injection (de Jong)**: PNS- or paraesthesia-guided insertion of needle above or below the artery depending on the surgical site (e.g. above the artery for median territory and below the artery for radial/ ulnar territory). The entire drug is injected now; however, the disadvantage is that sparing is quite frequent.

▶ **Multi-injection**: two, three or four injections have been advocated. First, the median nerve is sought above the artery followed by injection of 5–10 mL of local anaesthetic. Subsequently, the needle is redirected obliquely into coracobrachialis muscle to stimulate musculocutaneous (elbow flexion), and 5 mL is deposited here. The needle is then inserted below the artery, stimulating the ulnar and then the radial nerves with 5–10 mL injectate at each location. Total volume used is 20–40 mL.

▶ **Transarterial (Urquhart)**: half injection made posterior to the artery (after puncturing it) and half superficial to it.

▶ **Perivascular infiltration**: 10–20 mL infiltrated above the artery and 10–20 ml below it in a fan-wise manner.

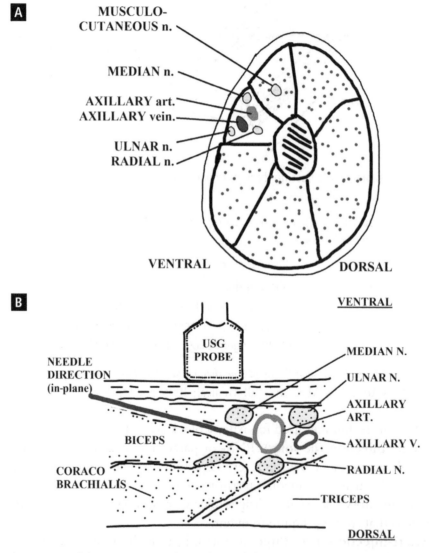

Figure 5.14 (A) Cross-section of arm showing the arrangement of nerves around the axillary artery; (B) ultrasound view of axillary approach for brachial plexus block

▶ **Paresthaesia guided**: usually single injection after paresthesia/fascial click.

▶ **Ultrasound guided**: high-frequency probe used to guide injections. The median nerve lies at the **11 o'clock** position, the ulnar at the **3 o'clock** (separated from the median by the axillary vein), while the radial nerve is at the **6 o'clock** position above the conjoint tendon. The musculocutaneous nerve can be blocked easily within the coracobrachialis muscle.

Mid-humeral block is similar to multistimulation technique but performed at the junction of the upper and middle thirds of the humerus.

- Hadzic A. *Textbook of Regional Anesthesia and Acute Pain Management*. 1st ed. New York, NY: McGraw-Hill Medical; 2006. pp. 444–7.
- Mulroy MF, Bernards CM, McDonald SB, *et al. A Practical Approach to Regional Anesthesia*. 4th ed. Philadelphia, PA: Lippincott Williams & Wilkins; 2008. pp. 192–9.

A31 **A** Salient features of axillary block are as follows.

▶ **Most common** and **easiest** upper-limb block.

▶ Best block for **ambulatory** surgery.

▶ Best suited for **hand surgery**.

▶ Not well suited for catheter because of frequent dislodgement.

▶ **Multistimulation** technique has higher success rate and shorter onset time.

▶ Best given as high in axilla as possible, as this allows proximal anaesthetic spread and less sparing.

▶ **Musculocutaneous sparing** is the most common inadequacy of single-injection technique.

▶ **Inadequate blocks** can be supplemented by relevant blocks at lower (elbow or forearm) levels.

▶ Excessive arm abduction (> 90°) is **not advocated**, as this obscures the axillary pulse and limits proximal spread of anaesthetic.

▶ **Tourniquet** use needs blocking of the medial cutaneous nerve of arm and intercostobrachial by subcutaneous infiltration of local anaesthetic at axillary floor.

- Cousins MJ, Bridenbaugh PO, Carr DB, *et al. Cousins and Bridenbaugh's Neural Blockade in Clinical Anesthesia and Pain Medicine*. 4th ed. Philadelphia, PA: Lippincott Williams & Wilkins; 2008. pp. 332–3.
- Hadzic A. *Textbook of Regional Anesthesia and Acute Pain Management*. 1st ed. New York, NY: McGraw-Hill Medical; 2006. pp. 444–7.
- Mulroy MF, Bernards CM, McDonald SB, *et al. A Practical Approach to Regional Anesthesia*. 4th ed. Philadelphia, PA: Lippincott Williams & Wilkins; 2008. pp. 192–9.

A32 **B** The correct way to assess adequacy of brachial plexus block is '**push-pull-pinch-pinch**' method. It involves checking adequacy of **four terminal nerve** actions as follows.

- Push: inability to push by elbow extension against resistance (indicates radial block – lack of elbow extension).
- Pull: inability to pull the forearm by flexing it against resistance (indicates **musculocutaneous** nerve block – lack of elbow flexion).
- Pinch: anaesthesia to pinch at palmar base of index finger (median block).
- Pinch: anaesthesia to pinch at palmar surface of little finger (ulnar block).

  - Cousins MJ, Bridenbaugh PO, Carr DB, *et al. Cousins and Bridenbaugh's Neural Blockade in Clinical Anesthesia and Pain Medicine.* 4th ed. Philadelphia, PA: Lippincott Williams & Wilkins; 2008. p. 317.

A33 **A** Tourniquet pain in non-anaesthetised volunteers occurs around **30 minutes**. General anaesthesia has little effect on this, but under regional anaesthesia this may be delayed up to **60–90 minutes**. It has been said that the pain may be mediated by local metabolite accumulation (due to ischaemia) and is transmitted by **C fibres**.

Various strategies have been tried, including:
- gabapentine premedication
- intravenous ketamine to reduce intraoperative hypertensive response;
- epidural clonidine (with bupivacaine)
- systemic opioids.

A34 **B** PNS technique:
- **Radial nerve**: blocked 1–2 cm above the brachial crease, between tendon of biceps and brachioradialis; 5–7 mL of local anaesthetic injected here after stimulating a radial nerve response (wrist/finger extension).
- **Median nerve**: blocked medial to brachial artery 2 cm above the brachial crease; 5–7 mL local anaesthetic is injected after stimulating a median nerve response (pronation, thumb opposition, finger flexion).
- **Ulnar nerve**: elbow is flexed to 30° and the ulnar nerve is blocked just above the groove between medial epicondyle and olecranon (excessive flexion may cause nerve to slip out of the groove). Local anaesthetic (5 mL) is injected, avoiding excessive pressure of injectate (this can injure the nerve, which rests against the bone here).

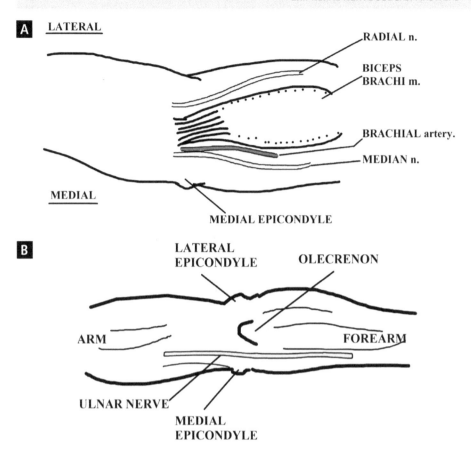

Figure 5.15 (A) Elbow block: radial and median nerve block; (B) elbow block: ulnar nerve block

Ultrasound techniques (using high-frequency probe): nerves can be blocked at the elbow, as shown in Figure 5.15, or as follows.

▶ **Radial nerve**: blocked at the **spiral groove** where the nerve is seen above humerus, but below triceps. As it proceeds distally, it divides into a **superficial and deep branch**, tracking anteriorly towards the cubital fossa and appears to be '**jumping off the cliff**'. It is ideally blocked away from the humerus to avoid any nerve damage.

▶ **Ulnar nerve**: ulnar artery is identified at the wrist, and tracked proximally until the ulnar nerve is seen separating from the artery near the **mid-forearm**. It can be blocked here. At this level, the ulnar nerve lies lateral to the ulnar artery.

▶ **Median nerve**: at the same level (**mid-forearm**), the ultrasound probe is moved laterally to identify the median nerve.

Note: spared nerves should be blocked by supplemental injection **distally and not proximally**.

- Mulroy MF, Bernards CM, McDonald SB, *et al. A Practical Approach to Regional Anesthesia*. 4th ed. Philadelphia, PA: Lippincott Williams & Wilkins; 2008. p. 213.
- www.usra.ca/midanatomy.php

A35 D Wrist block is performed just proximal to wrist crease (see Figure 5.16 on p. 159). It may be performed using a landmark technique, PNS or USG technique as follows.

- ▶ **Radial nerve**: since the radial nerve divides into many branches above the radial styloid, two or more separate injections in a **fan-wise manner** above the styloid process are needed to block it. Hence essentially it is a **field block**.
- ▶ **Median nerve**: blocked between the tendons of palmaris longus and flexor carpi radialis.
- ▶ **Ulnar nerve**: should be blocked medial to flexor carpi ulnaris.

Spared nerves should be blocked by supplemental injection distally (digital blocks). Epinephrine should not be added to these blocks, as they may cause ischaemia in these terminal digits.

Note: arteriovenous (AV) fistula may be created proximally at the level of the antecubital fossa (under axillary block) or distally at forearm level (by blocking medial and lateral cutaneous nerve of the forearm). Wrist block is not suitable for AV fistula surgery.

- Mulroy MF, Bernards CM, McDonald SB, *et al. A Practical Approach to Regional Anesthesia*. 4th ed. Philadelphia, PA: Lippincott Williams & Wilkins; 2008. p. 215.

A36 A Suprascapular nerve arises from the **upper trunk** of brachial plexus (**C4, C5 and C6**) and supplies:

- ▶ cutaneous supply to posterior shoulder joint capsule and scapular surface
- ▶ innervation of acromioclavicular joint and glenohumeral (shoulder) joint
- ▶ infraspinatus and supraspinatus (**external rotation**).

It is blocked 1–2 cm **lateral** to midpoint of spine of scapula, at a depth of 4–5 cm at the **suprascapular notch**. The nerve may be identified and blocked with ultrasound. Recently, shoulder arthroscopy has been performed under suprascapular and axillary block alone without an interscalene block.

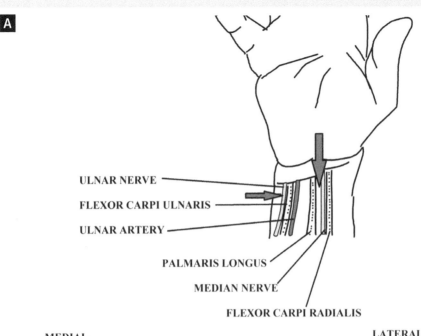

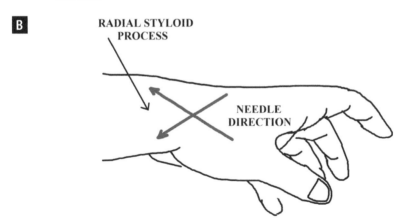

Figure 5.16 (A) Wrist block: ulnar and median nerve block; (B) wrist block: radial nerve block

- Harmon D, Hearty C. Ultrasound-guided suprascapular nerve block technique. *Pain Physician*. 2007; **10**(6): 743–6.
- Mulroy MF, Bernards CM, McDonald SB, *et al. A Practical Approach to Regional Anesthesia*. 4th ed. Philadelphia, PA: Lippincott Williams & Wilkins; 2008. pp. 211–12.
- Price DJ. Combined suprascapular and axillary (circumflex) nerve block: the shoulder block. *J NYSORA*. **15**.

A37 B The cervical plexus is formed by the **anterior primary rami of the C1–C4.** It lies deep to the internal jugular vein and the sternocleidomastoid muscle and superficial to scalenus medius and levator scapulae.

The main components of the cervical plexus are:

▶ **cutaneous branches** – lesser occipital, greater auricular (largest), transverse cervical, and supraclavicular nerves
▶ **ansa cervicalis** – innervates infrahyoid and geniohyoid
▶ **phrenic nerve** innervates the diaphragm
▶ contributions to the **accessory nerve (CNXI)** – innervates the sternocleidomastoid and trapezius muscles
▶ **muscular branches** – supply prevertebral neck muscles.

- Cousins MJ, Bridenbaugh PO, Carr DB, *et al. Cousins and Bridenbaugh's Neural Blockade in Clinical Anesthesia and Pain Medicine.* 4th ed. Philadelphia, PA: Lippincott Williams & Wilkins; 2008. p. 409.

A38 A

▶ The cutaneous branches are derived from **C2–C4** (as C1 gives only motor fibres to suboccipital muscles and has no sensory component) and form the superficial cervical plexus. This plexus emerges at the midpoint of the lateral border of sternocleidomastoid and can be blocked here by superficial infiltration of 10 mL of 1%–2% lignocaine along the **middle third** of the lateral border of sternocleidomastoid.

▶ A superficial cervical plexus block constitutes injection superficial to **investing fascia of the neck**, while the deep cervical plexus block is given deep to the **deep cervical fascia**. An injection between the two layers is called the **intermediate block**. Interestingly, any spillage between the two layers may result in phrenic nerve paresis, recurrent laryngeal nerve paresis (hoarseness) and Horner's syndrome (sympathetic block). Intravascular injection (external jugular vein) and deep cervical plexus occur infrequently.

▶ **Indications**: analgesia for tracheostomy, thyroidectomy, anterior neck surgery, mastoid surgery, parietal craniotomy and clavicular surgery.

▶ Carotid surgery may be performed under cervical plexus block, which offers benefits such as better cardiovascular stability, shorter critical care stay and financial savings when compared to general anaesthesia. **There is no consensus regarding the use of superficial or deep cervical plexus block for this.** A recent review concluded that deep/combined blocks were associated with a higher serious complication rate and higher conversion rate to general anaesthetic.

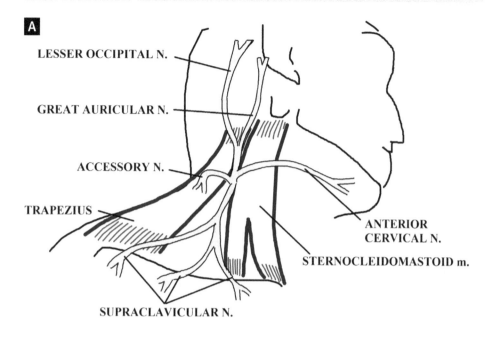

A

LESSER OCCIPITAL N.

GREAT AURICULAR N.

ACCESSORY N.

TRAPEZIUS

ANTERIOR
CERVICAL N.

STERNOCLEIDOMASTOID m.

SUPRACLAVICULAR N.

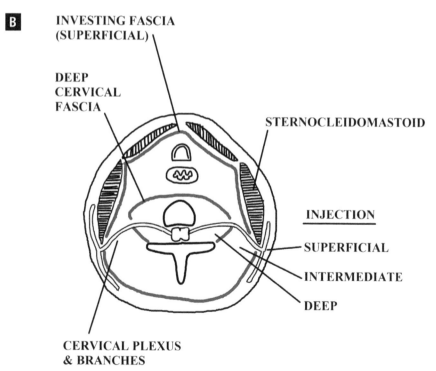

B

INVESTING FASCIA
(SUPERFICIAL)

DEEP
CERVICAL
FASCIA

STERNOCLEIDOMASTOID

INJECTION

SUPERFICIAL

INTERMEDIATE

DEEP

CERVICAL PLEXUS
& BRANCHES

Figure 5.17 (A) Cervical plexus – branches; (B) fascie of neck and relevant blocks

- Cousins MJ, Bridenbaugh PO, Carr DB, *et al. Cousins and Bridenbaugh's Neural Blockade in Clinical Anesthesia and Pain Medicine*. 4th ed. Philadelphia, PA: Lippincott Williams & Wilkins; 2008. p. 420.
- Pandit JJ, Satya-Krishna R, Gration P. Superficial or deep cervical plexus block for carotid endarterectomy: a systematic review of complications. *Br J Anaesth*. 2007; **99**(2): 159–69.

A39 D

▶ The deep cervical plexus block (anterior cervical paraverterbral block) is given under the **deep cervical fascial**. This can be accomplished by joining the tips of Chassaignac's tubercle (C6) and mastoid process. C2 tubercle is located 1.5 cm caudal to mastoid process, C3 tubercle 1.5 cm caudal to C2, and C4 tubercle 1.5 cm caudal to C3 tubercle. A 50-mm 22-G needle is inserted at C4, and directed caudally towards the tubercle; on contact with bone, it is 'walked off' and 3–5 mL of 1% lignocaine is injected at each level **from C2 to C4 (Moore technique)**.

▶ A single injection (**Winnie technique**) of 6–8 mL at a single level has also been described.

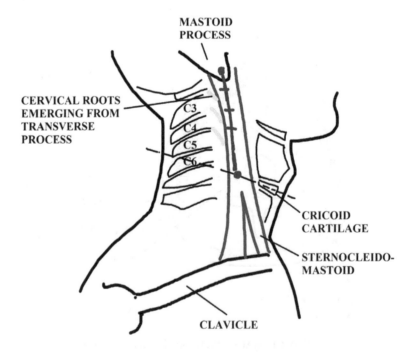

Figure 5.18 Landmarks for deep cervical plexus blocks

▶ Interestingly, any spillage above the deep cervical fascia may result in phrenic nerve paresis, recurrent laryngeal nerve paresis (hoarseness) and Horner's syndrome (sympathetic block). Other complications include vertebral artery injection, spinal injection, brachial plexus block, carotid body stimulation (bradycardia and hypotension) and haematoma formation.

▶ The **carotid sheath** needs to be infiltrated by the surgeon during carotid surgery, as it is supplied by cranial nerves (CN IX, X, XI and XII). **Trigeminal nerve block** may be required to allow surgical retraction near the submandibular area.

▶ Injections at C6 are made for **stellate ganglion** blockade.

• Cousins MJ, Bridenbaugh PO, Carr DB, *et al. Cousins and Bridenbaugh's Neural Blockade in Clinical Anesthesia and Pain Medicine*. 4th ed. Philadelphia, PA: Lippincott Williams & Wilkins; 2008. pp. 422–3.

A40 B

▶ The lumbosacral plexus is not a single plexus; it comprises two distinct and separate components: the lumbar and sacral plexus. The lumbar plexus is derived from the **anterior primary rami (ventral) T12–L4**, while the sacral plexus is derived from **anterior primary rami (ventral) L4–S3** spinal nerves. A single injection of the lumbosacral plexus cannot anaesthetise the whole lower extremity.

▶ The renewed popularity of lower-limb peripheral blocks has been attributed to techniques such as ultrasound guidance and continuous catheter techniques. It also avoids the potential risk of **epidural haematoma** in orthopaedic patients, where the use of venous thromboprophylaxis is routine.

▶ Continuous lumbosacral plexus block has been shown to be **superior** to morphine patient-controlled analgesia and **equally effective** as epidural analgesia, for post-operative analgesia.

Note: the posterior (dorsal) primary rami produce lateral and medial branches which innervate the back. The **medial branch** innervates the facet joint and is often targeted as a chronic pain procedure to treat **facet joint pain**.

• Campbell A, McCormick M, McKinlay K, *et al.* Epidural vs. lumbar plexus infusions following total knee arthroplasty: randomized controlled trial. *Eur J Anaesthesiol.* 2009; **26**(5): 439–40.

• Mulroy MF, Bernards CM, McDonald SB, *et al. A Practical Approach to Regional Anesthesia*. 4th ed. Philadelphia, PA: Lippincott Williams & Wilkins; 2008. p. 218.

A41 C The lumbar plexus is formed by the anterior primary rami of **T12–L4** spinal nerves. The lumbar plexus mainly supplies the **anterior part** of the thigh. The spinal nerve roots course laterally from their respective transverse processes and come to lie with the bulk of the **psoas muscle**. Here, they divide into anterior and posterior divisions and give rise to their most important branches: the lateral cutaneous nerve of the thigh (LCN) (lies laterally), the femoral nerve (FN) (lies in between) and the obturator nerve (ON) (lies medially) within the psoas muscle.

Note: there is evidence that the LCN and the FN may be separated from the ON by a muscular compartment, hence a fascia iliaca or femoral three-in-one block usually spares the obturator nerve.
* Mulroy MF, Bernards CM, McDonald SB, *et al. A Practical Approach to Regional Anesthesia*. 4th ed. Philadelphia, PA: Lippincott Williams & Wilkins; 2008. p. 218.

A42 A

Table 5.13 The branches of the lumbar plexus (T12–L4)

Nerves	Root value	Motor supply	Sensory supply
Iliohypogastric	T12–L1 (anterior rami)	Abdominal muscles	Inferior abdomen and buttock
Ilioinguinal	L1 (anterior rami)	Abdominal muscles	Medial thigh, external genitalia
Genitofemoral	L1–L2 (anterior rami)	Cremaster	Medial thigh, external genitalia
LCN	L2–L3 (posterior rami)	None	Lateral thigh
Femoral	L2–L4 (posterior rami)	Anterior thigh muscles	Anterior thigh and medial side of leg below knee up to medial malleolus **Hip and knee joint**
Obturator	L2–L4 (anterior rami)	Medial thigh muscle	Medial side of thigh, posterior lower thigh **Hip and knee joint**

The **femoral nerve** innervates iliacus, psoas, sartorius, quadriceps (rectus femoris and three vastus muscles), and pectinius. The **obturator nerve** innervates three adductor muscles, obturator externus, gracilis and pectinius.

Note: Additionally, the anterior rami of the L4 pass communicating branches, the lumbosacral trunk, to the sacral plexus.

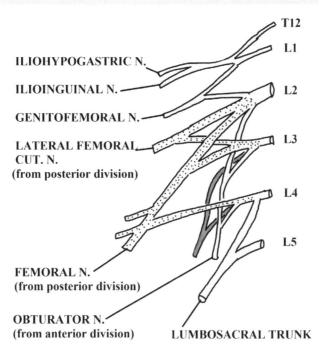

Figure 5.19 Lumbar plexus anatomy

- Cousins MJ, Bridenbaugh PO, Carr DB, *et al. Cousins and Bridenbaugh's Neural Blockade in Clinical Anesthesia and Pain Medicine.* 4th ed. Philadelphia, PA: Lippincott Williams & Wilkins; 2008. p. 344.
- Enneking FK, Chan V, Greger J, *et al.* Lower-extremity peripheral nerve blockade: essentials of our current understanding. *Reg Anesth Pain Med.* 2005; **30**(1): 4–35.

A43 **B** Lateral cutaneous nerve of the thigh has a cutaneous innervation only. The anterior divisions of both femoral and obturator nerve supply the **hip joint**, while their posterior branches supply the **knee joint**.
- Enneking FK, Chan V, Greger J, *et al.* Lower-extremity peripheral nerve blockade: essentials of our current understanding. *Reg Anesth Pain Med.* 2005; **30**(1): 4–35.

A44 **C** Lower-limb blocks are an efficacious way to provide post-operative analgesia.
- The **lumbar plexus** supplies the hip joint and part of the knee joint. Hence a lumbar plexus block offers good analgesia for hip surgery, while femoral nerve block often proves inadequate for knee surgery.
- The **sacral plexus** supplies the posterior part of knee joint and ankle as

well. Hence a combined lumbar plexus–sciatic nerve block is appropriate for a total knee replacement.

Only the medial malleolus of the ankle is supplied by the femoral nerve (via the saphenous nerve), while the remainder is innervated by the sciatic nerve.

A45 C

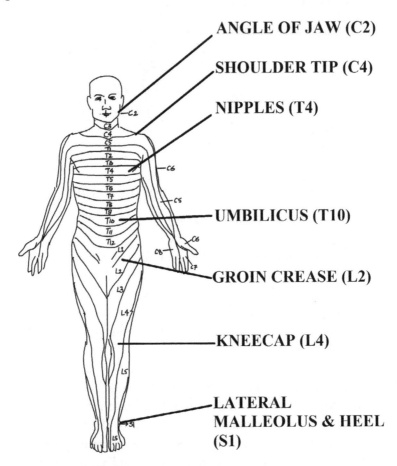

Figure 5.20 Body dermatomes

Table 5.14 Dermatomes of lower limbs

Level	Area
T12	At inguinal ligament
L1	Pubic area
L2	Anterior medial thigh
L3	At the medial epicondyle of the femur
L4	Over the medial malleolus
L5	On the dorsum of the foot
S1	On the lateral aspect of the calcaneus
S2	At the midpoint of the popliteal fossa
S3	Over the tuberosity of the ischium or infragluteal fold
S4, S5	Perianal area

A46 **A** The lumbar plexus block is performed at **L3–L5 level** where the lumbar plexus originates. The aim is to block the three main branches by depositing a large volume of local anaesthetic within the bulk of psoas

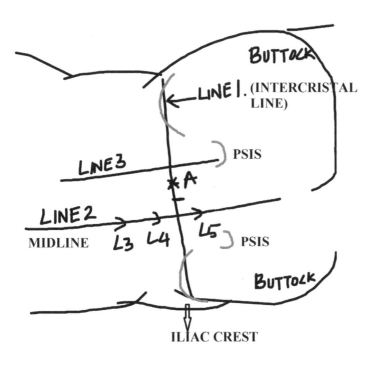

Figure 5.21 Landmarks for lumbar plexus block

muscle. The needle pierces skin, subcutaneous fat, erector spinae, quadratus lumborum and psoas major muscles.

The patient is positioned laterally (side to be blocked uppermost) and their hips and knees are flexed at right angles. The landmarks include:
- Line 1 – iliac crest and intercristal line/Tuffier's line (vertical).
- Line 2 – passing through spinous process of L4 and L5 (horizontal).
- Line 3 – parallel to the above line passing through the posterior superior iliac spine (PSIS) (horizontal).

Puncture point:
- **Winnie's**: junction of lines 1 and 3. Anatomical studies suggest that the location of this classic site is in fact too lateral.
- **Capdevila's**: the part of the intercristal line between lines 2 and 3 is divided into three parts. The **puncture point** is the junction between lateral and the middle third (as shown).
- **Chayen's**: caudal to Capdevila's puncture point at L5 level.
  - Mulroy MF, Bernards CM, McDonald SB, *et al. A Practical Approach to Regional Anesthesia*. 4th ed. Philadelphia, PA: Lippincott Williams & Wilkins; 2008. p. 223.

A47 D **Performing a lumbar plexus block**:
- The patient in placed in the lateral position (side to be blocked uppermost) and hips and knees flexed at right angles.
- A 100–150-mm 22-G needle is inserted perpendicular to the skin at Capdevila's puncture point. The PNS is set at 1–2 mA and 100 μsec pulse width.
- The needle contacts the transverse process at **6–8 cm** depth (varies with gender and body mass index). This depth is noted and the needle is withdrawn and reinserted by directing it 5° cranially or caudally, to pass its tip beyond the transverse process until evoked motor response (EMR) for lumbar plexus (**patellar twitch**) is obtained.
- The needle should not be advanced more than **2 cm** beyond the transverse process, as studies indicate the average distance between transverse process and plexus is 18 mm regardless of body mass index or gender.
- A successful lumbar plexus block will anaesthetise the FN, LFN and ON, and the lower abdominal nerves (iliohypogastric/ilioinguinal) in 70% of cases.
  - Hadzic A. *Textbook of Regional Anesthesia and Acute Pain Management*. 1st ed. New York, NY: McGraw-Hill Medical; 2006. p. 484.

A48 B

Table 5.15 Troubleshooting manoeuvres while performing a lumbar plexus block

Response	Interpretation	Manoeuvre
Twitch of erector spinae	Superficial muscles	Advance needle deeper
Needle contacts transverse process	An important landmark that serves as a guide; mark this distance	Redirect 5° cranially/caudally to proceed deeper
Quadriceps twitch (patellar tap)	Appropriate twitch	Inject solution in aliquots of 5 mL
Obturator twitch (thigh adduction)	Needle too medial	Redirect laterally at the same level
Hamstring twitch	Sacral plexus stimulation caudally or medially (lumbosacral twig)	Redirect needle cranially and laterally
Psoas twitch (thigh flexion)	Needle is too deep and is stimulating muscle directly	Withdraw needle

Note: obturator nerve stimulation is not a suitable end point, as it will lead to medial injection and inadequate block of the femoral nerve; however, a correctly placed lumbar plexus block will anaesthetise the obturator nerve consistently, as demonstrated by studies.

A49 D Precautions while performing lumbar plexus block:
- The patient should not be anticoagulated, since this is a deep block.
- The needle should not be advanced 2–3 cm beyond the transverse process.
- The needle should not be directed medially to avoid epidural or intrathecal injection.
- Rapid, forceful injections must be avoided, as this is a vascular area.
- For the same reason, epinephrine should be added to injectate to permit early recognition of intravascular injections.
- Avoid injection of local anaesthetic when a response is produced with a current < 0.5 mA, as this may lead to epidural or intrathecal spread.
- A continuous catheter should not be threaded beyond 3 cm, as it may migrate away from the plexus.

Note: this block is not considered amenable to ultrasound-guided techniques, as the plexus is located in deep tissue. Although ultrasound-guided lumbar plexus blocks have been described recently, considerable skill is required.

- Hadzic A. *Textbook of Regional Anesthesia and Acute Pain Management*. 1st ed. New York, NY: McGraw-Hill Medical; 2006. p. 486.
- Mulroy MF, Bernards CM, McDonald SB, *et al. A Practical Approach to Regional Anesthesia*. 4th ed. Philadelphia, PA: Lippincott Williams & Wilkins; 2008. p. 225.

A50 D

▸ The complications of the lumbar plexus block include renal and retro-peritoneal haematomas, intravascular injections (due to vascularity of this region), nerve damage and catheter placement in the abdomen or other unintended places.

▸ More serious complications include **unintended sympathetic block** (spread to sympathetic chain located anteriorly), epidural (15%–30% incidence due to medial injections or lateral extension of dural sleeves) or even intrathecal anaesthesia. In fact, the epidural spread may even be bilateral.

  - Cousins MJ, Bridenbaugh PO, Carr DB, *et al. Cousins and Bridenbaugh's Neural Blockade in Clinical Anesthesia and Pain Medicine*. 4th ed. Philadelphia, PA: Lippincott Williams & Wilkins; 2008. p. 348.
  - Mannion S. Psoas compartment block. *Contin Educ Anaesth Crit Care Pain*. 2007; **7**(5): 162–6.

A51 C The FN is formed by the **posterior divisions** of the **anterior rami of the L2–L4** spinal nerves. It first lies within the bulk of psoas muscle, emerging from its lateral border in a fascial compartment between the psoas and iliacus muscles and innervating both. It then enters the thigh under the inguinal ligament. Here it lies lateral to femoral artery. The femoral sheath contains the femoral artery and vein, which lie beneath the fascia lata but above the fascia iliaca. **The femoral nerve lies deep to the fascia iliaca**, which forms the iliopectineal ligament to separate the femoral nerve from the femoral vessels medially.

▸ The **anterior division** of the femoral nerve supplies the skin of the medial and anterior surfaces of the thigh, innervates sartorius and pec-tineus muscles and provides articular branches to the hip.

▸ The **posterior division** of the femoral nerve provides muscular branches to the quadriceps and articular branches to the knee; eventually it becomes the saphenous nerve. The saphenous nerve lies within the adductor canal under the sartorius muscle above the medial aspect of the knee.

- Mulroy MF, Bernards CM, McDonald SB, *et al. A Practical Approach to Regional Anesthesia.* 4th ed. Philadelphia, PA: Lippincott Williams & Wilkins; 2008. pp. 219–20.

A52 B

Table 5.16 Various techniques to block femoral nerve

Technique	Landmarks	Needling	End point
Peripheral nerve stimulator-guided femoral nerve block	Inguinal crease, 1–2 cm lateral to femoral artery	A 50-mm 22-G needle is inserted at this puncture point directed 60° cephalad	Patellar twitch; 15–20 mL local anaesthetic is injected
Femoral three-in-one block	Same as above	Same as above	Patellar twitch; higher volume and distal pressure applied
Fascia iliaca block	Line joining anterior superior iliac spine and pubic tubercle (inguinal ligament) is divided into three parts	Needle inserted 1 cm below the junction of lateral and middle third	20 mL local anaesthetic injected after two pops (signifying fascia lata and fascia iliaca)
Ultrasound guidance	Inguinal crease	Identifying femoral vessels, nerve and fascia iliaca	Patellar twitch if a nerve stimulator is used

Note: femoral three-in-one block does not consistently block obturator nerve. Ultrasound guidance may reduce the volume of local anaesthetic needed and the onset time of anaesthesia for femoral block, but no study has demonstrated a reduction in peripheral nerve injury.

- Mulroy MF, Bernards CM, McDonald SB, *et al. A Practical Approach to Regional Anesthesia.* 4th ed. Philadelphia, PA: Lippincott Williams & Wilkins; 2008. pp. 502, 512.

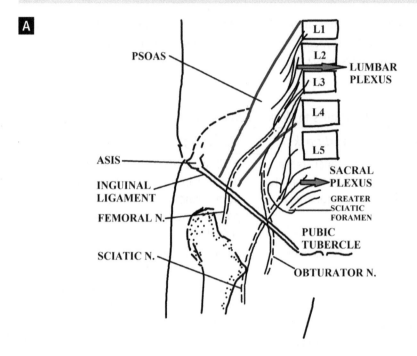

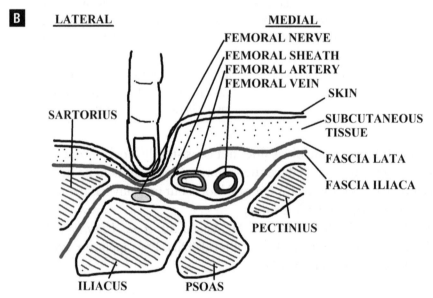

Figure 5.22 (A) Course of branches of lumbar plexus; (B) femoral nerve location

A53 B Indications for femoral nerve block include:
- **Single injections**: quadriceps biopsy, long saphenous vein stripping, knee arthroscopy (along with intra-articular LA), analgesia for primary total knee replacement (TKR) and analgesia for anterior cruciate ligament (ACL) reconstruction.
- **Continuous catheter**: analgesia for femoral shaft/femoral neck fractures (catheter placed upon initial presentation) and TKR.
- **Combined with sciatic block**: any surgery below mid-thigh level.

Salient features of PNS-guided femoral nerve block are as follows.
- Ideally performed at the inguinal crease, since:
  - The femoral nerve is widest and most superficial.
  - At inguinal ligament, needle directed cephalad can enter pelvis.
  - It is less painful than piercing through the inguinal ligament.
- Initially, a sartorial twitch is obtained (movement of lower medial thigh) due to stimulation of anterior branch of femoral nerve.
- The needle is then redirected slightly **deeper** (and laterally or medially) to stimulate **posterior branch** (supplying quadriceps), resulting in typical 'patellar twitch'. Local anaesthetic (15–20 mL) may be injected at this point.
- Femoral nerve catheters should not be passed more than **3–5 cm** beyond the tip, as the chances of migration away from the nerve are increased (i.e. medial or lateral rather than proximal).
  - Cousins MJ, Bridenbaugh PO, Carr DB, *et al. Cousins and Bridenbaugh's Neural Blockade in Clinical Anesthesia and Pain Medicine*. 4th ed. Philadelphia, PA: Lippincott Williams & Wilkins; 2008. p. 349.
  - Hadzic A. *Textbook of Regional Anesthesia and Acute Pain Management*. 1st ed. New York, NY: McGraw-Hill Medical; 2006. p. 500.
  - Mulroy MF, Bernards CM, McDonald SB, *et al. A Practical Approach to Regional Anesthesia*. 4th ed. Philadelphia, PA: Lippincott Williams & Wilkins; 2008. p. 227.

A54 B **Fascia iliaca block**:
- It is the simplest way to block the femoral nerve.
- A line joining ASIS and pubic tubercle (inguinal ligament) is divided into three parts; at 1 cm below the junction of the lateral and middle thirds, a 50-mm blunt-tipped needle is inserted angled at 60° cephalad,
- Two clicks or pops are detected as the needle pierces through the fascia lata and the fascia iliaca, and 20–30 mL local anaesthetic is injected.
- For a continuous catheter technique, the needle tip is directed **medially**

to allow catheter to migrate towards the medially situated femoral nerve at this point.

Femoral three-in-one block:
▶ Uses the same landmarks and technique as PNS-guided femoral nerve block, but a larger volume of local anaesthetic and distal pressure is used to encourage proximal migration block of the three main nerves of the lumbar plexus. However, studies have shown that this does not occur and local anaesthetic actually spreads laterally and medially rather than proximally.
▶ The following nerves are inconsistently anaesthetised during a three-in-one block: the LCN of the thigh, the FN and the anterior branch of the ON. However, the posterior branch of the ON and femoral branch of genitofemoral nerve are not blocked and it is unsuitable for surgery performed in the inguinal or popliteal areas. Also, because of inconsistent block of anterior branch of the ON, surgery of medial aspect of the thigh may also need supplementation in some form.

Continuous catheters:
▶ They may be inserted either using the **PNS or ultrasound**. The femoral nerve lies deep to fascia iliaca, and therefore the **catheter tip should lie below this layer**.
▶ Catheters may be inserted along the long axis (using the out-of-plane approach) or **perpendicular to the long axis** of the nerve (using the in-plane approach).
▶ Catheters may be **non-stimulating or stimulating**. Theoretically, stimulating catheters should improve secondary block success rate; however, recent reviews have only been able to demonstrate a limited benefit.
  • Gandhi K, Lindenmuth DM, Hadzic A, *et al*. The effect of stimulating versus conventional perineural catheters on postoperative analgesia following ultrasound-guided femoral nerve localization. *J Clin Anesth*. 2011; **23**(8): 626–31.
  • Tran de QH, Muñoz L, Russo G, *et al*. Ultrasonography and stimulating perineural catheters for nerve blocks: a review of the evidence. *Can J Anaesth*. 2008; **55**(7): 447–57.

A55 C The saphenous nerve is the **terminal branch** of the **posterior** division of femoral nerve. It has **no motor supply** and provides sensory innervations to the anterior thigh, medial aspect of knee and leg down to the **medial malleolus**. It may be blocked in the following locations.
▶ Above the knee:
  – subcutaneous infiltration above knee

- **subsartorial injection** 5 cm above knee – blind or PNS/ultrasound guided.
▶ Below the knee:
  - subcutaneous infiltration along the medial tibia and the media popliteal fossa;
  - paravenous technique (along the long saphenous vein) just distal to knee;
  - infiltration above medial malleolus.

The highest success rate is achieved by **sub-sartorial injections**. The patient is positioned supine, with the chosen leg slightly abducted and external rotated. The sartorius muscle is identified (above the medial aspect of the knee) by asking the patient to elevate the leg slightly. A 50-mm 22-G needle is inserted through the belly of sartorius to enter the **subsartorial plane**, and paraesthesia is elicited in the saphenous distribution. Local anaesthetic (10 mL) may be injected here. Using utrasound guidance, the saphenous nerve may be identified in the subsartorial plane, sandwiched between the sartorius and the vastus medialis initially and the sartorius and the gracilis distally. Distally it lies next to the **descending genicular artery**, which serves as a landmark for identification under ultrasound.

- • Mulroy MF, Bernards CM, McDonald SB, *et al. A Practical Approach to Regional Anesthesia*. 4th ed. Philadelphia, PA: Lippincott Williams & Wilkins; 2008. pp. 231–2.

A56 C The obturator nerve originates from the **ventral (anterior) divisions of anterior primary rami of L2–L4** spinal nerve roots. It is formed within the substance of psoas muscle and travels near its medial border, emerging from the **obturator foramen** to enter the thigh.

▶ Here it divides into an **anterior division**, which lies between the adductor longus and pectinius above and the adductor brevis below. It supplies these muscles and gracilis, articular branch to hip and a variable cutaneous branch to the medial side of the thigh.
▶ The **posterior division** passes deep to adductor brevis but lies above adductor magnus. It supplies adductor magnus and obturator externus; and an articular branch to the **knee** joint.

Note: an accessory obturator nerve (L3, L4) may occur in a third of individuals, and innervates the pectinius muscle.

- • Mulroy MF, Bernards CM, McDonald SB, *et al. A Practical Approach to Regional Anesthesia*. 4th ed. Philadelphia, PA: Lippincott Williams & Wilkins; 2008. pp. 220–1.

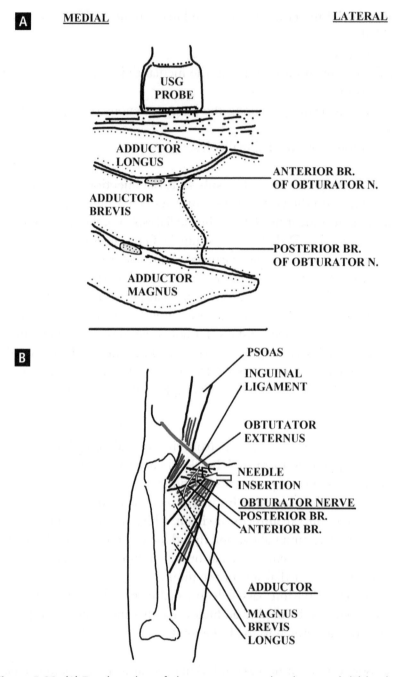

Figure 5.23 (A) Two branches of obturator nerve under ultrasound; (B) landmark-based classic approach

A57 D

Various techniques for blocking the obturator nerve:

▶ **Winnie's classic approach**: 2 cm lateral and 2 cm caudal to pubic tubercle, a stimulating needle is inserted perpendicular to the skin to contact the pubic ramus. Then it is walked off the inferior edge of ramus to enter the obturator foramen until an adductor EMR is observed. This approach is painful because of periosteal contact.

▶ **Inguinal approach**: a line is drawn from the femoral artery to the medial border of adductor longus on the inguinal crease. At the midpoint of this line, a needle is inserted 30° cephalad in a parasagittal plane to elicit a medial adductor response (stimulation of adductor longus supplied by anterior branch of the ON) at a depth of about 4 cm, and 5 mL of local anaesthetic is deposited here. The needle is redirected caudal and lateral towards adductor magnus to elicit a posterior adductor twitch (stimulating posterior branch of ON) and a further 5 mL of local anaesthetic is injected.

▶ **Ultrasound guidance approach**: a high-frequency ultrasound probe is placed parallel to the inguinal crease. The anterior branch is identified between the adductor longus and the brevis, while the posterior branch can be seen lying between the adductor brevis and the magnus muscles.

Note: success of obturator block is assessed by **loss of motor block only**, since the anterior branch inconsistently supplies the medial thigh. In addition, adductor magnus is also innervated by the sciatic nerve; therefore, it is not completely paralysed with an isolated ON block.

- Mulroy MF, Bernards CM, McDonald SB, *et al. A Practical Approach to Regional Anesthesia.* 4th ed. Philadelphia, PA: Lippincott Williams & Wilkins; 2008. pp. 234–5.

A58 D

▶ The LCN of the thigh is derived from the **dorsal division** of **anterior rami** of **L2–L3**.

▶ It originates within the body of psoas and emerges from the lateral border of the muscle to lie on the **iliacus muscle**.

▶ The nerve proceeds towards the ASIS, passing **under the inguinal ligament** medial to the ASIS. The LCN of the thigh may be blocked here by injecting local anaesthetic **2 cm medial and 2 cm caudal** to ASIS.

▶ It lies **under the fascia lata**, but above the fascia iliaca.

Note: in **meralgia paraesthetica**, the LCN may pass above the inguinal ligament and may need surgical decompression.

- Mulroy MF, Bernards CM, McDonald SB, *et al. A Practical Approach to Regional Anesthesia*. 4th ed. Philadelphia, PA: Lippincott Williams & Wilkins; 2008. pp. 220, 236.

A59 D The sacral plexus is derived from the **lumbosacral trunk** (anterior rami of L4, L5) and the **sacral nerves** (anterior rami of S1–S3). It is formed within the pelvis and exits it through the **greater sciatic foramen**. It is bounded by **piriformis posteriorly** and the **iliac vessels anteriorly**.

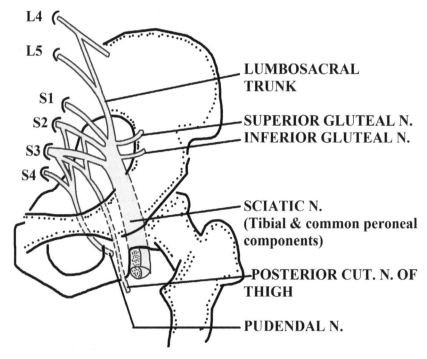

Figure 5.24 Branches of sacral plexus

Note: sciatic nerve is the main terminal branch of the sacral plexus (the other being the posterior cutaneous femoral nerve (PCFN)). It is the largest (2 cm wide) and longest nerve of the body (approx 45 cm till division).

- Cousins MJ, Bridenbaugh PO, Carr DB, *et al. Cousins and Bridenbaugh's Neural Blockade in Clinical Anesthesia and Pain Medicine*. 4th ed. Philadelphia, PA: Lippincott Williams & Wilkins; 2008. p. 349.

Table 5.17 Branches of sacral plexus

Nerves	Motor supply	Cutaneous supply
Gluteal nerves (L4–S2)	Superior gluteal nerve: gluteus medius and minimus Inferior gluteal nerve: gluteus maximus Nerve to quadratus femoris Nerves to the piriformis and obturator internus muscles	Upper medial buttock
Sciatic nerve (L4–S3)	Common peroneal: see Answer 66 (Chapter 5) Tibial nerve: see Answer 66 (Chapter 5)	See Answer 66 (Chapter 5)
Posterior femoral cutaneous nerve (S1–S3)	**None**	Inferior cluneal nerves and perineal branches: lower medial buttock and posterior thigh
Pudendal nerve (S2, S3, S4)	Muscles of the pelvic structures	External genitalia

A60 B Sciatic nerve course and branches and relevant blocks:

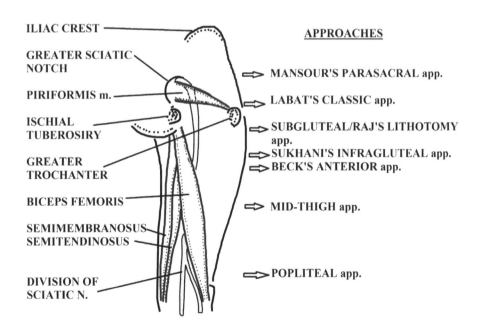

Figure 5.25 Course of sciatic nerve and various blocks

Table 5.18 Various blocks of sciatic nerve

Course	Appropriate block (positioning)
Sciatic nerve exits the greater sciatic foramen, **deep** to the piriformis	Mansour's parasacral block (lateral) Labat's classic sciatic nerve block (lateral decubitus)
Enters the thigh **midway** between the greater trochanter and the ischial tuberosity	Subgluteal approach (lateral decubitus) Raj's approach (lithotomy)
Passes **medial** to the lesser trochanter	Beck's anterior approach (supine)
Upper thigh: lies **lateral** to the tendon of biceps femoris	Sukhani's infragluteal approach (prone)
Mid-thigh: **under** the belly of biceps femoris	Guardini's subtrochanteric block (supine)
Popliteal fossa: divides into a **medial tibial nerve and lateral common peroneal nerve (fibular nerve)**; bounded by biceps femoris laterally, and semitendinosus and semimembranosus medially	Popliteal block (prone/supine/lateral/lithotomy)

Note: tibial and common peroneal nerves are **two distinct nerves** from the **very start** contained within the **same common sheath**, as shown by anatomical studies. Sciatic nerve divides into its two main branches generally at **lower thigh level**, although this is very variable (**0–13 cm** from popliteal crease).

- Vloka JD, Hadzić A, April E, *et al.* The division of the sciatic nerve in the popliteal fossa: anatomical implications for popliteal nerve blockade. *Anesth Analg.* 2001; **92**(1): 215–17.
- Vloka JD, Hadzić A, Lesser JB, *et al.* A common epineural sheath for the nerves in the popliteal fossa and its possible implications for sciatic nerve block. *Anesth Analg.* 1997; **84**(2): 387–90.

A61 A

Table 5.19 Innervation of the hip joint

Hip joint capsule area	Innervation by branches of
Anterior aspect	Femoral nerve
Anteromedially	Obturator nerve
Posterior aspect	Superior gluteal nerve
Posteromedially	Nerves to quadratus femoris and sciatic nerve

- Birnbaum K, Prescher A, Hessler S, *et al.* The sensory innervation of the hip joint: an anatomical study. *Surg Radiol Anat.* 1997; **19**(6): 371–5.

A62 C

- The parasacral approach (Mansour's) is the **most proximal approach** to block the sacral plexus. It **consistently blocks** the two terminal branches of the sacral plexus (sciatic and PCNF); however, it may also block the gluteal, pudendal and obturator nerves.
- The patient is positioned in the lateral position and a line is drawn between the **PSIS** and **ischial tuberosity (IT)**. A 100-mm insulated 22-G needle is inserted at a point **6 cm caudal from the PSIS** on this line in horizontal plane.
- Initially a gluteal muscle contraction may be obtained, and the needle should be inserted deeper, where usually contact with the greater sciatic notch is made. Slight caudal redirection results in a sciatic nerve EMR (tibial nerve, common peroneal nerve or hamstring contractions).
- Out of these, **a tibial nerve EMR (planterflexion and inversion)** provides the highest success rate.
- Compared with distal sciatic approaches (popliteal block), the parasacral approach is **advantageous** for knee or above-knee surgery, as it may block the entire sacral plexus. However, this is a **disadvantage** for below-knee procedures because of adductor weakness (obturator block) causing interference with patient mobilisation.
  - Hagon BS, Itani O, Bidgoli JH, *et al.* Parasacral sciatic nerve block: does the elicited motor response predict the success rate? *Anesth Analg.* 2007; **105**(1): 263–6.
  - Mulroy MF, Bernards CM, McDonald SB, *et al. A Practical Approach to Regional Anesthesia.* 4th ed. Philadelphia, PA: Lippincott Williams & Wilkins; 2008. pp. 243–4.

A63 C

- Parasacral block (Mansour's approach) is a relatively easy block to perform and has a high success rate.
- As sacral outflow is predominantly parasympathetic, sacral nerve blockade causes parasympathetic blockade, hence is **unlikely to cause hypotension**.
- Obturator nerve can be reliably blocked either by a lumbar plexus block or specific obturator block. It is **not reliably and consistently blocked by** either a fascia iliaca or sacral plexus block.
- The PCFN has **no motor or articular supply**. It provides sensory

innervations to the lower buttock and posterior thigh and therefore is important for prevention of thigh tourniquet pain, in combination with femoral nerve and LCN of thigh. The PCFN may be blocked by proximal approaches only (Mansour's parasacral block, Labat's gluteal, Beck's anterior approach). However, a randomised study of proximal and distal block has **not revealed any statistical difference** in thigh tourniquet tolerance for below-knee surgery.

▶ Along with **lumbar psoas compartment block** (not femoral nerve block) it may be used for unilateral lower-limb anaesthesia.

- Cousins MJ, Bridenbaugh PO, Carr DB, *et al. Cousins and Bridenbaugh's Neural Blockade in Clinical Anesthesia and Pain Medicine*. 4th ed. Philadelphia, PA: Lippincott Williams & Wilkins; 2008. pp. 356–7.
- Fuzier R, Hoffreumont P, Bringuier-Branchereau S, *et al*. Does the sciatic nerve approach influence thigh tourniquet tolerance during below-knee surgery? *Anesth Analg*. 2005; **100**(5): 1511–14.
- Ripart J, Cuvillon P, Nouvellon E, *et al*. Parasacral approach to block the sciatic nerve: a 400-case survey. *Reg Anesth Pain Med*. 2005; **30**(2): 193–7.

A64 D Various approaches can block the sciatic nerve proximally. These approaches are as follows.

▶ **Posterior transgluteal (Labat's) approach**: a line is drawn connecting greater trochanter (GT) and PSIS (line 1) and another between GT and sacral hiatus (line 2). From the midpoint of line 1, a perpendicular is dropped to intersect line 2 at **point A**. This point corresponds to the lateral border of the sciatic notch, where the sciatic nerve emerges from the sciatic foramen. The patient is placed in **lateral decubitus** with slight forward tilt and the hips flexed with the side to be blocked uppermost. A 100–150-mm 22-G needle is inserted at this point perpendicular to all planes. The initial gluteal response is ignored and the needle directed deeper to elicit a sciatic nerve response.

▶ **Subgluteal approach (lateral)**: with the patient in **lateral decubitus**, a line connecting GT and the ischial tuberosity (IT) is drawn. The sciatic nerve lies roughly at the midpoint of this line, having emerged from the inferior border of gluteus muscles. A 100-mm 22-G needle is inserted perpendicularly at the midpoint of this line to elicit sciatic twitches.

▶ **Lithotomy subgluteal (Raj's) approach**: with the patient **supine**, both hip and the knee are flexed at 90°. A line connecting GT and IT is drawn. The sciatic nerve traverses superficially at the midpoint of this line. A 100-mm 22-G needle is inserted perpendicularly at the midpoint of this line to elicit sciatic twitches.

▶ **Infragluteal (Sukhani's) approach**: with the patient **prone**, the lateral border of the biceps femoris (BF) muscle is palpated. The point where its tendon intersects the infragluteal crease is the point of insertion of the needle. A 100-mm 22-G needle is inserted perpendicularly at the midpoint of this line to elicit sciatic twitches. BF twitches should not be accepted.

▶ **Anterior (Beck's) approach**: with the patient **supine** and the leg in neutral position, a line joining ASIS and pubic tubercle is divided into thirds (line 1). A line parallel to this line is drawn from GT (line 2). A perpendicular is dropped from the junction of the middle and medial thirds of line 1, to intersect line 2 at point A. Here, a 150-mm needle is inserted perpendicularly, initially to hit the femur, and directed medially subsequently to pass the lesser trochanter. The sciatic nerve is located deep to adductors but anterior to gluteus maximus. Deeper passage elicits the sciatic nerve EMR. This approach has seen resurgence with ultrasound guidance allowing identification of sciatic nerve behind lesser trochanter.

▶ **Subtrochanteric (Guardini's) approach**: with patient **supine**, GT is palpated. The puncture site is 2 cm inferior and 4 cm distal to the GT. A 100-mm 22-G needle is inserted perpendicularly in horizontal plane to elicit sciatic twitches.

- Cousins MJ, Bridenbaugh PO, Carr DB, *et al. Cousins and Bridenbaugh's Neural Blockade in Clinical Anesthesia and Pain Medicine.* 4th ed. Philadelphia, PA: Lippincott Williams & Wilkins; 2008. pp. 356–60.

- Mulroy MF, Bernards CM, McDonald SB, *et al. A Practical Approach to Regional Anesthesia.* 4th ed. Philadelphia, PA: Lippincott Williams & Wilkins; 2008. pp. 243–53.

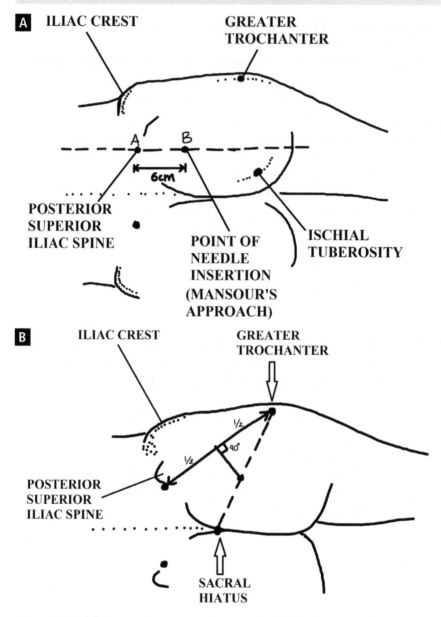

Figure 5.26 (A) Mansour's parasacral approach; (B) Labat's approach

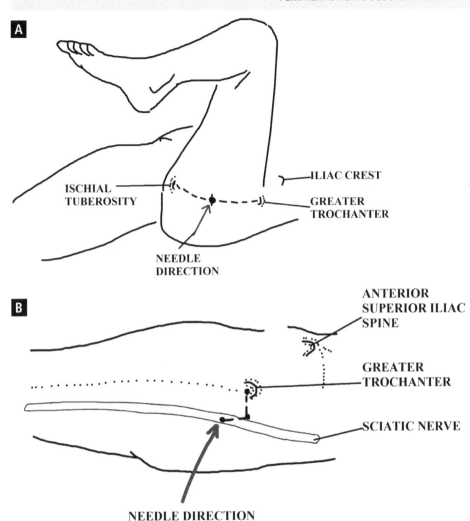

Figure 5.27 (A) Raj's lithotomy approach; (B) Guardini's subtrochanteric approach

A65 C

Table 5.20 Comparison of various proximal sciatic nerve approaches

Approach	Advantage	Disadvantage
Mansour's parasacral	Simple landmarks Easy to perform High success rate	Lateral positioning needed
Labat's posterior transgluteal	Proximal approach	Lateral positioning needed Difficult landmarks Painful needle insertion Ultrasound guidance difficult since nerve is deeper at this level
Subgluteal	Sciatic nerve is not covered by gluteus Reliable landmarks even in obese individuals Ultrasound guidance easier to do	Lateral positioning needed Anisotropy of sciatic nerve
Raj's lithotomy	Supine positioning Reliable landmarks	Procedural difficulty (someone needs to hold the leg, and limb moves with stimulation)
Sukhani's infragluteal	Simple landmarks	Prone positioning needed Landmarks may be variable (only bony landmarks are fixed) Spares the posterior cutaneous femoral nerve
Beck's anterior	Supine positioning Resurgence with ultrasound guidance approach	Deeper insertions, hence painful Technically challenging
Guardini's subtrochanteric	Supine positioning	Not a favoured approach

A66 A

▶ The sciatic nerve is composed of two components, the tibial and the common peroneal. The tibial nerve (TN) is **larger and lies medially**, while the common peroneal nerve (CPN) is **smaller and lies laterally**.

▶ The TN supplies gastronemius, soleus and plantaris in the leg; and flexor hallucis longus and flexor digitorum longus in the foot through medial and lateral plantar nerves. Stimulation of TN causes **plantar flexion.**

▶ The CPN divides into a superficial and a deep branch. The superficial peroneal nerve supplies peroneus brevis and longus, which **evert** the ankle.

▶ The deep peroneal nerve supplies branches to muscles of the anterior leg (tibialis anterior, extensor digitorum longus, peroneus tertius, and extensor hallucis propius) and extensors of ankle (extensor hallucis longus and extensor digitorum longus). This causes **dorsiflexion** upon stimulation.

▶ The **inversion** of the foot is caused by tibialis anterior (deep peroneal nerve) and tibialis posterior (the TN). Hence, such a response suggests a central needle-tip location and stimulation of both TN and CPN components. This has been the reason suggested for a higher success rate and a shorter onset time of anaesthesia with inversion EMR.

- Sukhani R, Nader A, Candido KD, *et al.* Nerve stimulator-assisted evoked motor response predicts the latency and success of a single-injection sciatic block. *Anesth Analg.* 2004; **99**(2): 584–8.

A67 **B** Popliteal approach to the sciatic nerve is the **most common**, as it is located most superficially at this level (2–4 cm). As the sciatic nerve descends into the thigh, it separates into its two components: medial tibial nerve (TN) and lateral common peroneal nerve (CPN). This division occurs variably above the popliteal crease from **0 to 13 cm** and is a frequent cause of sparing of one of these components in PNS-guided single-injection blocks. Hence, multistimulation or ultrasound guidance techniques enhance success rates. Two approaches to PNS-guided popliteal block are in vogue.

▶ **Posterior approach**: the patient is positioned prone; a triangle is drawn over the posterior aspect of the knee where the popliteal crease forms the base, biceps femoris tendon the lateral border and semimembranosus tendon the medial border. A perpendicular line (P) is dropped from the apex to the popliteal crease bisecting it. A point **7–8 cm above the popliteal crease** on this perpendicular line is chosen, and a **50-mm 22-G needle** is inserted 1 cm lateral to this point. In most people, the sciatic nerve has not divided at this point. **Inversion** EMR yields best results followed by plantar flexion, dorsiflexion and eversion. A **volume of 25–40 mL** of local anaesthetic may be used. The same landmark technique may be performed with the patient in lithotomy position.

▶ **Lateral approach**: the groove between biceps femoris and vastus lateralis is palpated, and a **100-mm needle** is inserted perpendicularly **7–8 cm above the popliteal crease**. The needle is walked off the femur

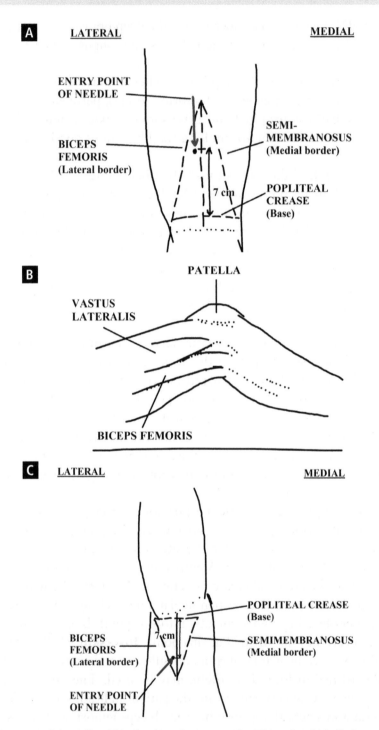

Figure 5.28 (A) Popliteal block, posterior approach; (B) popliteal block, lateral approach; (C) popliteal block, lithotomy approach

at an angle of **30° dorsal** to stimulate the sciatic nerves. Common peroneal nerve is commonly stimulated here, and the drug is injected subsequently.

- Mulroy MF, Bernards CM, McDonald SB, *et al. A Practical Approach to Regional Anesthesia*. 4th ed. Philadelphia, PA: Lippincott Williams & Wilkins; 2008. pp. 253–8.

A68 D Ultrasound-guided popliteal block:

▶ This uses a high-frequency array (6–13 MHz), as sciatic nerves are located superficially.

▶ The sciatic nerve is **anisotropic**, hence the beam needs to be aligned at 90° to obtain the best view. This can be achieved by a cranial tilt of the probe at the proximal thigh, vertical positioning at mid-thigh and a caudal tilt at the lower-thigh level.

▶ The probe is placed parallel to popliteal crease, and moved upward until the pulsatile popliteal artery is seen. The sciatic nerve components can be seen **superficial and lateral** to the artery at this level.

▶ They may be traced upwards, where they are seen joining to form a single sciatic nerve. This is the **best location for injection** as well as catheter placement.

▶ At this point, local anaesthetic is deposited in a circumferential manner to enclose **hyperechoic** nerve all around (the **doughnut sign**).

- Mulroy MF, Bernards CM, McDonald SB, *et al. A Practical Approach to Regional Anesthesia*. 4th ed. Philadelphia, PA: Lippincott Williams & Wilkins; 2008. pp. 255–7.
- www.usra.ca/popclinic.php

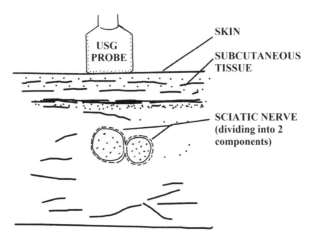

Figure 5.29 Ultrasound image of division of sciatic nerve at popliteal fossa

A69 **B** Cutaneous nerve supply of the ankle is important; it is derived from **five nerves**, and ankle blocks usually show some sparing. The nerve supply is shown in Figure 5.30.

Table 5.21 Nerve supply of ankle

Landmark	Nerve
Lateral malleolus	Sural
	Superficial peroneal
Medial malleolus	Saphenous
Dorsum of foot	Mostly superficial peroneal
Plantar surface of foot	Medial and lateral plantar (branches of tibial)
Lateral margin of foot	Sural
Medial margin of foot	Saphenous
Web space between the first and second toes	Deep peroneal
Fifth toe	Superficial peroneal
Heel	Posterior tibial

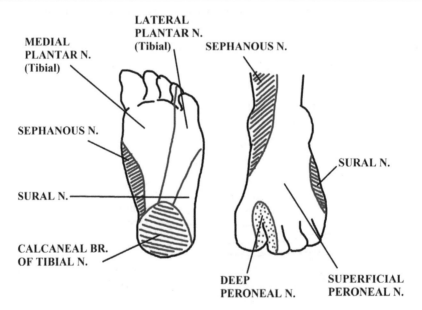

Figure 5.30 Nerve supply of ankle

A70 **D** The ankle is innervated by five nerves: three nerves are superficial (superficial peroneal, sural and saphenous), and two are located deep (deep peroneal and posterior tibial). Remember: **S** is **s**uperficial.

A71 A

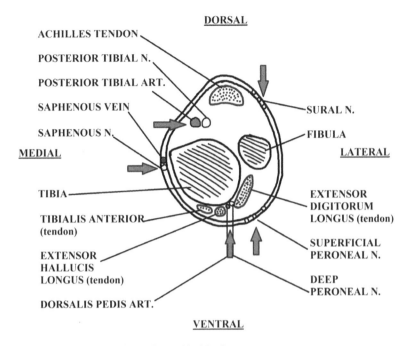

Figure 5.31 Injection landmarks for ankle block

Table 5.22 Injection landmarks for ankle block

Nerve	Landmarks	Volume (mL)
Deep peroneal	Peripheral nervous system: lateral to the tendon of the extensor hallucis longus muscle (between extensor hallucis longus and extensor digitorum longus) Ultrasound: nerve is immediately lateral to the **dorsalis pedis artery**	5
Posterior tibial	Behind medial malleolus, deep to **posterior tibial artery**	5
Saphenous	Subcutaneously at medial malleolus near **great saphenous vein**	5
Sural	Subcutaneously in the groove between lateral malleolus and calcaneum (behind **short saphenous vein**)	5
Superficial peroneal	Subcutaneously between anterior tibial and lateral malleolus	5–10

- www.nysora.com/peripheral_nerve_blocks/classic_block_tecniques/3035-ankle_block.html

A72 C

▶ The duration of analgesia provided for foot surgeries is **6 hours** by subcutaneous infiltration, **11 hours** by ankle block and **18 hours** by popliteal block.

▶ Mayo block is an alternative to ankle block for bunion or hallux surgery, as it anaesthetises the first metatarsal only.

▶ Adrenaline should ideally be avoided in ankle blocks because of the risk of vascular compromise.

- McLeod DH, Wong DH, Claridge RJ, *et al.* Lateral popliteal sciatic nerve block compared with subcutaneous infiltration for analgesia following foot surgery. *Can J Anaesth*. 199; **41**(8): 673–66.

- McLeod DH, Wong DH, Vaghadia H, *et al.* Lateral popliteal sciatic nerve block compared with ankle block for analgesia following foot surgery. *Can J Anaesth*. 1995; **42**(9): 765–9.

- Worrell JB, Barbour G. The Mayo block: an efficacious block for hallux and first metatarsal surgery. *AANA J*. 1996; **64**(2): 146–52.

A73 D

▶ Uncontrolled acute pain is related to the development of **chronic pain syndromes, post-operative myocardial ischemia and post-operative cognitive decline**. Post-operative pain relief after thoracic surgery can be provided by intercostal, interpleural, paravertebral and epidural block.

▶ Compared with opioid analgesia, intercostal block results in **higher peak expiratory flows**.

▶ Although epidural and paravertebral block (PVB) provides comparable analgesia after thoracic surgery, PVB has a **better side-effect profile**.

- Cousins MJ, Bridenbaugh PO, Carr DB, *et al. Cousins and Bridenbaugh's Neural Blockade in Clinical Anesthesia and Pain Medicine*. 4th ed. Philadelphia, PA: Lippincott Williams & Wilkins; 2008. pp. 383–4.

A74 B The thoracic nerves T1–T12 emerge from their respective intervertebral foramina, and divide into the:

▶ paired gray and white rami communicantes (passing to the sympathetic chain anteriorly)

▶ posterior primary rami (supplying paravertebral muscles)

▶ anterior primary rami (forming the ICN).

The ICN divides into a lateral and an anterior cutaneous branch. T12 is actually a **subcostal nerve** rather than an intercostal nerve.

▶ **In the paravertebral region**, ICN overlies the parietal pleura and fat.
▶ **Medial to the angle of the ribs**, ICN is sandwiched between the parietal pleural and posterior intercostal membrane (fascia of internal intercostals).
▶ **At the angle of the rib**, the ICN lies between the intercostalis intimus (innermost intercostals) and internal intercostals.

The ICN lies in the **intercostal groove** (along with intercostal vein and artery) below the **inferior edge** of the rib.
▶ T1 lacks lateral and anterior branches.
▶ T2–T3 contribute to intercostobrachial nerve.
▶ T12 (subcostal nerve) joins L1 to form iliohypogastric, ilioinguinal and genitofemoral nerves.
  • Cousins MJ, Bridenbaugh PO, Carr DB, *et al. Cousins and Bridenbaugh's Neural Blockade in Clinical Anesthesia and Pain Medicine*. 4th ed. Philadelphia, PA: Lippincott Williams & Wilkins; 2008. p. 386.
  • Hadzic A. *Textbook of Regional Anesthesia and Acute Pain Management*. 1st ed. New York, NY: McGraw-Hill Medical; 2006. p. 600.

A75 D
▶ A systemic review has shown that ICN block provides equieffective analgesia as an epidural and significantly better than opioids alone.
▶ It provides **excellent analgesia** for fractured ribs, and pain relief after chest and upper-abdominal surgeries (thoracotomy, thoracostomy, breast surgery, gastrostomy and cholecystectomy).
▶ Chronic pain from post-mastectomy pain, post-thoracotomy pain, herpes zoster and tumour-related pain may also be treated.

ICNs are performed **proximally to the mid-axillary line**, as the lateral cutaneous nerve arises beyond that point. However, they are best performed at the **angle of the ribs**, where the ribs and intercostal spaces are thicker, allowing a larger margin of safety before pleura is contacted. ICN may be performed with patient in supine or lateral position (for mid-axillary injections), but is **best** performed in **prone** position (for injection at the angle of the rib) with arms hanging by the sides to allow scapulae to rotate laterally, and a pillow under the abdomen to accentuate intercostal spaces posteriorly. The skin over the intercostal area is retracted up and over the rib and a 23–25-G needle is introduced **20° cephalad** to come in contact with rib. The needle is walked off the inferior edge, **maintaining the angulation**, and advanced 2–4 mm into the intercostal groove. Between 3 and 5 mL of local anaesthetic (LA) (0.5% bupivacaine) is injected after aspiration.

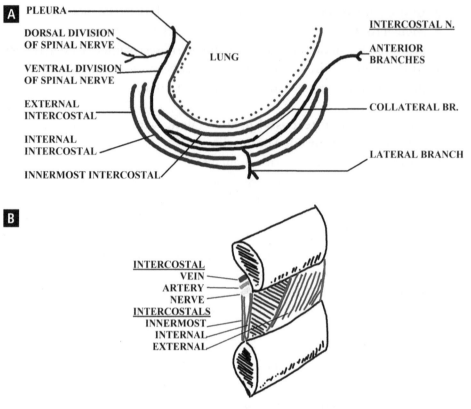

Figure 5.32 (A) Origin and branches of intercostal nerve; (B) intercostal nerve in the intercostal groove

- Cousins MJ, Bridenbaugh PO, Carr DB, *et al. Cousins and Bridenbaugh's Neural Blockade in Clinical Anesthesia and Pain Medicine*. 4th ed. Philadelphia, PA: Lippincott Williams & Wilkins; 2008. p. 388.

A76 A

- ▶ The intercostal nerve block **does not block visceral pain**, for which coeliac or splanchnic plexus block may be needed.
- ▶ Usually, multiple level injections are needed due to **overlap** of ICN from above and below segments.
- ▶ Injection at a single level may spread to segments above and below due to medial spread. CT images have shown that the LA spreads medially along the intercostal groove to the **paravertebral space**.
- ▶ Complications may include pneumothorax (< 1%), LA toxicity due to rapid drug absorption and spread to subarachnoid space (because dural cuff may extend up to **8 cm** laterally).

- Cousins MJ, Bridenbaugh PO, Carr DB, *et al. Cousins and Bridenbaugh's Neural Blockade in Clinical Anesthesia and Pain Medicine*. 4th ed. Philadelphia, PA: Lippincott Williams & Wilkins; 2008. pp. 386–90.
- Hadzic A. *Textbook of Regional Anesthesia and Acute Pain Management*. 1st ed. New York, NY: McGraw-Hill Medical; 2006. pp. 600–6.

A77 C

▶ Interpleural block provides anaesthesia to the thorax and upper abdomen. Anaesthesia is attained by diffusion of LA to the nerves in proximity (intercostals nerves **anteroposterolaterally**, inferior roots of brachial plexus **superiorly** and the sympathetic chain, splanchnic, phrenic and vagus nerves **medially**). The epidural and subarachnoid spaces are distant and not felt to be the site of anaesthesia generally.

▶ The block may be performed in an **awake or anaesthetised spontaneously breathing patient** (since positive-pressure ventilation may lead to positive intrapleural pressures), in sitting, lateral or prone position; at least 8–10 cm lateral to the midline (to avoid dural cuff), overlying the **top edge** of a rib.

▶ After contacting the rib, a 16–18-G Tuohy needle is walked off **cephalad** to the top edge of the rib, using a loss-of-resistance technique to enter the intrapleural space.

▶ Nitrous oxide should be subsequently discontinued if under general anaesthetic.

▶ Because the spread of LA in the interpleural space is governed by **gravity** (besides volume injected and catheter position), operative side up may produce sympathetic blockade, supine positioning results in intercostals block and head down may anaesthetise the inferior roots of the brachial plexus.

- Cousins MJ, Bridenbaugh PO, Carr DB, *et al. Cousins and Bridenbaugh's Neural Blockade in Clinical Anesthesia and Pain Medicine*. 4th ed. Philadelphia, PA: Lippincott Williams & Wilkins; 2008. pp. 390–2.

A78 D

▶ Interpleural technique may be best used for open cholecystectomy, renal surgery and unilateral breast procedures.

▶ **Thoracotomy is a controversial indication**, since duration of the block is significantly reduced when parietal pleura is open and a thoracostomy tube is placed.

▶ Although producing hemithoracic analgesia and sympathetic block, apart from minimising number of injections require, the analgesia is less intense and of shorter duration when compared to intercostal blocks.

▶ Complications may include **pneumothorax (2%)**, phrenic nerve paresis, Horner's syndrome, ipsilateral bronchospasm and cholestasis.

- Cousins MJ, Bridenbaugh PO, Carr DB, *et al. Cousins and Bridenbaugh's Neural Blockade in Clinical Anesthesia and Pain Medicine*. 4th ed. Philadelphia, PA: Lippincott Williams & Wilkins; 2008. pp. 390–2.

A79 **C** Rectal sheath blocks provide analgesia for abdominal surgery requiring a midline incision. The midline area from xiphoid to pubis is innervated by the **anterior cutaneous branches of T7–T11 nerves**. These terminal branches of ICN enter the rectus sheath at its **posterolateral** border, and pierce the **posterior sheath** to cross rectus abdominis muscle, eventually terminating by supplying the overlying skin.

▶ A 5-cm 22-G needle is passed through skin and subcutaneous tissue until it meets resistance by the anterior rectus sheath. The needle is carefully advanced to pierce this sheath, through the belly of the muscle.

▶ As the needle approaches the **posterior rectus sheath**, a firm resistance is felt, and 10 mL LA is deposited over it. The block requires injections **bilaterally** due to overlap in innervations across the midline.

▶ Also, **tendinous insertions** of rectus abdominis prevent supraumbilical LA to spread to infraumbilical regions, mandating inferior injections. It may be difficult to identify posterior rectus sheath infraumbilically,

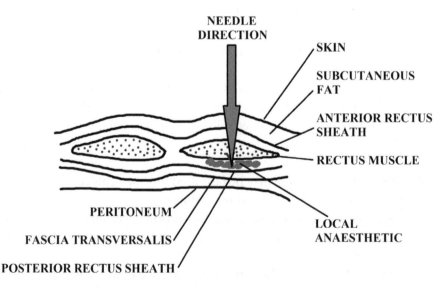

Figure 5.33 Rectus sheath anatomy and its block

and injection after loss of resistance of anterior sheath may be safer and sufficient.

▶ The block is widely used in paediatrics, and easily performed by ultrasound.

▶ It is difficult to perform in **obese, cachexic, elderly (poor abdominal tone) and distended abdomen**. Deeper injections may lead to bowel perforation or injury to underlying organs.

- Cousins MJ, Bridenbaugh PO, Carr DB, *et al. Cousins and Bridenbaugh's Neural Blockade in Clinical Anesthesia and Pain Medicine*. 4th ed. Philadelphia, PA: Lippincott Williams & Wilkins; 2008. pp. 396–7.

A80 D

Table 5.23 Nerves supplying the inguinal area

Nerve (root value) and its course	Supplies
Subcostal (T12): Lies between internal oblique and external oblique at the anterior superior iliac spine	Area around iliac crest
Iliohypogastric (T12, L1): Emerges from lateral border of psoas and passes over quadratus lumborum to penetrate transverse abdominal muscle near the iliac crest It lies between internal oblique and external oblique at the anterior superior iliac spine	Skin over ilium, hypogastric and suprapubic region
Ilioinguinal (L1): Emerges from the lateral border of the psoas major just inferior to the iliohypogastric, and passes obliquely across the quadratus lumborum and iliacus It then perforates the transversus abdominis near the anterior part of the iliac crest, to lie between it and internal oblique initially, and then between internal oblique and external oblique medial to the anterior superior iliac spine Travelling through the spermatic, it emerges from the superficial inguinal canal	Skin over medial aspect of thigh Skin over the root of the penis and upper part of the scrotum (male) and skin covering the mons pubis and labium majus (female)
Genitofemoral (L1 and L2): In abdomen, it descends on anterior surface of psoas and then divides into genital and femoral branches The genital branch travels through the inguinal canal, along with the spermatic cord to emerge at the superficial inguinal ring	Genital branch innervates cremaster muscle and gives twigs to scrotum and adjacent thigh Femoral branch passes under inguinal ligament and supplies skin of femoral triangle

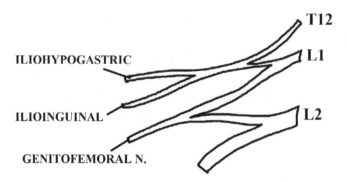

Figure 5.34 Origin of the inguinal region nerves

Note: the ilioinguinal nerve does not pass through the deep inguinal ring, and therefore it only travels through part of the inguinal canal. The genital branch of the genitofemoral nerve passes through both deep and superficial inguinal rings.

- Cousins MJ, Bridenbaugh PO, Carr DB, *et al. Cousins and Bridenbaugh's Neural Blockade in Clinical Anesthesia and Pain Medicine.* 4th ed. Philadelphia, PA: Lippincott Williams & Wilkins; 2008. pp. 397–9.
- Hadzic A. *Textbook of Regional Anesthesia and Acute Pain Management.* 1st ed. New York, NY: McGraw-Hill Medical; 2006. pp. 579–82.

A81 B

▶ The **inguinal block** constitutes blocking the subcostal, iliohypogastric, ilioinguinal and the genitofemoral nerves. The block may not provide total anaesthesia for inguinal herniorrhaphy if the last nerve is not blocked.

▶ The subcostal, iliohypogastric and ilioinguinal nerves are all blocked medial to anterior superior iliac spine (ASIS). A skin puncture point 1–2 cm medial and 1–2 cm inferior to ASIS is infiltrated with LA. A blunt needle is advanced at right angles to the skin in all planes.

 – As the needle pierces the external oblique, a characteristic **'click'** is felt, and 6–8 mL of LA is incrementally deposited to anaesthetise the **iliohypogastric**.

 – Advancing the needle pierces the internal oblique, resulting in **a second 'click'**. A further 6–8 mL of LA is injected incrementally to block the **ilioinguinal**.

 – Redirecting the needle towards ilium at this point will allow infiltration of LA (3–5 mL) to lateral **branches of subcostal nerve**. A subcutaneous infiltration made towards the midline blocks the **medial branches of subcostal nerve**.

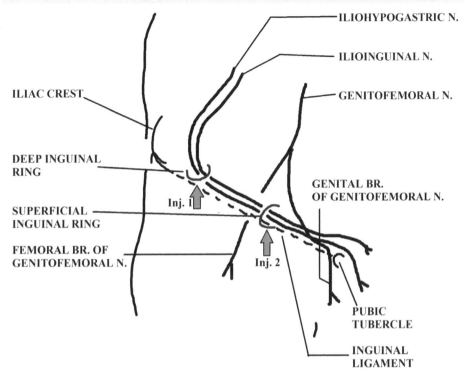

Figure 5.35 Landmarks for inguinal block (injection 1: iliohypogastric and ilioinguinal nerve block; injection 2: genitofemoral nerve block)

- **Genitofemoral nerve** is blocked by inserting the needle 2–3 cm above the mid-inguinal point to a depth of 3–5 cm, injecting 10–15 mL of LA. This may also be done by the surgeon after exposing the spermatic cord.
▶ This block may be used for inguinal herniorrhaphy, groin surgery and post-operative analgesia for lumbar spinal canal stenosis (bilateral ilioinguinal block). Complications may include haematoma formation, LA toxicity, **femoral nerve block (5%)** and rare bowel perforation.
  • Cousins MJ, Bridenbaugh PO, Carr DB, *et al. Cousins and Bridenbaugh's Neural Blockade in Clinical Anesthesia and Pain Medicine.* 4th ed. Philadelphia, PA: Lippincott Williams & Wilkins; 2008. pp. 397–9.
  • Hadzic A. *Textbook of Regional Anesthesia and Acute Pain Management.* 1st ed. New York, NY: McGraw-Hill Medical; 2006. pp. 579–82.

A82 A
▶ The transversus abdominis plane (TAP) exists between internal oblique and transversus abdominis muscles in the abdominal wall. The TAP block

was first described as a **landmark-guided technique** involving needle insertion at the **triangle of Petit** by **McDonnell** et al. This is an area bounded by the latissimus dorsi muscle posteriorly, the external oblique muscle anteriorly and the iliac crest inferiorly (the base of the triangle).

▶ A needle is inserted perpendicular to all planes, looking for a tactile end point of two pops. The **first pop** indicates penetration of the external oblique fascia and entry into the plane between external and internal oblique muscles. The second pop signifies entry into the TAP plane between internal oblique and transversus abdominis muscles. Deposition of LA (**large volume, 20–30 mL each side**) at this plane leads to anaesthesia of nerves supplying the anterior abdominal wall (T7–L1).

▶ It has been shown to provide good post-operative analgesia for a variety of procedures. Nerves of **T6–T9** enter the TAP medial to the anterior axillary line. Nerves running in the TAP lateral to the anterior axillary line, on the other hand, originate from segmental nerves T9–L1. This may explain the observation of some authors that the TAP block is only suitable for **lower-abdominal surgery**. Therefore, TAP injections are made **posterior to the mid-axillary line** in the landmark-based technique. Such injections are thought to act by tracking **paravertebrally**. However, injections made **anterior to the mid-axillary line** may behave as **field blocks** (and therefore have limited duration and effect).

▶ More recently, **ultrasound-guided techniques** of TAP block have been described. A variation of the classic TAP block, the **subcostal TAP block,** has also been described; it is designed to provide more reliable coverage of the upper abdominal wall.

▶ The **quadratus lumborum block** is an ultrasound-guided block into the quadratus lumborum space. It describes a space posterior to the abdominal wall muscles and lateral to the quadratus lumborum muscle. It has been used in abdominoplasties, Caesarean sections and lower abdominal operations, providing complete pain relief in the distribution area from T6 to L1 dermatomes.

- Cousins MJ, Bridenbaugh PO, Carr DB, *et al. Cousins and Bridenbaugh's Neural Blockade in Clinical Anesthesia and Pain Medicine.* 4th ed. Philadelphia, PA: Lippincott Williams & Wilkins; 2008. pp. 400–2.
- McDonnell JG, O' Donnell BD, Tuite D, Farrell T, Camillus P. The regional abdominal field infiltration (R.A.F.I.) technique: computerised tomographic and anatomical identification of a novel approach to the transversus abdominis neuro-vascular fascial plane. *Anesthesiology.* 2004;101:A899.
- http://usra.ca/tapanatomy.php

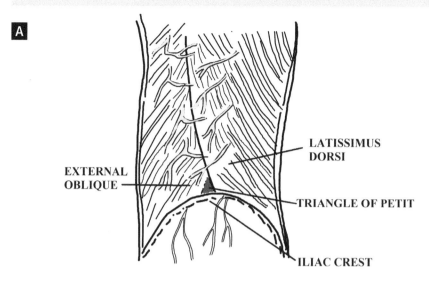

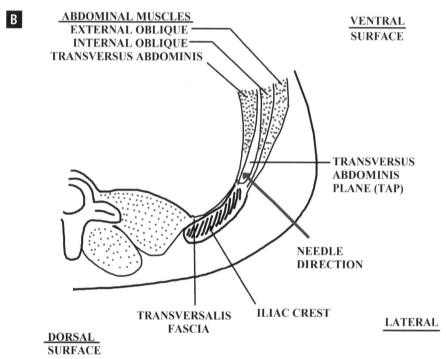

Figure 5.36 (A) Distribution of intercostal and lumbar spinal nerves; (B) injection of local anaesthetic into the transversus abdominis plane

A83 D

▶ As discussed above in Answer 74 (Chapter 5), the intercostal nerves lie in the intercostal groove **below** the inferior edge of the corresponding ribs.

▶ Performing the inguinal block needs the ASIS to be identified and then injection 2 cm medial and 2 cm inferior to it.

▶ TAP block is performed at the **triangle of Petit** above the iliac crest posterior to the mid-axillary line.

▶ The **transverse process** of the vertebrae is the critical bony structure required to perform paravertebral block.

• Mulroy MF, Bernards CM, McDonald SB, *et al. A Practical Approach to Regional Anesthesia*. 4th ed. Philadelphia, PA: Lippincott Williams & Wilkins; 2008. p. 147.

A84 B

▶ Paravertebral block (PVB) refers to the blockade of spinal nerves as they exit the intervertebral foramen.

▶ The thoracic paravertebral space is a **wedge-shaped area** on either side of the spine. It is bounded **posteriorly** by superior costotransverse ligament, **laterally** by posterior intercostal membrane, **anteriorly** by parietal pleura and **medially** by the posterolateral aspect of vertebral body, disc and intervertebral foramen. The **endothoracic fascia** divides this space into two potential fascial compartments: the anterior **extra-pleural paravertebral** compartment and the posterior **subendothoracic paravertebral** compartment. Its **contents** are ventral ramus (intercostal nerve), dorsal ramus, rami communicantes, sympathetic chain (anteriorly) and fatty tissue. It is contiguous with epidural space medially and intercostal space laterally.

▶ The lumbar paravertebral space **lacks costotransverse ligaments**. It is bound anterolaterally by psoas muscle, medially by vertebral body, disc and intervertebral foramen, and posteriorly by transverse process and its ligaments. It is primarily occupied by psoas muscle.

• Cousins MJ, Bridenbaugh PO, Carr DB, *et al. Cousins and Bridenbaugh's Neural Blockade in Clinical Anesthesia and Pain Medicine*. 4th ed. Philadelphia, PA: Lippincott Williams & Wilkins; 2008. p. 392.

• Hadzic A. *Textbook of Regional Anesthesia and Acute Pain Management*. 1st ed. New York, NY: McGraw-Hill Medical; 2006. pp. 579, 584, 594.

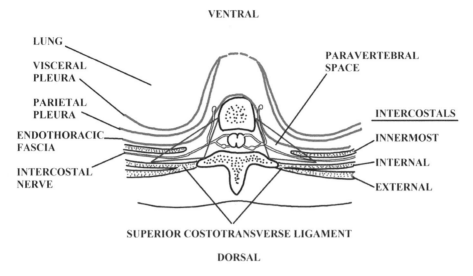

VENTRAL

LUNG

VISCERAL
PLEURA

PARAVERTEBRAL
SPACE

PARIETAL
PLEURA

INTERCOSTALS

ENDOTHORACIC
FASCIA

INNERMOST

INTERNAL

INTERCOSTAL
NERVE

EXTERNAL

SUPERIOR COSTOTRANSVERSE LIGAMENT

DORSAL

Figure 5.37 Paravertebral space anatomy

A85 A

▶ In thoracic and lumbar regions, the spinal nerves leave the intervertebral foramen **inferior** to the transverse process of its corresponding vertebra. For example, the L4 spinal nerve exits between the L4 and L5 vertebrae.

▶ Performing a PVB requires insertion of a **Tuohy needle** (18 G) at the level of a spinous process, 3 cm lateral to the midline to contact the transverse process at a depth of 2–4 cm. It is then walked off (caudally or cephalad) by 1–2 cm to reach the paravertebral space. This may be identified by LOR as the needle pierces the superior costotransverse ligament. The lumbar paravertebral space **lacks costotransverse ligaments**, rendering this technique useless.

▶ In the thoracic region, the tip of the spinous process lies at the level of the transverse process **below** it, due to its steep downward angulation. Hence the needle must be directed **cephalad** to walk off the transverse process to block the corresponding spinal nerve, whereas in the lumbar region, the tip of the spinous process lies at the level of the transverse process of the **same** vertebrae as it is almost horizontally directed. Hence the needle is directed **caudally** to walk off the transverse process to block the corresponding spinal nerve.

▶ In the thoracic region, a single large-volume injection may **spread cephalad or caudad** to reach one or more spinal nerves. No such communications exist between different levels in lumbar region. Therefore, multiple injections are needed. However, when a reliable multiple-level anaesthesia is desired, multiple small-volume injections are preferred over a single large-volume injection. This may slightly increase the chances of pneumothorax.

- Mulroy MF, Bernards CM, McDonald SB, *et al. A Practical Approach to Regional Anesthesia*. 4th ed. Philadelphia, PA: Lippincott Williams & Wilkins; 2008. pp. 147–55.
- Hadzic A. *Textbook of Regional Anesthesia and Acute Pain Management*. 1st ed. New York, NY: McGraw-Hill Medical; 2006. pp. 579, 584, 594.

A86 B

▶ Indications for PVB are breast surgery, thoracotomy, cholecystectomy, renal and ureteric surgery, inguinal hernia, appendicectomy, video-assisted thoracic surgery and minimally invasive cardiac surgery. It may be used to provide analgesia for fractured ribs, flail chest and herpes zoster neuralgia.

▶ PVB can be performed using a landmark, nerve stimulator or an ultrasound-based technique. It is also suited for catheter techniques. However, unlike the epidural space, catheter advancement in the paravertebral space is met with **significant resistance**. If a catheter threads **'easily'**, one should be concerned that the needle has entered the thorax. **Air aspiration** during needle insertion may indicate lung puncture.

▶ Complications may include ipsilateral epidural spread (up to 70%), contralateral epidural spread (7%), intravascular injections, subarachnoid injections, haematoma formation, pneumothorax (0.5%), hypotension and systemic toxicity. Post-dural puncture headache has been reported.

▶ **Medial angulation** of the needle increase chances of epidural/subarachnoid spread, but **lateral angulation** may increase chances of pneumothorax.

- Cousins MJ, Bridenbaugh PO, Carr DB, *et al. Cousins and Bridenbaugh's Neural Blockade in Clinical Anesthesia and Pain Medicine*. 4th ed. Philadelphia, PA: Lippincott Williams & Wilkins; 2008. pp. 392–4.
- Mulroy MF, Bernards CM, McDonald SB, *et al. A Practical Approach to Regional Anesthesia*. 4th ed. Philadelphia, PA: Lippincott Williams & Wilkins; 2008. p. 153.

A87 D

▶ **August Bier** was the first to introduce intravenous regional anaesthesia (IVRA, also called **the Bier block**), in 1908.

▶ Lignocaine and procaine are the most commonly employed local anaesthetics.

▶ IVRA is appropriate for surgeries and manipulations of the extremities requiring anaesthesia for up to **an hour**. It has been successfully used in the paediatric population as well.

- The block is easier to perform in upper extremity than the lower; with the latter needing larger volumes of LA and higher occlusion pressures for an adequate block.
- Although the block is **relatively contraindicated** in crush injuries, compound fractures, peripheral vascular disease and sickle-cell disease, the only **absolute contraindication** is patient refusal.
- Bier block is an acceptable form of regional anaesthesia in anticoagulated patients.
- IVRA has been also used for treatment of complex regional pain syndrome (CRPS) (guanethidine) and hyperhydrosis (botulinum toxin).
  - Hadzic A. *Textbook of Regional Anesthesia and Acute Pain Management*. 1st ed. New York, NY: McGraw-Hill Medical; 2006. p. 566.

A88 C The correct sequence of events for IVRA is: intravenous cannulation, exsanguination, proximal cuff inflation, LA injection, distal cuff inflation, proximal cuff deflation.
  - Mulroy MF, Bernards CM, McDonald SB, *et al. A Practical Approach to Regional Anesthesia*. 4th ed. Philadelphia, PA: Lippincott Williams & Wilkins; 2008. p. 570.

A89 B

- **Bupivacaine should be avoided** because of its cardiotoxicity.
- Although any vein may be cannulated, fast injections through **antecubital veins** may lead to escape of LA under the cuff. Injections should be made **slowly (over 90 seconds)** to produce a peak venous pressure that is not greater than the occluding pressure of the cuff.
- Cuff should not be deflated before 20 minutes. If less than 45 minutes have passed, the cuff is deflated in a **two-stage release**, first deflated for 10 seconds and then reinflated for a minute before release.
- After 45 minutes, the risk of systemic toxicity is minimal.
  - Mulroy MF, Bernards CM, McDonald SB, *et al. A Practical Approach to Regional Anesthesia*. 4th ed. Philadelphia, PA: Lippincott Williams & Wilkins; 2008. pp. 204–7.

A90 A Although opioids, α2 agonists (clonidine and dexmetomidine), muscle relaxants, dexamethasone and neostigmine have all shown some promise, only **non-steroidal anti-inflammatory drugs** (ketorolac) have shown good evidence as adjuncts in systemic review.

Dosages:

Upper limb: 0.5% lignocaine 30–50 mL or 2% lignocaine 12–15 mL. Lower limb: 0.5% lignocaine 50–100 mL or 2% lignocaine 15–30 mL ± ketorolac 20 mg.

- Hadzic A. *Textbook of Regional Anesthesia and Acute Pain Management.* 1st ed. New York, NY: McGraw-Hill Medical; 2006. p. 572.
- Reuben SS, Steinberg RB, Kreitzer JM, *et al.* Intravenous regional anesthesia using lidocaine and ketorolac. *Anesth Analg.* 1995; **81**(1): 110–13.

A91 D

▶ The optic foramen, the superior and the inferior orbital fissures are the most important fissures in the orbit.
▶ The **optic foramen** transmits the optic nerve and ophthalmic artery.
▶ The **superior orbital fissure** transmits the following:
    – lacrimal (V_1), frontal (V_1) and trochlear (IV): lie outside the annulus of Zinn.

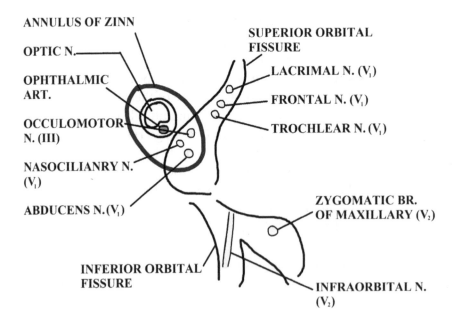

Figure 5.38 Structures passing through orbital fissures and optic foramen

– oculomotor (III), abducens (VI) and nasociliary (V₁): lie inside the annulus of Zinn.

▶ The inferior orbital fissure transmits the zygomatic branch of the maxillary nerve (V₂).

▶ The annulus of Zinn (tendinous ring) encircles the optic nerve, ophthalmic artery, superior branch of the oculomotor nerve, abducens nerve, nasociliary nerve and inferior branch of the oculomotor nerve. Importantly, the trochlear nerve lies outside the annulus of Zinn.

A92 D

Table 5.24 Motor supply of the eye muscles

Extraocular muscles (mnemonic: SO4, LR6)

Muscle	Nervous supply	Actions
Medial rectus	Oculomotor nerve	**Adduction**
Inferior rectus		**Depression**, adduction, extortion
Superior rectus		**Elevation**, adduction, intortion
Inferior oblique		**Extorsion**, elevation, abduction
Superior oblique	Trochlear nerve	**Intorsion**, depression, abduction
Lateral rectus	Abducens nerve	**Abduction**

Intraocular muscles

Iris sphinter muscles (pupillary sphincter)	Parasympathetic (M3 rec) via short ciliary nerves	Circular muscle contraction – **pupillary constriction**
Iris radial muscles (pulpillary dilator)	Sympathetic (α1 rec) via long ciliary nerves	Radial muscle contraction – **pupillary dilatation**
Ciliary body	Parasympathetic (M3 rec) via short ciliary nerves	Ciliary body contraction, lens relaxation, **loss of accommodation**
Ciliary body	Sympathetic (β2 rec) via short ciliary nerves	Ciliary body relaxation, lens contraction, **accommodation of eye**

Facial muscles

Levator palpebrae	Ciliary nerves (striated muscle fibres) and parasympathetic (smooth muscle fibres)	**Opens** the eye (elevates eyelids)
Orbicularis oculi	Upper and lower zygomatic branch	**Closes** the eye (lowers eyelids, blink)
Frontalis		Elevates eyebrows

The **sensory supply** of the eye is derived from the **trigeminal nerve** through its ophthalmic (V_1) division (frontal, nasociliary and lacrimal branches) and maxillary (V_2) division (infraorbital and zygomatic branches).

▸ **Retrobulbar (intraconal) block** provides for sensory anaesthesia, motor block of extraocular muscles and levator palpebrae, but does not block orbicularis oculi. This requires a separate facial nerve block. Because the trochlear nerve lies outside the cone, it may be spared and allow intortion, depression and abduction.

▸ **Peribulbar (periconal) block** often results in diffusion of LA to orbicularis oculi, rendering the facial nerve block **unnecessary**. It blocks the trochlear as well.

  • Cousins MJ, Bridenbaugh PO, Carr DB, *et al. Cousins and Bridenbaugh's Neural Blockade in Clinical Anesthesia and Pain Medicine*. 4th ed. Philadelphia, PA: Lippincott Williams & Wilkins; 2008. pp. 445–50.

A93 C Ophthalmic anaesthesia requires:

▸ **Anaesthesia of cornea and conjunctiva** (topical anaesthesia or bulbar blocks)

▸ **Akinesia of the eyeball** (retrobulbar, peribulbar or sub-Tenon's block)

▸ **Akinesia of levator palpebrae** (oculomotor and sympathetic) **and orbicularis oculi** (facial nerve block).

Topical anaesthesia is frequently employed to eliminate corneal and conjunctival reflexes, for eye surgeries and diagnostic procedures. Surgical advances and less invasive techniques have made this possible.

▸ Although cocaine was the first agent used for this purpose (**Koller**), it is very **toxic**. Hence other safer LAs like proparacaine, tetracaine and lignocaine are commonly used.

▸ Cocaine toxicity manifests as biphasic CNS effects (stimulation followed by depression), sympathetic stimulation, hyperthermia, **pupillary dilatation** and feeling of **crawling insects on the skin**.

▸ The hypertension is best controlled by an **alpha and beta blocker** like labetalol. Unopposed alpha action resulting from only beta blockade (propranalol) has caused lethal hypertensive exacerbation.

▸ All agents have some degree of **corneal epithelium toxicity**, cocaine being most toxic. The dose should be restricted to **200 mg in a 70-kg man (3 mg/kg)** to minimise risk of toxicity.

  • Cousins MJ, Bridenbaugh PO, Carr DB, *et al. Cousins and Bridenbaugh's Neural Blockade in Clinical Anesthesia and Pain Medicine*. 4th ed. Philadelphia, PA: Lippincott Williams & Wilkins; 2008. pp. 443–4.

A94 B

▶ Retrobulbar block is an **intraconal** injection; that is, it is given in the cone of extraocular muscles producing their akinesia with anaesthesia of cornea and conjunctiva. Combined with a facial nerve block for akinesia of orbicularis oculi, it permits eye surgery under local anaesthesia. Intraconal injection site produces **faster onset, denser block and requires less anaesthetic** than periconal injections.

▶ After anaesthetising the eye topically, a **1.25-inch 23-G non-cutting-edge blunt needle** is inserted **inferotemporally** through the lower eyelid, **directed superonasally** with the eye in **inferonasal or neutral gaze**, injecting **3–4 mL** of LA after negative aspiration.

▶ The traditional Atkinson position of superonasal gaze during inferotemporal needle placement is **not** recommended, as it results in rotation of the posterior pole of the globe into the path of the advancing needle, increasing chances of optic nerve damage, globe perforation or piercing of the meningeal sheath.

▶ Non-cutting-edge blunt needles (23 G) have **higher** scleral perforation pressures than those with a cutting edge of a smaller gauge (25 G), as well as potential for more serious retinal damage should the perforation occur.

▶ As the trochlear nerve and superior oblique lie outside the annulus of Zinn, a residual intortion after the block may need a separate trochlear injection.

▶ Ocular complications include perforation of the globe (0.1%), retrobulbar haemorrhage (1%–3%) and optic nerve damage. Systemic complications include intra-arterial injection, optic nerve sheath injection and oculocardiac reflex.

▶ **Risk factors for globe perforation** include an anteroposterior length of > 26 mm (high myopes), severe enophthalmos, previous scleral buckle, repeated surgeries, posterior staphyloma, repeated injections and an uncooperative moving patient. It presents as **intense and immediate pain with sudden loss of vision**. Surgery may need to be postponed and retinal treatment undertaken.

- Cousins MJ, Bridenbaugh PO, Carr DB, *et al. Cousins and Bridenbaugh's Neural Blockade in Clinical Anesthesia and Pain Medicine.* 4th ed. Philadelphia, PA: Lippincott Williams & Wilkins; 2008. pp. 453–5.
- Mulroy MF, Bernards CM, McDonald SB, *et al. A Practical Approach to Regional Anesthesia.* 4th ed. Philadelphia, PA: Lippincott Williams & Wilkins; 2008. pp. 289–91.

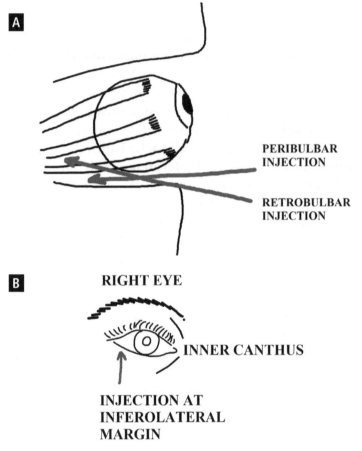

Figure 5.39 (A) Retrobulbar block and peribulbar block; (B) inferolateral injection

A95 A

- ▶ Retrobulbar haemorrhage (1%–3%) is the **most common** complication following retrobulbar injection. It presents with **pain, increasing proptosis and frequently subconjunctival or eyelid ecchymosis**.
- ▶ Following its occurrence, the intraocular pressure and central retinal artery pulsations should be monitored by an ophthalmologist for signs of impending retinal artery occlusion.
- ▶ Because **oculocardiac reflex** (trigeminal afferent, vagus efferent) can be triggered several hours after its occurrence, **ECG monitoring** is a must.
- ▶ Treating high pressures may require a deep lateral canthotomy, and if needed an anterior chamber paracentesis.
- ▶ Postponing the surgery is prudent, with a general anaesthetic planned for rescheduled surgery.

❱ **Risk factors** may be previous retrobulbar bleeds, vascular or haematological disorder.

- Cousins MJ, Bridenbaugh PO, Carr DB, *et al. Cousins and Bridenbaugh's Neural Blockade in Clinical Anesthesia and Pain Medicine.* 4th ed. Philadelphia, PA: Lippincott Williams & Wilkins; 2008. pp. 455–6.

A96 B

❱ Peribulbar (periconal) block is made **outside** the cone of extraocular muscles, theoretically **reducing** the chances of retrobulbar haemorrhage and globe perforation. But the onset is **slower** and **reinjections** are frequently needed. After topical anaesthesia, two injections are made, first **inferotemporally** and then **superonasally**, injecting **4–5 mL** of LA at each site. The needle is directed **parallel** to floor of the orbit and advanced only **1 inch (25 mm)** just behind the equator of the globe. Sometimes a medial transconjunctival injection may also be made. It is associated with **the same incidence** of post-operative ptosis as retrobulbar block, but **eyelid ecchymosis** is more common.

❱ Sub-Tenon's block makes use of an anatomical fascial plane called **Tenon's capsule**. After topical anaesthesia, with patient looking outward and upward, the **inferonasal quadrant** of conjunctiva is nicked with blunt Wescott scissors, and a curved cannula is inserted onto the bare sclera below the Tenon fascia. Then 4–5 mL of LA is injected, resulting in rapid akinesia proportional to the volume injected. The use of longer rigid metallic cannulae is associated with higher complication rate (globe perforation, haemorrhage, muscle trauma, brainstem anaesthesia, and orbital cellulitis). Therefore, **shorter plastic cannulae** are preferable.

- Cousins MJ, Bridenbaugh PO, Carr DB, *et al. Cousins and Bridenbaugh's Neural Blockade in Clinical Anesthesia and Pain Medicine.* 4th ed. Philadelphia, PA: Lippincott Williams & Wilkins; 2008. pp. 457–62.

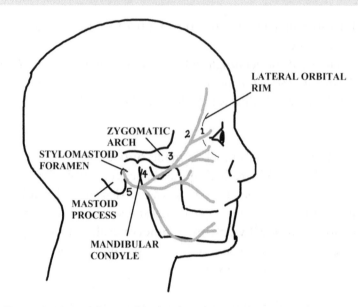

Figure 5.40 Facial nerve blocks along its course

A97 C

Facial nerve block is performed to attain **akinesia of orbicularis oculi** along with retrobulbar block and is not needed with peribulbar block. It may be performed **proximally** along its course (causing lower facial hemiparesis and anaesthesia) or **distally** (preferable). Various approaches are outlined in Table 5.25.

Table 5.25 Various approaches of facial nerve block for ocular surgery

Approach	Landmark	Needle direction	Side effects
Classic Van Lint	Lateral orbital rim	Subcutaneously superlaterally and inferolaterally	Lid oedema and periorbital ecchymosis
Classic Atkinson	Zygomatic arch	Superiorly and posteriorly along zygoma	
Modified Atkinson	2 cm away from lateral orbital rim	Subcutaneously superlaterally and inferolaterally	Less periorbital ecchymosis
O'Brien	Mandibular condyle	Injection over condyle and then redirected inferiorly along posterior edge of ramus	Total facial paralysis
Nadbath–Rehman	Stylomastoid foramen	Between mastoid process and mandibular ramus, directed toward top of the opposite ear	Total facial paralysis

Note: Nadbath–Rehman block may also result in paralysis of glossopharyngeal, vagus and spinal accessory nerves, as they exit via jugular foramen 1 cm medial to the stylomastoid foramen.

- Cousins MJ, Bridenbaugh PO, Carr DB, *et al. Cousins and Bridenbaugh's Neural Blockade in Clinical Anesthesia and Pain Medicine.* 4th ed. Philadelphia, PA: Lippincott Williams & Wilkins; 2008. pp. 450–3.
- Mulroy MF, Bernards CM, McDonald SB, *et al. A Practical Approach to Regional Anesthesia.* 4th ed. Philadelphia, PA: Lippincott Williams & Wilkins; 2008. pp. 287–9.

A98 A Scalp is supplied by the following nerves.

▶ **Cervical nerve (C2)**:
  - greater occipital nerve (C2) posteriorly up to the vertex
  - lesser occipital nerve (C2) behind the ear.

▶ **Trigeminal nerve**:
  - ophthalmic division – supratrochlear and supraorbital nerve
  - maxillary division: zygomaticotemporal nerve
  - mandibular division: auriculotemporal nerve.

A99 D Blockade of nerves supplying the scalp (**scalp block**) is used for awake craniotomy. The landmarks for blocking these are outlined in Table 5.26.

Table 5.26 Nerve supply of the scalp

Nerves	Landmarks
Greater occipital	2–3 cm lateral to occipital protuberance
Greater and lesser occipital	Along line joining occipital protuberance and mastoid process
Lesser occipital	Superficial cervical plexus block along posterior border of sternocleidomastoid, on its middle third; or posterior to the auricle, above mastoid
Auriculotemporal	At the temporal fossa (in front of auricle)
Zygomaticotemporal	Against the zygomatic arch
Supraorbital	Above the supraorbital notch
Supratrochlear	Between the eyebrows (blocks both sides)

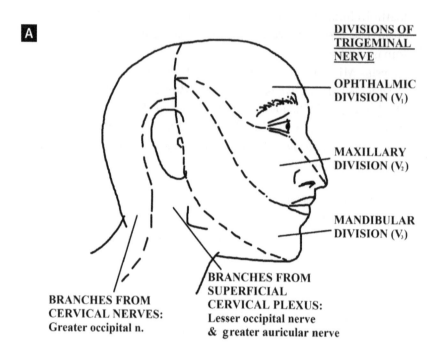

A

DIVISIONS OF TRIGEMINAL NERVE

OPHTHALMIC DIVISION (V₁)

MAXILLARY DIVISION (V₂)

MANDIBULAR DIVISION (V₃)

BRANCHES FROM CERVICAL NERVES:
Greater occipital n.

BRANCHES FROM SUPERFICIAL CERVICAL PLEXUS:
Lesser occipital nerve & greater auricular nerve

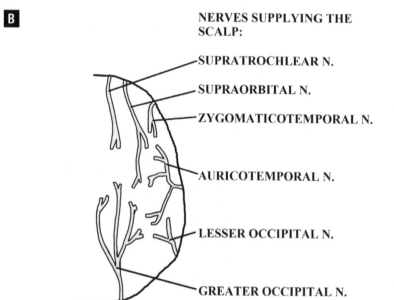

B

NERVES SUPPLYING THE SCALP:

SUPRATROCHLEAR N.

SUPRAORBITAL N.

ZYGOMATICOTEMPORAL N.

AURICOTEMPORAL N.

LESSER OCCIPITAL N.

GREATER OCCIPITAL N.

Figure 5.41 (A) Trigeminal nerve and its branches; (B) nerve supply of the scalp

Scalp block using 0.5% bupivacaine has been shown to be successful in blunting the haemodynamic response to head pinning.

- Pinosky ML, Fishman RL, Reeves ST, *et al*. The effect of bupivacaine skull block on the hemodynamic response to craniotomy. *Anesth Analg*. 1996; **83**(6): 1256–61.

A100 D Nerve supply of face is by trigeminal nerve and C2 spinal nerve is outlined in Table 5.27.

Table 5.27 Nerve supply of the face

Nerve	Area of face
Ophthalmic division (V_1)	Forehead, nose, upper eyelid
Maxillary division (V_2)	Cheeks, lower eyelid, upper lip
Mandibular division (V_3)	Lower lip, chin, most of jaw
Cervical nerve (C2)	Angle of jaw

The facial nerve gives motor but not sensory supply to face.

A101 B

- ▶ The trigeminal nerve (CNV) is the **largest cranial nerve**.
- ▶ It supplies sensory, proprioceptive and pain nerve fibres to the head and face, and the motor supply to the muscles of mastication.
- ▶ It emerges from the **side of the pons**, near its upper border, by **a small motor and a large sensory root**.
- ▶ It passes laterally to join the **Gasserian (semilunar) ganglion** in **Meckel's cave**. The Gasserian ganglion gives three branches: ophthalmic (V_1), maxillary (V_2) and mandibular (V_3).
- ▶ The ophthalmic and maxillary branches comprise sensory fibres exclusively, while the mandibular branch carries motor fibres as well.
- ▶ Four small parasympathetic ganglia are associated with the three divisions of the trigeminal nerve:
  - **ciliary ganglion** – ophthalmic nerve
  - **sphenopalatine ganglion (pterygopalatine)** – maxillary nerve
  - **otic and submaxillary ganglia** – mandibular nerve

Table 5.28 Characteristic cranial nerves

Characteristic	Nerve
Largest CN	Trigeminal
Longest CN	Vagus
CN with longest intracranial course	Abducens
CN emerging from posterior surface of brainstem	Trochlear

A102 C

Table 5.29 Trigeminal nerve branches and foramen

Branches	Exits cranium through	Associated foramen
Ophthalmic nerve	Superior orbital fissure	Supraorbital notch (supraorbital nerve)
Maxillary nerve	Foramen rotundum	Inferior orbital fissure Infraorbital foramen (infraorbital nerve)
Mandibular nerve	Foramen ovale	Mental foramen (mental nerve)

A103 D The ophthalmic nerve is the **first and smallest branch** of the trigeminal nerve. It traverses along the **lateral wall** of the cavernous venous sinus and exits the skull through the **superior orbital fissure**, dividing into three branches: frontal, lacrimal and nasociliary.

- Frontal nerve: (largest branch of the V_1):
  - supraorbital nerve – exits skull through the supraorbital notch. It supplies upper lid and the scalp up to the lambdoid suture. It is blocked at the **supraorbital notch** in the middle of the upper margin of orbit.
  - supratrochlear nerve – emerges from the upper medial quadrant of the orbit. It supplies medial eyelid and medial forehead. A single injection in the midline **between the eyebrows** blocks this nerve from both sides.
- Lacrimal nerve: passes in the **lateral part** of the superior orbital fissure. It supplies the lacrimal gland, conjunctiva and upper lid.
- Nasociliary nerve: passes in the **central part** of the superior orbital fissure. Its branches include the anterior ethmoid nerve, posterior ethmoid nerve, internal nasal branch, external nasal branches and two to three long ciliary nerves. The nasal branches are blocked by placing nasal pellets soaked with local anaesthetic.

Note: only the **extracranial** part of V₁ can be blocked.

- Cousins MJ, Bridenbaugh PO, Carr DB, *et al. Cousins and Bridenbaugh's Neural Blockade in Clinical Anesthesia and Pain Medicine.* 4th ed. Philadelphia, PA: Lippincott Williams & Wilkins; 2008. p. 406.

A104 C The maxillary nerve (V_2) is a **purely sensory nerve**. It passes at the lateral wall of the cavernous sinus, leaves the skull through the **foramen rotundum**, then crosses the **pterygopalatine fossa** and enters the orbit through the **inferior orbital fissure**. It traverses the **infraorbital groove** and canal in the floor of the orbit, and appears upon the face at the **infraorbital** foramen as the **infraorbital** nerve. Its main branches are as follows.

- Zygomatic: zygomaticofacial (cheek) and zygomaticotemporal (temple). The latter is blocked at the zygomatic arch for **scalp block**.
- Sphenopalatine nerve: supplies nerves to the orbit, nasal branches, nasopalatine nerve, greater palatine nerve, lesser palatine nerve and pharyngeal branches. The nasopalatine and greater palatine branches are blocked for **palatal surgery**.
- Posterior alveolar nerve: supplies posterior upper alveolus. It is blocked for **molar tooth extraction**.

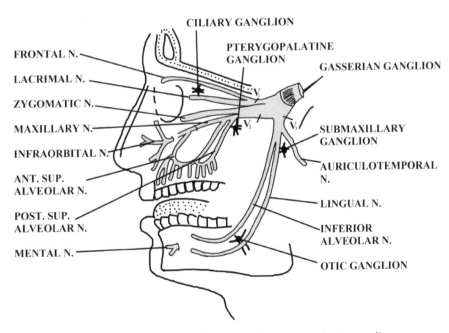

Figure 5.42 Branches of the trigeminal nerve and parasympathetic ganglia

Infraorbital nerve is the **terminal branch** of maxillary nerve and exits through the **infraorbital foramen**. It divides into inferior palpebral, lateral nasal and superior labial branches. It is blocked at the infraorbital foramen (intramucosal or extramucosal approach) for cleft lip surgery (analgesia to upper lip) and **upper-incisor dental surgery**.

- Hadzic A. *Textbook of Regional Anesthesia and Acute Pain Management*. 1st ed. New York, NY: McGraw-Hill Medical; 2006. pp. 342–3.

A105 C The mandibular nerve (V₃) is the **largest** branch of the trigeminal nerve. It is made up of a **large sensory root** and a **small motor root** (supplies the muscles of mastication). They exit through the **foramen ovale** and unite to form the main trunk of V₃. The main trunk gives two branches before it divides into anterior and posterior divisions, which give more branches again. Of interest are its three branches of posterior division.

▶ Auriculotemporal nerve: ascends upwards behind the temporomandibular joint (TMJ) innervating the auricle, external auditory meatus, tympanic membrane and **TMJ**. It is blocked at **temporal fossa** for **scalp block**.

▶ Lingual nerve: supplies sensory innervation to the anterior two-thirds of the tongue, floor of mouth and gingival mucosa.

▶ Inferior alveolar nerve: traverses the mandibular canal to emerge as the **mental nerve** at the mental foramen. It supplies the chin and lower lip.

- Hadzic A. *Textbook of Regional Anesthesia and Acute Pain Management*. 1st ed. New York, NY: McGraw-Hill Medical; 2006. pp. 345–6.

A106 B All of the options in the question are terminal nerves of CNV.

Table 5.30 Blockade of terminal branches of trigeminal nerve

Nerve	Landmark
Supraorbital	Supraorbital notch
Supratrochlear	Just above the medial end of eyebrows or between eyebrows to block bilaterally
Infraorbital nerve	Infraorbital foramen
Mental nerve	Mental foramen

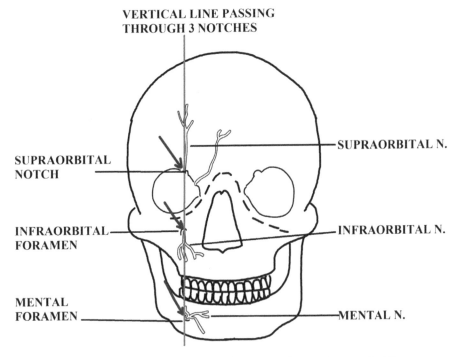

VERTICAL LINE PASSING
THROUGH 3 NOTCHES

SUPRAORBITAL N.

SUPRAORBITAL
NOTCH

INFRAORBITAL
FORAMEN

INFRAORBITAL N.

MENTAL
FORAMEN

MENTAL N.

Figure 5.43 Blockade of terminal branches of trigeminal nerve in a vertical line

A107 A The maxillary nerve can be blocked after it exits the foramen rotundum. For this, a lateral approach through the **infratemporal fossa** is used. An 8-cm 22-G needle is passed below the midpoint of zygomatic arch, overlying the **coronoid notch** of mandible. As it is advanced deeper, it contacts the **lateral pterygoid plate** at a depth of 5 cm. It is then redirected anteriorly to walk off the edge of the lateral pterygoid plate, to enter the **pterygopalatine fossa**. Paraesthesias/radiological confirmation can be used to access placement. Local anaesthetic (5 mL) is injected here.

Indications for the maxillary block:

▶ surgery – lower eyelid, the nose (with the nasal nerve), the cheek, the zygomatic area, the upper lip, superior dental surgery, palate and maxillary bone surgery

▶ trigeminal neuralgias

▶ refractory headaches (sphenopalatine ganglion origin).

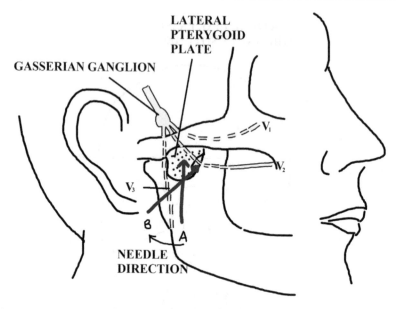

Figure 5.44 Maxillary block: needle direction

Spread of local anaesthetic here may cause **transient blindness**. For the same reason, neurolytic blocks are avoided through this approach; rather, they are performed at the **Gasserian ganglion**.

- Cousins MJ, Bridenbaugh PO, Carr DB, *et al. Cousins and Bridenbaugh's Neural Blockade in Clinical Anesthesia and Pain Medicine*. 4th ed. Philadelphia, PA: Lippincott Williams & Wilkins; 2008. p. 414.

A108 C The mandibular nerve can be blocked after it exits the foramen ovale. For this, a lateral approach through the **infratemporal fossa** is used. An 8-cm 22-G needle is passed below the midpoint of zygomatic arch, overlying the **coronoid notch** of mandible. As it is advanced deeper, it contacts the **lateral pterygoid plate** at a depth of 5 cm. It is then redirected **posteriorly** to walk off the edge of the lateral pterygoid plate to stimulate V_3 near the foramen ovale. Paraesthesias, motor stimulation or radiological confirmation can be used to access placement. Local anaesthetic (5 mL) is injected here.

Indications for the mandibular block:

- surgery – lower lip, mandible, temple surgery, inferior dental surgery and wound of the anterior two thirds of the tongue
- pain syndromes
- TMJ pain.

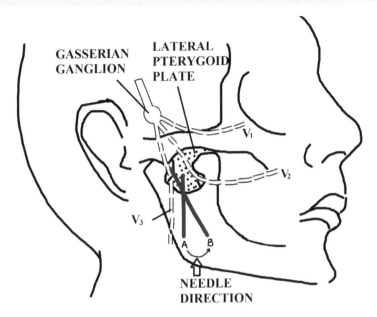

Figure 5.45 Mandibular block: needle direction

Deeper placement of the needle can result in piercing the **pharynx**. Neurolytic blocks can affect the otic ganglion, resulting in **xerostomia**. They are best performed at the Gasserian ganglion.

- Cousins MJ, Bridenbaugh PO, Carr DB, *et al. Cousins and Bridenbaugh's Neural Blockade in Clinical Anesthesia and Pain Medicine*. 4th ed. Philadelphia, PA: Lippincott Williams & Wilkins; 2008. p. 415.

A109 D **Indications** for airway blocks:

- for awake intubation in patients with airway compromise, trauma to the upper airway, or cervical instability
- to allow tolerance of nasal endotracheal tube, oral endotracheal tube or tracheal tubes in critically ill patients in intensive care (sometimes)
- transoesophageal echocardiography in an awake patient.

This acts by abolishing the gag reflex, glottis closure reflex and the cough reflex. Stapedial reflex involves the facial nerve (not blocked in airway blocks).

Table 5.31 Airway reflexes

Reflex	Afferent	Efferent
Gag	Glossopharyngeal	Vagus
Glottis closure	Superior laryngeal nerve	Vagus
Cough	Superior and recurrent laryngeal nerves	Vagus

A110 B

Table 5.32 Innervation of the airway (three neural pathways)

Nasal cavity and nasopharynx	Oropharynx	Larynx and trachea
Maxillary branches of the trigeminal nerve (V$_1$)	Glossopharyngeal nerve (CNIX)	Vagus nerve (CNX)

A111 B

▶ The **facial nerve** does not participate in airway reflexes and need not be blocked.

▶ The **mandibular nerve** supplies sensation to anterior two thirds of the tongue and need not be blocked.

▶ The **ophthalmic and maxillary divisions** of trigeminal nerves supply the nasal cavity and have to be blocked.

▶ Since the airway is supplied by three different cranial nerves, no single block can be used to anaesthetise them.

▶ However, local anaesthetic nebulisation (4% lignocaine for 10–15 minutes) usually anaesthetises the entire airway effectively.

- Hadzic A. *Textbook of Regional Anesthesia and Acute Pain Management*. 1st ed. New York, NY: McGraw-Hill Medical; 2006. p. 335.
- Kundra P, Kutralam S, Ravishankar M. Local anaesthesia for awake fibre-optic nasotracheal intubation. *Acta Anaesthesiol Scand*. 2000; **44**(5): 511–16.

A112 D

Table 5.33 Anaesthesia of the nasal cavity

Nerve	Derived from	Innervation	Location of applicator
Anterior ethmoidal nerves	Ophthalmic division (**V₁**)	Anterior part of nasal septum and lateral wall	Along the **superior turbinate**, resting against the cribriform plate
Sphenopalatine ganglion: nasopalatine, greater and lesser palatine nerves	Maxillary division (**V₂**)	Posterior and inferior parts of nasal septum and lateral wall	Along the **middle turbinate** resting against the sphenoid bone (*most important*)

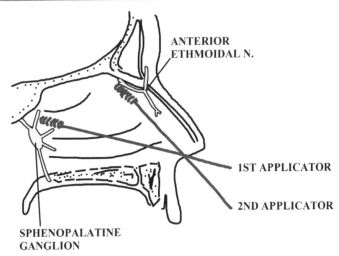

Figure 5.46 Nasal mucosal block by applicators

Drugs used:

Anaesthetic: 4% lignocaine (maximum **500 mg**)
Vasoconstrictor: cocaine is a 4% solution (maximum **200 mg**) or epinephrine (1:200 000) or 0.05% phenylephrine.

Technique: the patient is most comfortable when the head of the bed is **elevated approximately 30°**. Then 6–8-cm-long cotton-tipped applicators or wide cotton pledgets soaked in the drug solution are inserted into both nares as follows:

▶ first applicator along the **inferior turbinate** to rest against the posterior nasopharyngeal wall

 ‣ second applicator is placed in a cephalad angulation along the **middle turbinate**, against the sphenoid bone (**most important**, as it anaesthetises branches of the sphenopalatine ganglia)
 ‣ third applicator may be placed along the **superior turbinate**, resting against the cribriform plate, anaesthetising the anterior ethmoid nerve.

The applicators/pledgets are left in place for **5 minutes**. Next, nasal cavity is dilated with nasal airways bilaterally (in increasing sizes) by lubricating with 2%–5% lignocaine jelly.

Instillation technique: with the patient's head low, or with a pillow under the patient's shoulder, LA is instilled in the nasal cavity (10 minutes for each side). It can lead to total spinal anaesthesia, as it involves injection into the nasal cavity near the cribriform plate.

Complications are epistaxis, systemic toxicity and increased risk for aspiration.

 • Cousins MJ, Bridenbaugh PO, Carr DB, *et al. Cousins and Bridenbaugh's Neural Blockade in Clinical Anesthesia and Pain Medicine*. 4th ed. Philadelphia, PA: Lippincott Williams & Wilkins; 2008. p. 413.

A113 B Oropharyngeal anaesthesia requires blocking the **glossopharyngeal nerve**. This can be accomplished by atomisation or CNIX block (bilateral).

Atomisation:
 ‣ 10% lignocaine spray (each puff has 20 mg).
 ‣ 2% viscous lignocaine (10 mL) gargles for 10 minutes.
 ‣ 4% lignocaine (5–10 mL) with 1:200 000 epinephrine nebulisation for 15–20 minutes.
 ‣ Cetacaine spray (mix of 14% benzocaine and 2% tetracaine): more toxicity.

Advantages are that it is simple, easy and comfortable for patient, with no special skill needed. Disadvantages are **variable anaesthesia** and risk of neurological depression in compromised patients. *Note:* maximum safe plasma levels of lignocaine are **5 mg/L**.

Glossopharyngeal nerve (lingual branch): blocked bilaterally intraoral approach. Initially, topical anaesthesia is provided to oral cavity by above-mentioned methods. Next the tongue is depressed (with a tongue depressor) and a spinal needle (9–10 cm 25 G) is used to inject 0.5% lignocaine (2 mL) 0.5 cm below the mucosa of the base of anterior tonsillar pillar after aspiration. It is repeated on the other side. Although it is more effective, it is more discomforting than atomisation.

- Mulroy MF, Bernards CM, McDonald SB, *et al. A Practical Approach to Regional Anesthesia*. 4th ed. Philadelphia, PA: Lippincott Williams & Wilkins; 2008. p. 268.

A114 D Superior laryngeal nerve (SLN) block: the internal branch of the superior laryngeal nerve originates from the SLN **lateral to the greater cornu of the hyoid bone**. It travels along inferior to the greater cornu, then pierces the thyrohyoid membrane and travels under the mucosa in

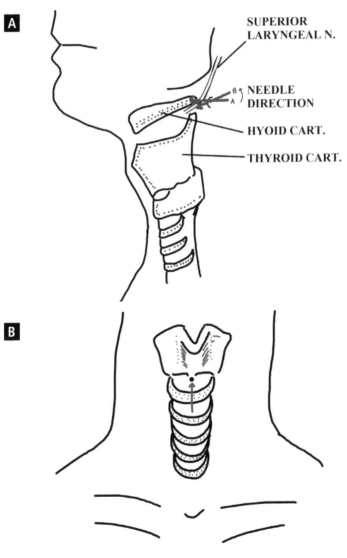

Figure 5.47 (A) Superior laryngeal nerve block; (B) recurrent laryngeal nerve block

the pyriform recess. The internal branch of the SLN provides sensory innervation to the **base of the tongue, superior epiglottis, aryepiglottic folds, arytenoids and laryngeal mucosa** (above the vocal cords). The external branch of the SLN supplies the motor innervation to the cricothyroid muscle. The SLN can be anaesthetised non-invasively by keeping anaesthetic-soaked gauze in the **pyriform sinuses** bilaterally (using right-angle forceps). Alternatively, it can be blocked invasively at the **greater cornu** of the hyoid bone bilaterally by walking the needle off it, into the thyrohyoid membrane. At a depth of 1–2 cm, 2 mL of 2% lignocaine (with epinephrine) is injected (after negative aspiration) between the thyrohyoid membrane and pharyngeal mucosa. The block is repeated on the opposite side.

Recurrent laryngeal nerve (RLN) block (transtracheal or translaryngeal block): the mucosa below the vocal cords receives innervation from the RLN. With the patient supine and the neck hyperextended, a 20-G intravenous cannula is inserted into the **cricoid membrane**. After tracheal entry is confirmed by air aspiration, stellate is removed and 4 mL of 2% lignocaine (with epinephrine) is injected as the patient inspires. This initiates a **cough reflex** and spreads the LA to both below and above the vocal cords (SLN and RLN territory).

- Hadzic A. *Textbook of Regional Anesthesia and Acute Pain Management*. 1st ed. New York, NY: McGraw-Hill Medical; 2006. pp. 336–8.

6

Regional anaesthesia in specific populations

Questions

> **Distribution**
>
> *Questions 1–9: Obstetrics*
>
> *Questions 10–26: Paediatrics*
>
> *Questions 27–31: Geriatrics*
>
> *Questions 32–42: Patients with systemic disease*

Choose one best answer for each of the following questions.

Q1 Which of the following changes is **not** seen in pregnancy?
   a. There is increased sensitivity to local anaesthetics due to oestrogen
   b. Minimum alveolar concentration of volatile anaesthetics is decreased due to progesterone
   c. There is a decrease in albumin, altering the unbound drug concentration
   d. Fibrinogen levels are elevated

Q2 Concerning the transfer of local anaesthetics in foetus, which of the following statements is **false**?
   a. Accumulation of bupivacaine may occur in a foetus with acidosis
   b. Accumulation of 2-chloroprocaine may occur in a foetus with acidosis
   c. Regional anaesthesia in the mother may lead to behavioural changes in the newborn
   d. The local anaesthetics can be excreted from the foetus back in the mother, even when total drug concentrations are higher in the mother

Q3 Regarding pain relief during labour, which of the following statements is **incorrect**?
   a. Blocking T10–L1 dermatomes provides analgesia for the first stage of labour
   b. Blocking T10–S4 provides analgesia for the second stage of labour
   c. Prolongation of the first stage of labour occurs with epidural analgesia
   d. Dysfunctional labour may be converted to a normal labour by epidural analgesia

Q4 Which of the following statements about pain relief during labour is **false**?
   a. Combined spinal epidural is ideal for labour analgesia
   b. There are transient changes in foetal heart rate following combined spinal epidural in mother
   c. Incidence of post-dural puncture headache with combined spinal epidural is similar to epidural block
   d. Paracervical block reduces pain of second stage of labour

Q5 Which is the **false** statement among the following?
   a. Paravertebral sympathetic block can be used for pain relief during the first stage of labour
   b. Pudendal nerve block can be used for analgesia during repair of episiotomy
   c. Paracervical block can be used for analgesia during uterine curettage
   d. Pudendal nerve is blocked near ischial tuberosity

Q6 Which of the following statements is **correct**?
   a. A long-acting morphine preparation that is lipid-encapsulated can be used epidurally for analgesia after Caesarian section
   b. In the past, 2-chloroprocaine was not used because the ethylene-diamine-tetra-acetic-acid (EDTA) present in it was neuorotoxic
   c. The most reliable test to identify proper position of epidural catheter is aspiration of catheter for blood for cerebrospinal fluid
   d. Maternal mortality with general anaesthesia is the same as with regional anaesthesia

Q7 Which of the following statements about pregnancy-induced hypertension (PIH) is **false**?
a. Oedema is one of the diagnostic criteria for PIH
b. Epidural anesthesia is considered to be better than spinal in women with pre-eclampsia
c. Pre-eclamptic patients require lower dose of ephedrine to maintain their blood pressure after central neuraxial blocks
d. Severe PIH is associated with rise in systolic blood pressure > 15%

Q8 Which of the following statements about innervations of the perineum is **false**?
a. The skeletal muscles of the pelvic floor are supplied by pudendal nerve
b. The genital branch of genitofemoral nerve innervates anterior perineum
c. The ilioinguinal nerve innervates the lateral part of the perineum
d. The perineum is also innervated by the posterior femoral cutaneous nerve

Q9 Regarding pharmacological management of pain in pregnant women or mothers, which of the following statements is **incorrect**?
a. NSAIDs can be safely prescribed during pregnancy
b. Opioids are safe for use in breastfeeding mothers
c. NSAIDs are safe in breastfeeding mothers
d. Phenytoin can be safely prescribed for neuropathic pain in breastfeeding mothers

Q10 Which of the following statements about paediatric regional anaesthesia is **false**?
a. It is mostly done under general anaesthesia
b. The dose in mg/kg is same as adults
c. Complications are less common than in adults
d. Ester local anaesthetics have to be used with caution in neonates and infants

Q11 Which of the following is a **false** statement about local anaesthetics in neonates?

    a. There is greater risk of toxicity with bupivacaine in neonates than adults

    b. First sign of local anaesthetic toxicity in neonates is cardiovascular changes and not central nervous system changes

    c. Maximum recommended dose of lignocaine with adrenaline is 7 mg/kg

    d. Maximum recommended dose of 2-chloroprocaine is 3 mg/kg

Q12 Concerning anatomy of vertebral column in neonates, which is the **correct** statement?

    a. Tuffier's line passes through L5 in neonates

    b. The spinal cord reaches adult level of L1 by 8 years of age

    c. The sacral vertebrae ossify and form sacrum by 10 years of age

    d. There is densely packed fat in epidural space in neonates

Q13 Which of the following is a **true** statement about use of local anaesthetics in epidural space in children?

    a. Spread of local anaesthetic is better predicted with body weight

    b. Spread of local anaesthetic is better predicted with age

    c. For single-shot caudal, 0.7% ropivacaine 1 mL/kg can be used

    d. Use of opioids in epidural space is relatively safe for day-case surgeries

Q14 Which of the following is an **incorrect** statement about adjuvants used in epidural space in children?

    a. The most common adjuvant used is epinephrine

    b. Ventilatory response to carbon dioxide is blunted by epidural clonidine

    c. Neostigmine produces high incidence of nausea and vomiting

    d. None of the above

Q15 Which of the following statements about complication of epidural block in children is **correct**?
  a. The most common organism colonised on caudal epidural catheter is *Staphylococcus aureus*
  b. Use of blood patch for post-dural puncture headache (PDHP) in children should use blood 1 mL/kg
  c. Cardiovascular instability occurs with general anaesthesia and thoracic epidural anaesthesia
  d. Hypotension may indicate local anaesthetic toxicity

Q16 Which of the following is **not** a method to confirm epidural catheter position?
  a. Ultrasonography
  b. ECG
  c. Electrical stimulation
  d. Loss of resistance to saline

Q17 Which of the following statements about epidural block is **false**?
  a. Nerve stimulators used for peripheral nerve blocks can be used for epidural stimulation test used to confirm position of epidural catheter
  b. During insertion, epidural-stimulating catheter with stylet forms a J-shaped tip
  c. Epidural catheters containing a metal element are beneficial
  d. The ground electrode must be placed on the arms for lumbar epidurals

Q18 Which of the following is a **false** statement about epidural ECG as a method to confirm proper placement of epidural catheter?
  a. Epidural ECG can be reliably used to identify intrathecal placement of epidural catheter
  b. The right-arm electrode is connected to the epidural catheter
  c. Epidural ECG cannot be used to identify intravascular placement of epidural catheter
  d. Epidural ECG can be used to confirm proper placement of catheter in epidural space when local anaesthetic has been administered in the epidural space

Q19 Which of the following statements about caudal block is **correct**?
a. Needles with stylet are not useful
b. Angiocaths are useful, as they help in locating intravascular placement
c. An equilateral triangle is formed by joining the two posterior superior iliac spines, and sacral cornua
d. Skin is punctured at an angle of 20°–30° for caudal block

Q20 Which of the following statements about caudal block is **incorrect**?
a. Cannula over a needle technique is better
b. Needle over a cannula technique is better
c. The sensitivity to predict needle location in caudal space approaches 100% with nerve-stimulator technique
d. The specificity to predict needle location in caudal space approaches 100% with nerve-stimulator technique

Q21 Which of the following statements about epidural block in paediatric patients is **false**?
a. The tactile sensation of needle puncturing the ligamentum flavum is less distinct in neonates
b. The distance of epidural space from the skin is less than adults
c. There is no significant change in heart rate or blood pressure after epidural block in children
d. The mean depth of epidural space in neonates is 2 cm

Q22 Which of the following is a **false** statement about epidural block in children?
a. The tip of epidural catheter must be at the surgical site
b. For thoracic epidural, midline approach must be used
c. Thoracic placement of catheter from lumbar insertion site is usually easy in children
d. The depth of epidural space from skin may be dependent on age and weight of the child

Q23 Which of the following statement about spinal anaesthesia in children is **false**?
a. Cerebrospinal fluid (CSF) volume in neonates in mL/kg is larger than adults
b. The duration of spinal anaesthesia is shorter than in adults
c. Hypobaric solutions are not routinely used in infants
d. Neck flexion for proper positioning for spinal block, as for adults, must be done

Q24 Which of the following statements about spinal anesthesia in children is **true**?
a. Bromage scale can be used to assess spinal block in children under 2 years of age
b. Fluid preloading (10 mL/kg) is beneficial in children before spinal anaesthesia
c. Hypotension commonly occurs after spinal anesthesia in children
d. In children, the incidence of PDPH is less than adults

Q25 Regarding paediatric spinals, which of the following is a **false** statement?
a. Spinal anaesthesia is relatively contraindicated in preterm infants
b. Spinal anaesthesia is relatively contraindicated in patients with ventriculoperitoneal shunts
c. Spinal anaesthesia is relatively contraindicated in patients with degenerative neuromuscular disease
d. Spinal anaesthesia does not eliminate risk of postoperative apnoea

Q26 Which of the following statements about peripheral nerve blocks in paediatrics is **incorrect**?
a. Interscalene block is not preferred in children
b. Parascalene approach is preferred in children
c. Axillary approach is most commonly used in children
d. Complications are more common, as the blocks are performed under general anaesthetic

Q27 Which of the following physiological changes is **not** seen in elderly patients?
a. A decrease in myelinated nerves
b. Dura is more permeable to local anaesthetics
c. CSF volume decreases with age
d. CSF-specific gravity decreases with age

Q28 Which of the following statements about epidural anaesthesia in elderly is **incorrect?**
a. There is faster onset of motor block
b. There is greater cephalad spread of local anaesthetic
c. The use of epidural test-dose lignocaine with epinephrine is unreliable in elderly
d. There is a linear relationship between dose of local anaesthetic/segment and spread of analgesia

Q29 Which of the following is a **true** statement about pharmacokinetics of local anaesthetic?
a. There is biphasic absorption of local anaesthetics after central neuraxial anaesthesia
b. There is initial slower phase of absorption of local anaesthetic due to decreased vascularity in elderly
c. There is faster phase of absorption later due to decreased fat in epidural space
d. All of the above

Q30 Which of the following is a **true** statement about use of drugs in the elderly?
a. The clearance of lignocaine decreases because of a decrease in enzyme activity of hepatocytes
b. The clearance of bupivacaine decreases due to decrease in hepatic blood flow
c. The top-up doses and frequency of epidural local anaesthetics must be decreased
d. Intrathecal opioids are very safe in elderly

Q31 Which of the following is a **false** statement about neuraxial anaesthesia in elderly?
a. The incidence of PDPH in elderly is lower
b. Taylor's approach to neuraxial anaesthesia may be helpful in patients with osteoarthritis
c. There is a decrease in post-operative cognitive dysfunction in elderly with central neuraxial anaesthesia as compared to general anaesthesia
d. There is a decrease in 1-month mortality in elderly with central neuraxial anaesthesia as compared with general anaesthesia

Q32 Which of the following respiratory parameters is **not** decreased by lumbar epidural anaesthesia?
a. Forced vital capacity (FVC)
b. Peak expiratory flow rate (PEFR)
c. Resting minute ventilation
d. Forced expiratory volume during first second (FEV_1)

Q33 All of the following statements about respiratory parameters during blocks are true **except**:
a. Interscalene block reduces FVC and FEV_1
b. Preservation of pulmonary functions after thoracotomy is better with paravertebral blockade than epidural analgesia
c. Supraclavicular block may reduce FVC and FEV_1
d. Infraclavicular block does not reduce FVC and FEV_1

Q34 Which of the following is a **correct** statement about regional anaesthesia in patients with chronic renal failure?
a. Neuraxial block up to T10 level causes significant decrease in renal blood flow
b. In renal transplant patients, graft function is affected by central neuraxial anaesthesia
c. Chronic renal failure patients have higher plasma levels of local anaesthetic after a peripheral nerve block than normal patients
d. In uremic patients, there is decrease in free fraction of bupivacaine, requiring higher doses to produce effect

Q35 Which of the following statements about anaesthetic technique for arteriovenous fistula is **incorrect**?
a. General anaesthetic increases blood flow through fistula
b. Brachial plexus block increases blood flow through fistula
c. Local anaesthetic infiltration increases blood flow through fistula
d. The differences in outcome after operation for arteriovenous fistula due to different technique of anaesthesia are negligible

Q36 Which of the following statements about regional anaesthesia in patients with hepatic disease is **incorrect**?

a. Dose adjustment of local anaesthetic is required for single-shot peripheral nerve block

b. Dose adjustment of local anaesthetic is required for continuous catheter techniques for peripheral nerve blocks

c. High levels of neuraxial block reduce portal blood flow to liver

d. High levels of neuraxial block maintain hepatic arterial blood flow to liver

Q37 Which of the following is a **false** statement about regional anaesthesia in diabetic patients?

a. The hyperglycaemic response following surgery is prevented by regional anaesthesia

b. Lower intensity of stimulating current must be used to locate nerves via nerve stimulator during peripheral nerve blocks to prevent nerve damage

c. Perioperatively, blood glucose levels must be tightly controlled

d. Regional anaesthesia inhibits gluconeogenesis in liver

Q38 Which of the following statements about regional anaesthesia in patients with hypothyroidism is **incorrect**?

a. Higher intensity of stimulating current must be used to locate nerves via nerve stimulator during peripheral nerve blocks

b. 'Double crush syndrome' may occur in patients with hypothyroidism

c. There is increased risk of neurological injury following regional anaesthesia

d. Thyroid neuropathy usually does not respond to thyroxine

Q39 Which of the following statements about nerve injury and anaesthesia is **correct**?

a. Incidence of brachial plexus injury is higher with regional anaesthesia than with general anaesthesia

b. Incidence of ulnar nerve injury is higher with general anaesthesia than with regional anaesthesia

c. In patients with mononeuropathy, general anaesthesia is safer than regional anaesthesia

d. Spinal cord injury is the most common injury reported due to anaesthesia

Q40 Which of the following is a **false** statement about regional anaesthesia in patients with neurological disease?
a. Regional anaesthesia is preferred over general anaesthesia in patients with Parkinsonism
b. Opioids must be used with caution in patients with Parkinsonism
c. Peripheral nerve block must be avoided in patients with multiple sclerosis
d. Lumbar paravertebral block may have a prolonged duration of action in patients with multiple sclerosis

Q41 Which of the following statements about anaesthesia in patients with spinal cord injury is **correct**?
a. General anaesthesia is avoided in patients during acute phase of spinal cord injury
b. Regional anaesthesia is safe in patients during chronic phase of spinal cord injury
c. Autonomic dysreflexia is seen if level of injury is above T4
d. There is no risk of haemodynamic instability if level of spinal cord injury is below T8

Q42 Which of the following is a **true** statement in patients with myasthenia gravis?
a. Thymectomy can be done under general anaesthesia or high-thoracic epidural anaesthesia
b. All local anaesthetics are safe
c. Supraclavicular brachial plexus blocks are safe for upper-limb surgeries
d. Benzodiazepines and opioids are safe to use for sedation during peripheral nerve block

Answers

A1   A

Table 6.1 Physiological changes seen in pregnancy, Part 1

System	Increase	Decrease	Unchanged
Cardiovascular system	Blood volume Plasma volume Cardiac output Heart rate	Systemic vascular resistance Pulmonary vascular resistance Pulmonary artery pressure	Central venous pressure Pulmonary capillary wedge pressure
Respiratory system	**Minute ventilation** Alveolar ventilation Tidal volume Inspiratory capacity	**Functional residual capacity** **Minimum alveolar concentration of volatile anaesthetics** Residual volume Total lung capacity	Respiratory rate Forced vital capacity

Table 6.2 Physiological changes seen in pregnancy, Part 2

Other changes	Significance
Delayed gastric emptying	Consider patients as non-fasting
Fall in albumin concentration	Higher free fraction of most protein-bound drugs, leading to toxicity
Higher increase in plasma volume than in red blood cell mass	Physiological anaemia
Decrease in serum cholinesterase activity	Prolonged action of suxamethonium
Progesterone-mediated increased sensitivity to local anaesthetics	Use lower doses
Decrease in minimum alveolar concentration of volatile anaesthetics	Use lower minimum alveolar concentration values

Note: fibrinogen levels are raised.

- Hadzic A. *Textbook of Regional Anesthesia and Acute Pain Management*. 1st ed. New York, NY: McGraw-Hill Medical; 2006. p. 698.

A2   **B** The protein binding in the foetus is less than that in the mother. This results in **higher ionised fraction** of local anaesthetics in the foetus. This free fraction further increases with foetal acidosis, resulting in **ion trapping**. Drugs like bupivacaine which are highly protein-bound may accumulate in this way. 2-Chloroprocaine is an ester local anaesthetic. It does not accumulate in foetus during acidosis, as it undergoes rapid hydrolysis by **pseudocholinesterase**. Transient neurobehavioural changes may be seen in newborn after regional anaesthesia.

- Hadzic A. *Textbook of Regional Anesthesia and Acute Pain Management*. 1st ed. New York, NY: McGraw-Hill Medical; 2006. p. 702.

A3   **C**

Table 6.3 Pain during different stages of labour

Stage of labour	Cause of pain	Dermatomes involved
First stage	Cervical dilatation Lower uterine segment distension	**T10–L1** (Pain afferents via superior hypogastric plexus)
Second stage	Vaginal vault and perineum	**S2–S4** (pudendal nerves)

Epidural analgesia relieves pain. This decreases the catecholamine levels in the mother and may change dysfunctional labour to normal labour. It also decreases the maternal hyperventilation and prevents left shift in oxygen–haemoglobin dissociation curve. Epidural analgesia may delay the second stage of labour. It may not affect the first stage of labour.

- Hadzic A. *Textbook of Regional Anesthesia and Acute Pain Management*. 1st ed. New York, NY: McGraw-Hill Medical; 2006. p. 704.
- Cousins MJ, Bridenbaugh PO, Carr DB, *et al. Cousins and Bridenbaugh's Neural Blockade in Clinical Anesthesia and Pain Medicine*. 4th ed. Philadelphia, PA: Lippincott Williams & Wilkins; 2008. p. 540.

A4   **D**

▶ Combined spinal epidural: combines the benefit of both spinal and epidural anaesthetics. It results in rapid onset of analgesia, and its action can be prolonged with the help of an epidural catheter. Due to instantaneous pain relief, it results in fall in maternal catecholamine and **transient changes in foetal heart rate (bradycardia)**. The incidence of post-dural puncture headache is similar to epidural block.

▶ Paracervical block: involves injection of local anaesthetic at vaginal fornix. It was mainly used to **reduce pain of first stage of labour.** It is not commonly used, due to its association with constriction of uterine artery and foetal asphyxia. It is not effective for second stage of labour, as it does not block the sensory fibres arising from the perineum.

  - Hadzic A. *Textbook of Regional Anesthesia and Acute Pain Management.* 1st ed. New York, NY: McGraw-Hill Medical; 2006. p. 706.
  - Cousins MJ, Bridenbaugh PO, Carr DB, *et al. Cousins and Bridenbaugh's Neural Blockade in Clinical Anesthesia and Pain Medicine.* 4th ed. Philadelphia, PA: Lippincott Williams & Wilkins; 2008. p. 541.

A5   D

▶ Paravertebral lumbar sympathetic block: can be used for pain relief during first stage of labour. However, it is not popular, as it is technically difficult and there is higher risk of intravascular injection.

▶ Paracervical block: involves blocking the nerve fibres to uterus by depositing the local anaesthetic near vaginal fornix. Uterine curettage can be done under paracervical block. It is not popular for labour analgesia because of its association with **foetal asphyxia** secondary to uterine artery vasoconstriction.

▶ Pudendal nerve block: pudendal nerves are blocked around **ischial spines** and not ischial tuberosity. It can be used for analgesia during repair of **episiotomy** as well as delivery of foetus with forceps.

  - Hadzic A. *Textbook of Regional Anesthesia and Acute Pain Management.* 1st ed. New York, NY: McGraw-Hill Medical; 2006. pp. 706–7.

A6   A

▶ 2-Chloroprocaine, which is used intrathecally, is a **preservative-free** solution. In the past, it was formulated with a preservative **sodium bisulphite** which was shown to be neurotoxic. Later it was replaced with **EDTA,** which caused severe back pain.

▶ A new morphine formulation (**lipid-encapsulated**) for epidural use has been approved for analgesia after lower-segment Caesarean section.

▶ Positive aspiration of blood or cerebrospinal fluid from an epidural catheter identifies intravascular or intrathecal location. A negative aspiration still does not rule out a partial intravascular or intrathecal placement. Hence it may not be able to identify the correct location of the catheter.

▶ **Other tests** that may be used to identify catheter location are:
  – test dose with lignocaine 45 mg with epinephrine 15 mcg

   – epidural hanging drop technique

   – meniscus fall sign

   – injection of air through the epidural catheter and precordial Doppler monitoring.

▶ The maternal mortality with general anaesthesia is **16.7 times more** than regional anaesthesia, according to studies between 1979 and 1990 in the United States.

   • Hadzic A. *Textbook of Regional Anesthesia and Acute Pain Management.* 1st ed. New York, NY: McGraw-Hill Medical; 2006. p. 710.

A7   A Hypertensive disorders in pregnancy are classified as:

▶ **Gestational hypertension**: a rise in blood pressure (> 140/90 mmHg) after 20 weeks of gestation without proteinuria.

▶ **Pre-eclampsia**: a rise in blood pressure **after 20 weeks** of gestation **with proteinuria**. Oedema may or may not be present in pre-eclampsia.

Table 6.4 Features of preeclampsia

Pre-eclampsia	Features
Mild	BP > 140/90 mmHg
	Protienuria > 0.3 g/24 hours
Severe	BP > 160/110 mmHg
	Systolic BP > 15% above baseline
	Diastolic BP > 15% above baseline
	Proteinuria > 5 g/24 hours
	Headache
	Epigastric pain
	Oliguria
	Visual disturbances

▶ **Eclampsia**: pre-eclampsia associated with convulsions.

▶ **Chronic hypertension**: hypertension detected **before 20 weeks** of gestation. It can be primary or secondary.

In pre-eclamptic patients, intravascular volume is depleted. Hence **spinal anaesthesia** is associated with **severe hypotension** in such patients. Epidural anaesthesia results in **gradual fall** in blood pressure and is easy to titrate by small boluses of local anaesthetic. Lower doses of vasopressors are required in patients with pre-eclampsia, as they have increased sensitivity to them.

   • Hadzic A. *Textbook of Regional Anesthesia and Acute Pain Management.* 1st ed. New York, NY: McGraw-Hill Medical; 2006. pp. 713–14.

A8 C The nerve supply to the perineum is as follows.

▶ **Genitofemoral nerve** (L1, L2) – innervates the anterior part of perineum.

▶ **Ilioinguinal nerve** – innervates the anterior part of perineum.

▶ **Pudendal nerve** arises from the anterior rami of S2–S4. These form a trunk before leaving the pelvis via the greater sciatic foramen. It passes immediately behind the ischial spine and swings forward to enter the perineum via the lesser sciatic foramen. The nerve passes through the ischiorectal fossa, where it gives off its terminal branches, which are:

  – **Inferior rectal nerve** – innervates the external anal sphincter and the perineal skin

  – **Perineal nerve** – deep branch innervates the sphincter urethrae and other muscles of the anterior compartment

  – **Superficial branch** – and the skin of the perineum posterior to the clitoris

  – **Dorsal nerve of the clitoris** – supplies the skin surrounding this structure.

▶ **Perineal branch of the posterior femoral nerve** – innervates the lateral part of perineum.

  • Cousins MJ, Bridenbaugh PO, Carr DB, *et al. Cousins and Bridenbaugh's Neural Blockade in Clinical Anesthesia and Pain Medicine.* 4th ed. Philadelphia, PA: Lippincott Williams & Wilkins; 2008. pp. 539–40.

A9 A

Table 6.5 Analgesics in pregnancy

Pregnancy	Breastfeeding
Safe	*Safe*
paracetamol	non-steroidal anti-inflammatory drugs and
opioids	paracetamol
	opioids
	antiepileptics (neuropathic pain)
	tricyclic antidepressants: amitryptyline, imipramine
	selective serotonin reuptake inhibitors
Unsafe	*Unsafe (caution advised)*
non-steroidal anti-inflammatory drugs	ketorolac
foetus: renal dysfunction and patent ductus arteriosus	aspirin (up to 100 mg/day)
mother: haemorrhage	

- Cousins MJ, Bridenbaugh PO, Carr DB, *et al. Cousins and Bridenbaugh's Neural Blockade in Clinical Anesthesia and Pain Medicine.* 4th ed. Philadelphia, PA: Lippincott Williams & Wilkins; 2008. p. 558.

A10 B

▶ Regional anaesthesia in children is usually done under **general anaesthesia or sedation**.

▶ In **neonates**, the liver enzymes and metabolic processes are **immature**, hence there is less metabolism of local anaesthetics and greater chances of toxicity as compared to adults. In neonates, $\alpha 1$ acid glycoprotein levels are 20%–40% of adult levels, hence higher plasma levels of unbound free drug contributes to toxicity as well.

▶ Around **3 months of age**, the conjugation of local anaesthetics reaches adult value, whereas full maturation and clearance equivalent to adults occur by around **8 months**.

▶ In children, there may be **higher vascular absorption** of local anaesthetics and higher plasma concentration.

▶ As myelination is incomplete up to the age of 12 years, local anaesthetic can penetrate better in the nerves. Because of greater sensitivity and potential for toxicity, the dose of local anaesthetic in children (mg/kg) is **less** than adults. Because of loose fascial layers, volume of LA is a key factor for spread than dose.

▶ Ester local anaesthetics do not depend on liver for their metabolism and have more rapid clearance than amide local anaesthetics in neonates. However, because of **low levels of plasma cholinesterases** in neonates, ester local anaesthetics should be used with caution.

- Hadzic A. *Textbook of Regional Anesthesia and Acute Pain Management.* 1st ed. New York, NY: McGraw-Hill Medical; 2006. pp. 722–4.

A11 D

Table 6.6 Local anaesthetics with their recommended doses

Local anaesthetic	Maximum dose
Lignocaine	7 mg/kg (with adrenaline) 5 mg/kg (without adrenaline)
Bupivacaine/ropivacaine/ levo-bupivacaine	2–4 mg/kg
Procaine	10 mg/kg
2-Chloroprocaine	20 mg/kg

There is greater risk of toxicity with bupivacaine in neonates than adults because of:

▶ Liver enzymes being immature – less metabolism of bupivacaine.

▶ Low levels of alpha-1 glycoprotein – higher free fraction of bupivacaine.

Regional blocks are usually done under sedation in paediatric patients. Therefore, the central nervous system signs of local anaesthetic toxicity are usually masked and the first sign usually detected is **cardiorespiratory arrest**.

• Hadzic A. *Textbook of Regional Anesthesia and Acute Pain Management*. 1st ed. New York, NY: McGraw-Hill Medical; 2006. p. 723.

A12 A Some anatomical facts in neonates and children:

▶ Spinal cord terminates at L3 and reaches adult level of L1 by 1 year of age.

▶ Dural sac ends at S4 in neonates and reaches adult level S2 by 1 year of age.

▶ Sacrum is formed by fusion of sacral vertebrae by 8 years of age.

▶ Tuffier's line passes through L5/S1 junction in neonates and lies at L4/L5 by 1 year.

▶ Epidural space may be found at 1 mm/kg body weight.

▶ There is easy passage of catheter in epidural space, as epidural fat is less densely packed than adults.

• Hadzic A. *Textbook of Regional Anesthesia and Acute Pain Management*. 1st ed. New York, NY: McGraw-Hill Medical; 2006. p. 727.

A13 A

▶ Spread of local anaesthetic correlates better with **body weight than age** in paediatric patients.

▶ Optimum doses for caudal block in children are: 0.2% ropivacine 1 mL/kg or 0.125%–0.175% bupivacaine 1 mL/kg.

▶ Epidural **opioids are avoided in day-case surgery** because of side effects like nausea, vomiting, respiratory depression and urinary retention.

• Hadzic A. *Textbook of Regional Anesthesia and Acute Pain Management*. 1st ed. New York, NY: McGraw-Hill Medical; 2006. p. 729.

A14 D

Table 6.7 Local anaesthetic adjuvants for epidural in children

Additives	Characteristics
Epidural opioids	Avoided in day-case surgeries Side effects like nausea, vomiting, respiratory depression and urinary retention
Clonidine 1–5 mcg/kg	Side effects: hypotension and sedation Ventilatory response to increasing levels of carbon dioxide is blunted
Ketamine 0.25–0.5 mg/kg	Preservative-free solution must be used Its safety for epidural use is not established There are few animal studies suggesting neurotoxicity Side effects: psychomimetic effects
Midazolam 0.05 mg/kg	Preservative-free solution must be used Its safety for epidural use is not established
Neostigmine 2 mcg/kg	Preservative-free solution must be used Its safety for epidural use is not established Side effects: nausea and vomiting

Note: the most common adjuvant used is epinephrine.

- Hadzic A. *Textbook of Regional Anesthesia and Acute Pain Management.* 1st ed. New York, NY: McGraw-Hill Medical; 2006. p. 729.

A15 D

▶ The predominant organism colonising epidural catheter is *Staphylococcus epidermidis.*

▶ The treatment of post-dural puncture headache in children involves **bed rest, sedation and analgesics** like non-steroidal anti-inflammatory drugs. Blood patch may be used if medications fail. The optimum dose of blood for blood patch is **0.3 mL/kg**.

▶ Unlike adults, use of epidural in children is cardiostable and presence of hypotension may indicate intrathecal location of catheter or local anaesthetic toxicity.

▶ Test dose must always be used for epidural catheter, with continuous ECG monitoring for T-wave changes.

- Hadzic A. *Textbook of Regional Anesthesia and Acute Pain Management.* 1st ed. New York, NY: McGraw-Hill Medical; 2006. pp. 730–1.

A16 D Confirmation of epidural catheter position can be done with:

▶ **Ultrasonography**: aids in identifying relevant anatomic structures and placement of epidural catheter. It is reliable only in children aged < 6 months, as calcification of vertebral bodies prevents visualisation after this age.

▶ **Epidural ECG**: T-wave changes help in identifying **intravascular location** of catheter. It may not identify intrathecal placement. The **right-arm electrode** is connected to the epidural catheter, and epidural ECG is compared with standard reference ECG. The amplitude of QRS complex in ECG obtained from epidural catheter increases as the tip reaches thoracic region, where it is comparable to the reference ECG. It can be used to confirm placement of epidural catheter after neuromuscular blockers have been given or local anaesthesia given in epidural space.

Table 6.8 Epidural stimulation test

Electrical current	Motor response	Interpretation (location of epidural catheter)
0–1 mA	Present	Intrathecal/subdural/adjacent to nerve
1–10 mA	Present	Epidural space
> 10 mA	Present	Skin/subcutaneous tissue

▶ **Electrical stimulation test (Tsui test)**: cathode attached to epidural catheter while the anode is attached to skin. Within the epidural space, after correct placement of local anaesthetic, there would be increase in the current threshold current required to produce the motor response. No change in threshold current indicates intravascular placement of catheter. It is not useful if neuromuscular blockers have been administered or local anaesthetics given in epidural space.

- Hadzic A. *Textbook of Regional Anesthesia and Acute Pain Management*. 1st ed. New York, NY: McGraw-Hill Medical; 2006. pp. 731–3.

A17 A

▶ Nerve stimulators used for epidural stimulation test must be able to deliver a current **up to 10 mA**. As the nerve stimulators used for peripheral nerve blocks usually deliver a current up to 5 mA, they are unsuitable.

▶ Epidural-stimulating catheter containing **metal element** helps in proper electrical conduction and decreases the resistance to flow of the current.

▶ The epidural catheter with stylet protects the tip and helps in **easy threading** of the catheter.

▶ The stylet ends 10 mm proximal to tip, forming a **J shape** during insertion.

▶ The ground electrode must be placed on upper limb and lower limb for lumbar and thoracic epidural catheter, respectively, to avoid any error from direct muscular stimulation by the electrical current.

- Hadzic A. *Textbook of Regional Anesthesia and Acute Pain Management*. 1st ed. New York, NY: McGraw-Hill Medical; 2006. pp. 733–4.

A18 A *See* Answer 16.

A19 B

▶ Caudal block can be done with **needles with stylet**, as they provide good tactile sensation and prevent contamination of epidural space with skin tags.

▶ **Intravenous cannulae** can be used, as they aid to detect placement in the blood vessel or bone.

▶ Caudal block can be performed in **prone (adults) or lateral decubitus position (children)**.

▶ Proper identification of sacral hiatus is done by drawing a line between the two posterior superior iliac spines. This line forms the base of an equilateral triangle whose apex is formed by the sacral hiatus.

▶ The needle for the skin puncture must be angulated at an angle of **70°–80°** and the angle must be **decreased to 20°–30°** once the sacrococcygeal ligament is punctured.

- Hadzic A. *Textbook of Regional Anesthesia and Acute Pain Management*. 1st ed. New York, NY: McGraw-Hill Medical; 2006. p. 737.

A20 A For caudal block, the **cannula-over-needle technique** aids in proper identification of the caudal space. The cannula **slides off easily** in the caudal space if the needle is in the right location. It also helps in identifying needle placement in the bone or blood vessel. It decreases the risk of intrathecal placement.

- Hadzic A. *Textbook of Regional Anesthesia and Acute Pain Management*. 1st ed. New York, NY: McGraw-Hill Medical; 2006. pp. 736–7.

A21 D

- The skin to epidural space distance in children is **less** than in adults.
- The mean distance in neonates is around **1 cm**.
- There is **less tactile sensation** on puncturing the ligamentum flavum as compared to adults.
- Sympathetic blockade is well tolerated in the paediatric population, and presence of hypotension must prompt suspicion of intravascular or intrathecal placement.
    - Hadzic A. *Textbook of Regional Anesthesia and Acute Pain Management*. 1st ed. New York, NY: McGraw-Hill Medical; 2006. p. 739.

A22 C

- The distance of the epidural space from skin may be dependent on **age and body weight** of the child.
- The tip of the catheter must be **at the surgical site**, as the distance in children between adjacent vertebrae is very small.
- Because of formation of lumbar curvature as the child grows, threading the catheter into a thoracic location from a lumbar insertion site becomes **difficult**.
- Thoracic epidural block is done via **median approach** in children, compared with paramedian approach in adults.
    - Hadzic A. *Textbook of Regional Anesthesia and Acute Pain Management*. 1st ed. New York, NY: McGraw-Hill Medical; 2006. p. 740.

A23 D

- Cerebrospinal fluid volume in infants is **4 mL/kg**, whereas in adults it is **2 mL/kg**.
- The duration of spinal anaesthesia is **shorter** than for adults and they require **higher dose** of local anaesthetic. Duration of block increases with age.
- For proper positioning in sitting position, **neck flexion**, required in adults, must be **avoided in infants**. Neck flexion may compromise the airway in infants and is not very helpful for spinal anesthesia.
- **Hypobaric** solutions are not routinely used in infants.
    - Hadzic A. *Textbook of Regional Anesthesia and Acute Pain Management*. 1st ed. New York, NY: McGraw-Hill Medical; 2006. pp. 747–8.

A24 D **Bromage scale** is used to assess the spinal blockade in children **> 2 years of age**.

Table 6.9 Original Bromage score

Grade	Criteria	Degree of block
I	Free movement of legs and feet	Nil
II	Just able to flex knees with free movement of feet	Partial (33%)
III	Unable to flex knees, but with free movement of feet	Almost complete (66%)
IV	Unable to move legs or feet	Complete

Table 6.10 Modified Bromage score (Breen *et al*)

Score	Criteria
1	Complete block (unable to move feet or knees)
2	Almost complete block (able to move feet only)
3	Partial block (just able to move knees)
4	Detectable weakness of hip flexion while supine (full flexion of knees)
5	No detectable weakness of hip flexion while supine
6	Able to perform partial knee bend

▶ In children, the incidence of PDPH is **less** than for adults.
▶ Sympathetic blockade is better tolerated in infants, and changes in heart rate and blood pressure are **rare**.
▶ **Preloading is rarely required** in infants prior to spinal blockade.
  • Breen TW, Shapiro T, Glass B, *et al*. Epidural anesthesia for labor in an ambulatory patient. *Anesth Analg*. 1993; **77**(5): 919–24.
  • Bromage PR. *Epidural Analgesia*. Philadelphia, PA: WB Saunders; 1978: pp. 301–20.
  • Hadzic A. *Textbook of Regional Anesthesia and Acute Pain Management*. 1st ed. New York, NY: McGraw-Hill Medical; 2006. p. 749.

A25 A
▶ Spinal anaesthesia is preferred in preterm infants, as it **reduces but does not eliminate** the risk of post-operative apnea.
▶ In their meta-analysis, Coté *et al* identified that the incidence of apnoea is strongly and inversely correlated with both gestational age (gA) post-conceptual age (pcA). Other strong correlations were found with anaemia and continuing apnoea at home. The risk of post-operative apnoea is ≈5% if the gA is < 35 weeks and pcA is < 48 weeks, and risk of

≈1% if gA 35 weeks and pCA 54 weeks.

▶ **Relative contraindications** to spinal anaesthesia include coagulation abnormalities, local infection, raised intracranial pressure, degenerative neurological disease, refusal by parents and presence of ventriculoperitoneal shunts.

- Coté CJ, Zaslavsky A, Downes JJ, *et al.* Postoperative apnea in former preterm infants after inguinal herniorrhaphy. A combined analysis. *Anesthesiology.* 1995; **82**: 809–21.
- Hadzic A. *Textbook of Regional Anesthesia and Acute Pain Management.* 1st ed. New York, NY: McGraw-Hill Medical; 2006. p. 750.

A26 D

▶ **Parascalene approach is preferred over interscalene** in children to reduce risk of complications.

▶ In parascalene approach, **roots and trunks** of brachial plexus are blocked. The needle is inserted at the junction of upper two thirds and lower one third of an imaginary line drawn from C6 to the midpoint of clavicle.

▶ **Axillary block is the most common approach** to brachial plexus block in the paediatric population.

▶ Despite performance of blocks under general anaesthetic, the incidence of complications is **not increased**.

- Hadzic A. *Textbook of Regional Anesthesia and Acute Pain Management.* 1st ed. New York, NY: McGraw-Hill Medical; 2006. pp. 754–7.

A27 D Physiological changes seen with ageing are as follows.

▶ **Central nervous system**:
  - the nerve fibres lose their myelin sheath and are **more sensitive** to local anaesthetics
  - there is **increased permeability** of the dura
  - there is a decrease in cerebrospinal fluid volume and an increase in specific gravity of cerebrospinal fluid, which may explain the **lower dose of local anaesthetic required** in the elderly.

▶ **Cardiovascular system**:
  - there is a decrease in sensitivity of the baroceptors
  - there is **physiological beta blockade**
  - there is increase in systemic vascular resistance as the arteries lose their elastic fibres (**leading to hypertension**)
  - there is left ventricular hypertrophy and **intolerance to volume overload** and a high incidence of ischaemic heart disease, atrial

fibrillation and sclerosis of the valves.

- Hadzic A. *Textbook of Regional Anesthesia and Acute Pain Management*. 1st ed. New York, NY: McGraw-Hill Medical; 2006. p. 789.

A28 D Changes in epidural space with age:
- decrease in fat
- sclerotic changes at intervertebral foramina (decrease in size)
- increase in compliance of epidural space
- decrease in resistance (hence higher cephalad spread).

All these changes lead to **faster onset** of block and **greater cephalad spread** of local anaesthetic. Due to physiologic beta blockade, **epidural test dose (lignocaine with epinephrine) is unreliable**. There is a **non-linear relationship** between local anaesthetic dose required per segment and spread of analgesia.

- Hadzic A. *Textbook of Regional Anesthesia and Acute Pain Management*. 1st ed. New York, NY: McGraw-Hill Medical; 2006. p. 791.

A29 A
- In geriatric patients, there is **biphasic absorption** of local anaesthetics from the epidural space.
- There is an **initial rapid absorption** phase from **increased vascularity** of the epidural space.
- This is followed by a **slower phase** of absorption because of uptake from the **epidural fat**.
- However, the initial absorption of local anaesthetic after **intrathecal injection** is slower because of poor perfusion of subarachnoid space.
  - Hadzic A. *Textbook of Regional Anesthesia and Acute Pain Management*. 1st ed. New York, NY: McGraw-Hill Medical; 2006. p. 793.

A30 C Depending on the clearance, local anaesthetics are classified as:
- high hepatic extraction ratio – clearance depends on **hepatic blood flow** (lignocaine)
- low hepatic extraction ratio – clearance depends on **enzymatic activity** (bupivacaine).

In geriatric patients, **both** the hepatic blood and hepatic enzyme activity are **reduced**. Therefore, the clearance of both lignocaine and bupivacaine is reduced in the elderly. This also explains the need for **reduced doses as well as frequency of doses**. There is **increased sensitivity to opioids**, and so their doses must be reduced.

- Hadzic A. *Textbook of Regional Anesthesia and Acute Pain Management*. 1st ed. New York, NY: McGraw-Hill Medical; 2006. p. 794.

A31 C Advantages of central neuraxial anaesthesia over general anaesthesia are:

- decrease in blood loss
- decrease in stress response
- decrease in thromboembolic phenomenon
- decrease in mortality immediate and at 1 month.

However, the incidence of **post-operative cognitive dysfunction** is **similar** with both.

- Hadzic A. *Textbook of Regional Anesthesia and Acute Pain Management*. 1st ed. New York, NY: McGraw-Hill Medical; 2006. p. 797.

A32 C

- Lumbar epidural anaesthesia paralyses the abdominal and intercostal muscles.
- Therefore the effort-dependent respiratory parameters are affected: **FEV_1 (forced expiratory volume in the first second), FVC (forced vital capacity) and PEFR (peak expiratory flow rate)**.
- Other respiratory parameters are unchanged: tidal volume, minute ventilation, respiratory rate, closing capacity and FRC (functional residual capacity).
  - Hadzic A. *Textbook of Regional Anesthesia and Acute Pain Management*. 1st ed. New York, NY: McGraw-Hill Medical; 2006. p. 830.

A33 D

- Brachial plexus blocks (supraclavicular, infraclavicular, interscalene) may paralyze the diaphragm and thereby **reduce FEV_1 and FVC**.
- Axillary block has **no effect on diaphragm** and therefore on any respiratory parameter.
- Various studies have shown that after thoracotomy, preservation of pulmonary function is **better with paravertebral blockade than epidural or intercostal** blockade.
  - Hadzic A. *Textbook of Regional Anesthesia and Acute Pain Management*. 1st ed. New York, NY: McGraw-Hill Medical; 2006. p. 832.

A34 C

▶ In patients with chronic renal disease, renal blood flow is **not affected by spinal and lower-thoracic anaesthesia**. However, **higher-thoracic blocks** up to T1 have decreased renal blood flow in various studies.

▶ Graft function in renal transplant patients is not affected by either general anaesthesia or central neuraxial anaesthesia.

▶ In uremic patients, there is hyperdynamic circulation, resulting in **increased absorption of local anaesthetic** following peripheral nerve blockade. **Acidosis** increases the free fraction of local anaesthetic like bupivacaine by **decreasing protein** binding. However, uremic patients have increase in levels of α1-acid glycoprotein, resulting in increase in protein binding and decreasing volume of distribution. Thus these two opposing effects try to balance each other, but the effect of acidosis predominates.

- Hadzic A. *Textbook of Regional Anesthesia and Acute Pain Management*. 1st ed. New York, NY: McGraw-Hill Medical; 2006. p. 833.

A35 C Creation of arteriovenous fistula is one of the commonest surgeries in patients with chronic renal failure. Various studies have shown that there is increased blood flow through fistula following brachial plexus block or general anaesthesia. Local anaesthetic infiltration has not shown similar increase in blood flow through the fistula. **The final outcome has remained almost the same, independent of the type of anaesthesia.**

- Hadzic A. *Textbook of Regional Anesthesia and Acute Pain Management*. 1st ed. New York, NY: McGraw-Hill Medical; 2006. p. 834.

A36 A

▶ Local anaesthetics depending on hepatic blood flow for their clearance are said to have **high hepatic extraction** ratio (e.g. etidocaine).

▶ Local anaesthetics depending on hepatic enzymatic activity for their clearance are said to have **low hepatic extraction** ratio (e.g. bupivacaine).

▶ Lignocaine is dependent on both hepatic blood flow and enzymatic activity and has **intermediate hepatic extraction** ratio.

In patients with severe hepatic disease, both mechanisms of clearance are affected and therefore the clearance of local anaesthetics is reduced. But plasma levels do not differ after a single dose of local anaesthetics due to altered volume of distribution. However, there is possibility of local anaesthetic toxicity with continuous infusions, and doses must be reduced. Liver has **dual blood supply**: hepatic artery (25%) and portal system (75%).

Autoregulation is present in hepatic arterial system, but not in portal venous system. Hepatic artery alters its blood supply depending upon portal venous blood flow. This is called hepatic arterial buffer response. A high level of neuraxial block is associated with decrease in the portal blood flow, but hepatic arterial blood flow is maintained.

- Hadzic A. *Textbook of Regional Anesthesia and Acute Pain Management*. 1st ed. New York, NY: McGraw-Hill Medical; 2006. p. 834.

A37 B

▶ Diabetic patients usually have peripheral neuropathy and **require higher stimulating current** to locate nerves via nerve stimulator during peripheral nerve blockade.

▶ Tight glucose control perioperatively is associated with **improved outcome** in diabetic patients.

▶ Regional anaesthesia prevents hyperglycaemic response to surgery by various mechanisms: inhibiting gluconeogenesis, inhibiting catecholamine and cortisol secretion (prevents stress response to surgery).

- Hadzic A. *Textbook of Regional Anesthesia and Acute Pain Management*. 1st ed. New York, NY: McGraw-Hill Medical; 2006. p. 836.

A38 D

▶ Thyroid **neuropathy** is common in hypothyroidism.

▶ It is characterised by a **delay in conduction velocity** on testing.

▶ **Higher intensity** of stimulating current may be required to locate the nerves via nerve stimulator during peripheral nerve blockade.

▶ **Nerve entrapment** is common – median nerve (carpal tunnel syndrome) and CNVIII involvement (deafness).

▶ There is increased risk of injury to nerves at one site if they are compressed or damaged at a different site. Therefore, hypothyroid patients with neuropathy are at **higher risk** of neurological damage following regional anaesthesia. Trivial trauma with the needle during block in patients can lead to neurological deficits: this is called '**double crush syndrome**'.

▶ **Thyroxine** helps in prompt correction of neuropathy, thereby reducing the risk of neurological injury.

- Hadzic A. *Textbook of Regional Anesthesia and Acute Pain Management*. 1st ed. New York, NY: McGraw-Hill Medical; 2006. p. 837.

A39 **B** The most common injuries reported from anaesthesia are in the following order:

Ulnar nerve injury > brachial plexus injury > lumbosacral nerve roots > spinal cord.

Incidence of brachial plexus and ulnar nerve injury is more with general anaesthesia than with regional anaesthesia. In the majority of cases, the cause of neurological injury is **ischaemia, prolonged tourniquet time, stretch, direct trauma and haematoma** compressing nerve or interfering with its blood supply. In patients with mononeuropathy, both regional and general anaesthesia are safe.

- Hadzic A. *Textbook of Regional Anesthesia and Acute Pain Management.* 1st ed. New York, NY: McGraw-Hill Medical; 2006. p. 844.

A40 **C** **Parkinsonism** is characterised by loss of dopaminergic neurons in substantia nigra clinically manifesting as tremor, rigidity and bradykinesia.
General anaesthesia is associated with:

- inhalational agents – may accelerate autonomic instability
- muscle relaxants, controlled ventilation – prolong post-operative ventilator support
- opioids – exacerbate muscle rigidity, post-operative nausea and vomiting
- increased incidence of post-operative cognitive dysfunction.

Regional anaesthesia offers:

- better control of autonomic instability
- avoidance of inhalation agents and muscle relaxants
- less impairment of respiratory function.

Therefore, **regional anaesthesia is always preferred over general anaesthesia** where feasible.

Multiple sclerosis (MS): involves only central nervous system (brain and spinal cord) and not the PNS. It is associated with **demyelination** in brain and spinal cord.

- Lumbar plexus blocks and paravertebral blocks may have a **prolonged duration** of action due to subarachnoid or epidural spread.
- Peripheral nerve block is safer where feasible.
- Patients with multiple sclerosis may have a relapse due to stress of surgery, irrespective of type of anaesthesia they receive.
    - Hadzic A. *Textbook of Regional Anesthesia and Acute Pain Management.* 1st ed. New York, NY: McGraw-Hill Medical; 2006. pp. 844, 848.

A41 **B** Acute spinal cord injury is associated with spinal shock. There are four phases of spinal shock:

- Stage 1: areflexia (0–1 days)
- Stage 2: return of reflexes (1–3 days)
- Stage 3: hyperreflexia (initial) (1–4 weeks)
- Stage 4: hyperreflexia, spasticity (1–12 months).

In the **acute phase** of spinal cord injury, **general anaesthesia is preferred** because of:

- the risk of airway compromise
- haemodynamic instability (relative contraindication for regional anaesthesia)
- the need for deep-vein thrombosis prophylaxis, as there is a high risk of thromoembolism.

However, succinylcholine use may lead to hyperkalaemia if used after 24 hours, because of proliferation of extrajunctional nicotinic acetylcholine receptors.

In the **chronic phase** of spinal cord injury, **regional anaesthesia is preferred** because:

- **Autonomic dysreflexia** is seen after the resolution of acute phase of spinal cord injury. It is seen when the level of injury is **at or above T7**. It is characterised by extreme haemodynamic instability from cutaneous or visceral stimulation below the level of spinal cord injury. If the injury is **below T7**, the risk of autonomic dysreflexia is reduced. Regional anaesthesia may be used in **chronic spinal cord injury**, as it **prevents autonomic dysreflexia**.
  - Hadzic A. *Textbook of Regional Anesthesia and Acute Pain Management*. 1st ed. New York, NY: McGraw-Hill Medical; 2006. p. 847.

A42 **A**

- Myasthenia gravis is an autoimmune disease characterised by weakness and progressive fatiguability.
- There are **antibodies** against the α-subunit of nicotinic ACh receptors at neuromuscular junction.
- Medical treatment includes anticholinesterases, steroids and immunosuppressants like cyclosporine, azathioprine, plasmapheresis and immunoglobulin.
- Surgical treatment includes thymectomy, which can be done under general anaesthesia or thoracic epidural anaesthesia.
- Full coagulation profile must be obtained prior to regional anaesthesia, as

platelet function might be affected by steroids and immunosuppressants.

▶ Bulbar and respiratory muscles may be affected in myasthenic patients hence **supraclavicular blocks should be avoided**.

▶ Metabolism of **ester local anaesthetics** is dependent on cholinesterase activity, and therefore they are best avoided.

▶ Myasthenic patients have increased **sensitivity to opioids and sedatives**, and so these should be used in **low doses**.

- Hadzic A. *Textbook of Regional Anesthesia and Acute Pain Management*. 1st ed. New York, NY: McGraw-Hill Medical; 2006. p. 854.

7

Pain therapy

Questions

Choose one best answer for each of the following questions.

Q1 Which of the following pain scales is **not** used for assessing acute pain?
a. Verbal rating scale
b. Visual analogue scale
c. Numerical rating scale
d. McGill Pain Questionnaire

Q2 Which of the following is not an advantage of simple pain rating scales?
a. They are simple, inexpensive and robust
b. They can be recorded quickly
c. They can be used for assessment of subtle differences
d. They can be used for audit

Q3 Which of the following is **not** a characteristic of the pain pathway?
a. It is an afferent pathway
b. It involves three neurons
c. It involves two ascending pathways
d. Modulation occurs mainly at supraspinal levels

Q4 The following process is **not** a part of the pain pathway:
a. Translation
b. Transduction
c. Transmission
d. Modulation

Q5 Which of the following is an inhibitory neurotransmitter in the pain pathway?
a. Glutamate
b. Substance P
c. Calcitonin gene–related peptide
d. Glycine

Q6 Regarding the 'gate control' theory of pain, which of the following is the **correct** statement?
a. It explains why sometimes we feel pain, while at other times we do not
b. It explains why local rubbing eases the pain
c. It explains why endogenous opioids decrease pain
d. It explains why after a certain threshold, a gate opens and acute pain transforms into chronic pain

Q7 Which of the following part is vital in the descending pain-modulating pathways?
a. Thalamus
b. Sensory cortex
c. Periaqueductal grey
d. Intermediate horn

Q8 Regarding intrathecal opioids for post-operative pain relief, which of the following is **false**?
a. Fentanyl undergoes ion trapping by binding to non-receptor sites, reducing the unionised fraction available for diffusion to receptor site
b. Morphine has a greater cephalad spread than fentanyl after intrathecal injection
c. Diamorphine is ideal for intraoperative and post-operative pain relief for Caesarean section
d. Morphine is suitable for day-case surgery, extending analgesia for 12 hours post-operatively

Q9 Regarding ethnic differences in pain perception and response, which of the following statements is **true**?
a. Ethnic minorities are at a higher risk of inadequate pain control
b. Caucasians have higher analgesic requirements than blacks, while Asians have the least analgesic requirement
c. Ethnicity of the clinician is also important
d. All of the above

Q10 Which of the following does **not** occur in stress response to surgery?
a. Increase in cortisol release
b. Increase in antidiuretic hormone release
c. Increase in insulin release
d. Increase in catecholamine release

Q11 Regarding pre-emptive analgesia, which of the following statements is **incorrect**?
a. It is based on the rationale of stopping pain before it happens
b. It reduces acute post-operative pain and prevents the development of chronic pain after surgery
c. It theoretically prevents central sensitisation
d. None of the above

Q12 Regarding the World Health Organization ladder for cancer pain relief, which of the following is **correct**?
a. Non-opioids are the first line in management, while opioids come next
b. To calm fears and anxiety, adjuvants such as benzodiazepines should be used
c. Analgesics should be given regularly rather than on demand
d. All of the above

Q13 Regarding perioperative pain management in opioid-dependent patients, which of the following statements is **false**?
a. Preoperative 24-hour opioid requirement should be established
b. Transdermal patches should always be removed, as they may interfere with calculation of amount of opioids to be given
c. Pentazocine should be avoided
d. Opioid rotation helps to reduce the dose needed

Q14 Which of the following statements regarding the autonomic nervous system is **false**?
a. They are not under voluntary control
b. Nerves may be myelinated or unmyelinated
c. They help mainly by sensing danger
d. They respond to internal stimuli

Q15 Which of the following statements regarding the autonomic nervous system (ANS) is **correct**?
a. The sympathetic and parasympathetic nervous systems are independent of each other
b. Parasympathetic system is active during rest
c. The effects of acetylcholine are stimulatory
d. The effects of norepinephrine are inhibitory

Q16 Which of the following organs lack a dual innervation from the ANS?
a. Eye
b. Salivary glands
c. Liver
d. Lacrimal glands

Q17 Which one of the following statements **correctly** reflects the difference between sympathetic and parasympathetic nervous systems?
a. Sympathetic systems have long preganglionic neurons, while those of parasympathetic are short
b. Sympathetic systems have long postganglionic neurons, while those of parasympathetic are short
c. Sympathetic postganglionic neurons always release norepinephrine, while those of parasympathetic always release acetylcholine
d. Sympathetic postganglionic neurons sometimes release norepinephrine while those of parasympathetic always release acetylcholine.

Q18 Regarding the organisation of the sympathetic nervous system, which of the following statements is **false**?

a. It originates from lateral grey horns of T1–L2 spinal segments

b. It is organised into two paraverterbral chains on either side of vertebrae

c. Each paraverterbral ganglia receives preganglionic fibres from the white ramus while it passes on the postganglionic fibres through the grey ramus

d. Suprarenal medulla is a modified sympathetic ganglion

Q19 After entering the white ramus, preganglionic fibres of the sympathetic division of the ANS course along which of the following paths?

a. Synapse in the corresponding paraverterbral ganglia

b. Ascend or descend in the sympathetic chain to relay in other paraverterbral ganglia

c. Pass through paraverterbral ganglia without relaying to synapse in the peripheral ganglia

d. Any of the above

Q20 Which of the following statements regarding the sympathetic nerve supply of body parts has both **incorrect**?

a. Head – C1–C4

b. Thoracic viscera – T1–T4

c. Abdominal viscera – T4–L2

d. Suprarenal medulla – T5–T8

Q21 Regarding the parasympathetic division of the ANS, which one of the following statements is **false**?

a. It is primarily craniosacral in origin

b. Preganglionic fibres are long, while the postganglionic fibres are short

c. Most of its supply is distributed through the hypogastric plexus

d. Most of the parasympathetic ganglia are located peripherally

Q22 Regarding the sensory nerve supply of the viscera (general visceral afferents), which of the following is **incorrect**?

a. Most are carried through the sympathetic division

b. They are not involved in referred pain

c. We are generally unaware of these afferent impulses

d. Visceral afferents conduct sensory information to higher centres, but do not relay in autonomic ganglia

Q23 Which of the following reflexes is mediated via the parasympathetic division of the ANS?
a. Direct light reflex
b. Cardioaccelerator reflex
c. Vasomotor reflex
d. Pupillary reflex

Q24 Regarding the performance of stellate ganglion block, which one of the following statements is **incorrect**?
a. It is performed at C6 level
b. Carotid artery is pushed medially
c. Nasal congestion is an undesirable complication of the block
d. Brachial plexus block may result

Q25 Of the following, all are indications for stellate ganglion block **except**:
a. Angina pain after recent myocardial infarction
b. Phantom limb pain
c. Frostbite
d. Raynaud's disease

Q26 Regarding the coeliac plexus, the following are true **except:**
a. It provides sympathetic supply to abdominal organs
b. It lies anterior to aorta at T12–L1 level
c. Block is performed mainly to block the sympathetic fibres
d. It receives parasympathetic supply through the vagus

Q27 Regarding the performance of coeliac ganglion block, which of the following is **true**?
a. Posterior retrocrural approach is inappropriate and hence least commonly practised
b. The solution is best deposited after hitting the transverse process
c. Transmitted aortic pulsations are a dangerous sign and needle should be redirected superficially
d. Landmarks can be the 11th or 12th rib

Q28 Which of the following is **not** a complication of coeliac plexus block?
a. Pneumothorax
b. Hypotension
c. Constipation
d. Kidney injury

Q29 Which one of the following blocks is **correctly matched** with the indication for its use?
a. Coeliac plexus block – lymphoedema
b. Hypogastric plexus block – pancreatic cancer pain
c. Ganglion impar block – coccydynia
d. Stellate ganglion block – hypohydrosis

Q30 Which one of the following terms is **correctly matched** with its definition?
a. Allodynia: an unpleasant abnormal sensation, whether spontaneous or evoked
b. Dysaesthesia: increased sensitivity to stimulation, excluding the special senses
c. Hyperaesthesia: pain due to a stimulus which does not normally provoke pain
d. Hyperalgesia: an increased response to a stimulus which is normally painful

Q31 Which of the following pain rating scales includes psychological assessment of the patient?
a. Brief Pain Inventory
b. Short Form – 36 Physical Function Scale
c. Galer Neuropathic Pain Score
d. McGill Pain Questionnaire

Q32 Which of the following mechanisms is involved in central sensitisation?
a. Increased sensitivity of nociceptor
b. Sympathetically mediated crosstalk
c. Wind-up phenomena
d. Spontaneous neuronal activity

Q33 Regarding the transition of acute to chronic pain, which of the following statements is **true**?
a. Persistent C-fibre activation causes wind-up or central sensitisation
b. Ion channel changes in neuromas following nerve injury
c. Phenotypic switching of $A\beta$ fibres occurs
d. All of the above

Q34 Regarding low-back pain, which of the following is **correct?**
a. Mechanical back pain is not common
b. Lumbar X-ray should always be taken to rule out serious pathology
c. Pain at night is a 'red flag' and should be evaluated further
d. Most are advised a 2-week bed rest

Q35 Which of the following statements regarding spinal disc prolapse is **incorrect?**
a. It is most common at L5–S1 level
b. Severe pain means nerve root compression
c. Most herniations are posterolateral
d. Intradiscal pressures are highest while sitting and bending forward

Q36 Which of the following is **not** a feature of L5–S1 disc prolapse (causing significant compression on the corresponding nerve roots)?
a. Inability to walk on toes
b. Inability to walk on heels
c. Loss of ankle reflex
d. Reduced sensation on lateral plantar foot surface

Q37 Which of the following is **not** a feature of C5–C6 disc prolapse (causing significant compression on the corresponding nerve roots)?
a. Inability to flex the elbow
b. Inability to extend the wrist
c. Inability to flex the wrist
d. Anaesthesia over index finger

Q38 Regarding lumbar facet arthropathy, which of the following is **false?**
a. Facet joints are innervated by the medial branches of dorsal rami
b. Radiation of pain below the knee is uncommon
c. A proper history and clinical examination reliably establishes diagnosis
d. Diagnostic blocks employ only local anaesthetics

Q39 Regarding lumbar canal stenosis, which of the following statements is **correct?**
a. Neurogenic claudication occurs immediately after starting to walk
b. There is an increase in pain after spine flexion
c. Walking uphill is easier than walking on a flat surface
d. Causes inability to ride a cycle

Q40 Regarding sacroiliac joint pain, which of the following is **true**?
  a. It is worse toward the end of the day
  b. Standing on the involved joint relieves the pain
  c. Lasègue's test is positive
  d. Intra-articular injections are an effective form of treatment

Q41 Regarding piriformis syndrome, which of the following is **false**?
  a. It may result from the splitting of piriformis muscle
  b. It leads to sciatica
  c. Pain decreases with hip flexion, adduction and internal rotation
  d. Neurological examination including straight leg raising may be normal

Q42 Which of the following is **not** used in intravenous drug infusion therapy for treatment of neuropathic pain?
  a. Lignocaine
  b. Magnesium
  c. Phentolamine
  d. Ketamine

Q43 Regarding fibromyalgia syndrome, which of the following is **false**?
  a. There are widespread tender points
  b. It is more common in females
  c. It is often associated with psychiatric complaints
  d. It responds best to analgesics

Q44 Regarding post-herpetic neuralgia, which of the following statements is **false**?
  a. It follows acute herpes zoster infection in most instances
  b. Non-steroidal anti-inflammatory drugs are very effective in relieving pain
  c. Amitryptiline is a first-line drug
  d. It is hard to treat once established, and therefore it is best prevented by vaccination

Q45 Which of the following has **not** been found to be effective for the treatment of painful diabetic neuropathy?
  a. Gabapentine
  b. Duloxetine
  c. Fluoxetine
  d. Caspacin cream

Q46 Regarding the neuropathic pain ladder, which of the following is a first-line drug?
a. A non-steroidal anti-inflammatory drug
b. An opioid
c. A tricyclic antidepressant or an antiepileptic
d. A tricyclic antidepressant and an antiepileptic

Q47 Regarding complex regional pain syndrome, which of the following is **false**?
a. Diagnosis is established by one sensory and one vasomotor symptom
b. Complex regional pain syndrome type I is not associated with known nerve damage
c. Injured nerve axons express α2 adrenoceptors
d. Physical therapy is a mainstay of treatment

Q48 Regarding phantom pain, which of the following statements is **true**?
a. It is the pain felt in the stump of the amputated body part
b. It occurs in less than half of amputees
c. It mostly causes persistent pain all the time
d. Mirror box therapy may relieve spasms

Q49 Regarding transcutaneous electrical nerve stimulation, which of the following statements is **false**?
a. It is based on the gate control theory of pain
b. It may be used in epileptic patients
c. It is used for treatment of chronic pain
d. It is contraindicated in patients with cardiac pacemakers

Q50 Concerning acupuncture, the following statement is **incorrect**:
a. It is based on maintaining the balance for a healthy body
b. Scientifically, it may act through the release of endogenous opioids
c. It is effective in the treatment of postoperative nausea and vomiting
d. Acupuncture is more effective than conventional treatments for lower-back pain

Q51 Concerning spinal cord stimulation, which of the following statements is **correct**?
   a. It is based on the gate control theory of pain
   b. The most common indication is failed back surgery
   c. It is contraindicated in patients with major psychological disturbances
   d. All of the above

Q52 Regarding intrathecal drug delivery, which of the following statements is **false**?
   a. It is used when oral or transdermal opioids are having intolerable side effects
   b. Its main indication is cancer pain
   c. Ziconitide is an Na+ channel blocker
   d. Morphine is the gold-standard drug used

Q53 Which of the following statements is **correct**?
   a. Opioid-induced hyperalgesia is a phenomenon associated with the short-term use of opioids
   b. Tolerance occurs because of rightward shift of the dose-response curve
   c. Pseudotolerance results from prescribing a higher opioid dose than is needed by the patient
   d. All of the above

Q54 Which of the following is **not** a risk factor for the development of chronic post-surgical pain?
   a. Increasing age increases the incidence of chronic post-surgical pain
   b. Preoperative anxiety and depression
   c. Invasive surgery
   d. Severe acute postoperative pain

Answers

A1   D Pain is defined by the International Association for the Study of Pain as 'An unpleasant sensory and emotional experience associated with actual or potential tissue damage, or described in terms of such damage'. It is **a multifaceted issue**, having sensory and affective (emotional) component. Hence objective assessment of pain is difficult. Therefore, pain rating scores or questionnaires are often used.

Table 7.1 Commonly used pain assessment modalities

Pain rating scales: unidimensional and more common in *acute* settings	
Verbal category rating scale	None, mild, moderate, severe, unbearable or 1–5
Visual analogue scale	10-cm line with anchor points of 'no pain' and 'worst pain imaginable' at either end; *most common simple scale used in pain research*
Numerical rating scale	Similar to a visual analogue scale, with the two anchors of 'no pain' and 'worst pain imaginable', but has numbers across the scale from 0 to 10 (making an 11-point scale)
Pain questionnaires: multidimensional and more common in *chronic* pain settings	
McGill Pain Questionnaire, Brief Pain Inventory, The Memorial Pain Assessment Card, Neuropathic Pain Scale, Pain diary and so forth	

- Apfelbaum JL, Chen C, Mehta SS, *et al.* Postoperative pain experience: results from a national survey suggest postoperative pain continues to be undermanaged. *Anesth Analg.* 2003; **97**(2): 534–40.

A2   C

Table 7.2 Simple pain rating scales

Advantages	Disadvantages
Simple and easy for the patient	Unable to detect subtle differences
Robust and reproducible	Less suitable for research (semiqualitative)
Rapidly recorded	Not suitable for parametric tests
Useful for audit	Non-parametric tests must be used (larger samples)
	Response can vary (in same and among different patients)
	Subjective measures (inaccurate)

- Coniam SW, Mendham J. *Principles of Pain Management for Anaesthetists*. 1st ed. London: Hodder Arnold Publication; 2005. p. 29.

A3   D Nociceptive or pain pathway is an **afferent** pathway involving:
 ‣ **Three neurons**:
   – First order: peripheral pain fibres (Aδ and C)
   – Second order: nociceptive specific neurons (Lamina I, II) and wide dynamic range neurons (WDR respond to both nociceptive and innocuous pain; lamina III–VI)
   – Third order: thalamic projections to somatosensory cortex.
 ‣ **Two pathways**:
   – Dorsal column–medial lemniscus pathway (touch and proprioception)
   – Anterolateral spinothalamic tract (pain and temperature).
 ‣ **Modulation**:
   – Spinal: most common and at dorsal horn of spinal cord
   – Supraspinal centres.
   - Barash PG, Cullen BF, Stoelting RK, *et al. Clinical Anesthesia*. 6th ed. Philadelphia, PA: Lippincott Williams & Wilkins; 2009. pp. 1474–5.

A4   A Pain processing involves:
 ‣ **Transduction**: conversion of noxious stimuli into action potentials.
 ‣ **Transmission**: conduction of action potential through neurons.
 ‣ **Modulation**: augmentation or attenuation of afferent transmission.
 ‣ **Perception**: sensory and affective by integration of inputs in the somato-sensory cortex and limbic system.
   - Barash PG, Cullen BF, Stoelting RK, *et al. Clinical Anesthesia*. 6th ed. Philadelphia, PA: Lippincott Williams & Wilkins; 2009. pp. 1475–6.

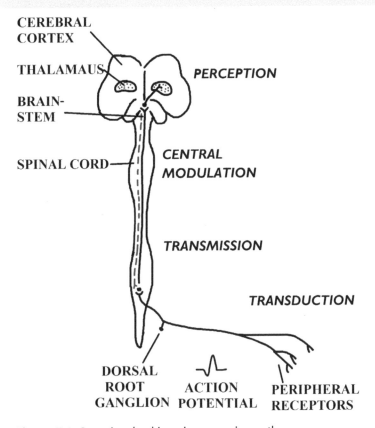

CEREBRAL CORTEX

THALAMAUS

PERCEPTION

BRAIN-STEM

SPINAL CORD

CENTRAL MODULATION

TRANSMISSION

TRANSDUCTION

DORSAL ROOT GANGLION

ACTION POTENTIAL

PERIPHERAL RECEPTORS

Figure 7.1 Steps involved in pain processing pathways

A5 D
- **Excitatory neurotransmitters** – glutamate, substance P, calcitonin gene–related peptide, neurokinins, histamine, serotonin, bradykinins, prostaglandins and so forth.
- **Inhibitory neurotransmitters** – in descending modulation system:
  - Cerebral – GABA, noradrenaline and serotonin
  - Spinal – GABA and glycine.
  - Smith T, Pinnock C, Lin T, *et al. Fundamentals of Anaesthesia*. 3rd ed. Cambridge: Cambridge University Press; 2009. p. 419.

A6 B The gate control theory was presented by Wall and Melzack (1965) to explain factors influencing pain perception. It states that pain is a function of the **balance** between the information through **large nerve fibres** (Aβ) and that through **small nerve fibres** (C). The collaterals of the large sensory fibers (Aβ) carrying cutaneous sensory input **activate inhibitory interneurons**, which inhibit (modulate) pain-transmission information

271

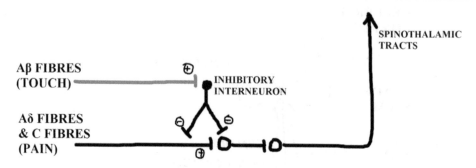

Figure 7.2 Model of 'gate control' theory of pain

carried by the small pain fibres (C). This means that non-noxious (sensory) input suppresses pain, or **'closes the gate'** to noxious input. This explains why rubbing or liniments (balms) reduces pain.

Note: transcutaneous electrical nerve stimulation is a clinical application of this theory.

- Smith T, Pinnock C, Lin T, *et al. Fundamentals of Anaesthesia*. 3rd ed. Cambridge: Cambridge University Press; 2009. p. 425.

A7 **C Descending pain-modulation pathways**: pain-modulating neurons from midbrain periaqueductal grey and rostral ventral medulla alter nociception in the dorsal horn of the spinal cord through inhibition of interneurons. This includes the **noradrenergic locus coeruleus pathway** and the **serotoninergic raphe magnus nuclei pathway**. It also involves endogenous opioid release.

Note: this is the site of action for tramadol, which inhibits norepinephrine and serotonin reuptake inhibition, mediating analgesia. Tricyclic antidepressants are also non-selective reuptake inhibitors, hence valuable in chronic pain management.

- Smith T, Pinnock C, Lin T, *et al. Fundamentals of Anaesthesia*. 3rd ed. Cambridge: Cambridge University Press; 2009. p. 425.

A8 D

Intrathecal fentanyl (acts up to 3 hours)

- ▶ **More lipophilic** but has high pKa of 8.4, resulting in 8% unionised fraction.
- ▶ Ionised fraction binds to non-receptor sites (epidural fat, myelin and white matter) resulting in **'ion trapping'** there.

▶ Lower amount of unionised fraction is available for action by binding to receptor sites in grey matter.

▶ Hence, cerebrospinal fluid (CSF) concentration falls rapidly, while epidural and plasma levels rise rapidly.

▶ This **limits the cephalad spread**, limiting segmental analgesia, but offers lower chances of late respiratory depression.

Intrathecal morphine (acts up to 12 hours)

▶ **More hydrophilic**, hence limited diffusion to non-receptor-binding sites.

▶ Means more is available within the CSF for cephalad spread, hence **greater segmental spread** and more chances of late respiratory depression.

▶ It is **unsuitable for day-case surgery** for the same reason, although it provides considerable duration of analgesia (12 hours).

Intrathecal diamorphine (acts for 6 hours)

▶ Up to 34% unionised drug available for binding to receptor sites.

▶ Characteristics **intermediate** between fentanyl and morphine.

▶ **Ideal** for intraoperative and post-operative analgesia for lower-segment Caesarean section.

▶ It is **unlicensed** for intrathecal use but is commonly used.

- Andrew H. Intrathecal opioids in the management of acute postoperative pain. *Contin Educ Anaesth Crit Care Pain.* 2008; **8**(3): 81–5.

A9 D Ethnic differences in pain perception and response:

▶ **Patient ethnicity** affects pain perception and pain responses to analgesics. In review of 250 consecutive patients hospitalised for open reduction and internal fixation of a limb fracture, analgesic consumption was found to be more in whites than blacks, while Asians needed the least.

▶ **Ethnicity of the clinician** also has an important role in both pain prescriptions and responses to pain relief.

▶ **Sharing a language** with caregivers improves analgesic care.

- Coniam SW, Mendham J. *Principles of Pain Management for Anaesthetists.* 1st ed. London: Hodder Arnold Publication: 2005. p. 67.
- International Association for the Study of Pain. Ethnicity and pain. *Pain: Clinical Updates.* 2001; **9**(4).

A10 C Stress of surgery leads to a **catabolic response** while suppressing the anabolic response. Hence all the catabolic mediators are released (cortisol, adrenocorticotropic hormone, catecholamines, growth hormone, antidiuretic hormone, glucagon, aldosterone), while that of anabolic mediators is suppressed (insulin and testosterone). This leads to hyperglycaemia, protein catabolism, lipolysis and ketogenesis, and water retention by body.

- Coniam SW, Mendham J. *Principles of Pain Management for Anaesthetists*. 1st ed. London: Hodder Arnold Publication: 2005. p. 67.

A11 B

▶ Pre-emptive analgesia is delivering analgesics **before painful stimulus** (surgical incision).

▶ It was first presented by **Crile** (1913) and subsequently developed by **Wall and Woolf**.

▶ Theoretically was based on the idea that preventing nociception early on would **reduce central sensitisation and receptive-field expansion**.

▶ However, most trials have not confirmed the promising principles of pre-emptive analgesia. At most, it may reduce acute post-operative pain, while others have **not found any benefit** for prevention of development of chronic pain following surgery.

▶ 'Anti-hyperalgesics' like NMDA antagonists and gabapentin are being evaluated for this role.

▶ Many have suggested that to be maximally effective, analgesics should be started before surgical incision, continue through the surgery and into the post-operative period until wound healing.

- Dahl JB, Møiniche S. Pre-emptive analgesia. *Br Med Bull*. 2004; **71**(1): 13–27.

A12 D **Regarding the World Health Organization pain ladder**:

▶ It is a three-step ladder.

▶ Non-steroidal anti-inflammatory drugs and other non-opioids (paracetamol) used as first step.

▶ Weak opioids (codeine and tramadol) added next.

▶ Strong opioids (morphine) are reserved for severe pain.

▶ Medications should be given regularly than on a per-need basis.

▶ Sedatives may be given to reduce pain-related anxiety.

- www.who.int/cancer/palliative/painladder/en/

A13 B Management of perioperative pain in an opioid-dependent patient:

‣ **Preoperative**
- Identifying 24-hour opioid dose needed.
- Liaising with chronic pain services and planning analgesia.
- Discussions with patient and reassuring them.
- Patients should continue their oral opioids in usual doses perioperatively.

‣ **Intraoperative**
- Transdermal patches can be **left as such** unless the surgery is major.
- Agonist-antagonists (pentazocine, butorphanol, nalbuphine) and full antagonists (naloxone and naltrexone) should be **avoided to prevent withdrawal**.
- Higher doses (30%–100%) of opioids used by patients may be needed due to tolerance.
- **Opioid rotation** may reduce doses needed by 50% in such instances.
- Neuromuscular reversal towards the end of the surgery allows assessment of respiratory rate. Titration of doses to allow a rate of **12–14 breaths per minute** (in adult) is an effective way of providing pain relief.

‣ **Post-operative**
- Intravenous opioids on an 'as per needed' basis to address initial pain relief.
- PCA subsequently best managed with **basal infusion, with incremental bolus** for breakthrough pain.
- Regular non-opioid analgesics added for opioid sparing if possible.
- Regional anaesthesia techniques help in reducing analgesic requirements.
- Watch out for risk of respiratory depression in patients receiving intrathecal and parenteral opioids.
  - Barash PG, Cullen BF, Stoelting RK, *et al. Clinical Anesthesia.* 6th ed. Philadelphia, PA: Lippincott Williams & Wilkins; 2009. p. 1498–500.

A14 C

Table 7.3 Differences between cerebrospinal and autonomic nervous systems

Cerebrospinal nervous system	Autonomic nervous system
Concerned with response to **external** stimuli	Concerned with response to **internal** stimuli
Subdivisions are: CNS: central (brain and spinal cord) PNS: peripheral nerves	Subdivisions are: Sympathetic Parasympathetic
Under voluntary/conscious control	Under involuntary/subconscious control
Mostly myelinated neurons	Both myelinated and unmyelinated neurons
No relay of fibres in ganglia	**Fibres relay** in peripheral ganglia before supplying target organs
Hence lowermost efferent in **CNS**	Lowermost efferent in **peripheral ganglia**

- Harold E. *Clinical Anatomy for Medical Students and Junior Doctors*. 11th ed. Malden, MA: Wiley-Blackwell; 2006. p. 393.

A15 B

▶ Although most often, the two divisions of the autonomic nervous system have **opposing actions**, this is not always the case. Many organs have **'dual innervation'**, and the two divisions, sympathetic and parasympathetic, work **synergistically to maintain homeostasis**.

▶ Parasympathetic division predominates in **resting conditions**, while the sympathetic division takes over during stress. While the former is usually **inhibitory**, the latter is usually **stimulatory**.

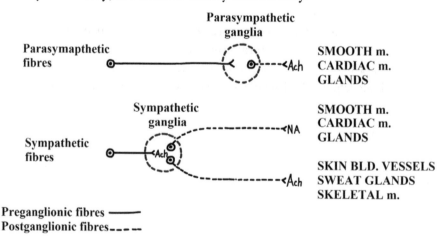

Figure 7.3 Simplistic representation of the two limbs of autonomic nervous system

▸ At preganglionic neurons, acetylcholine (ACh) is **always stimulatory**, while it can be **either stimulatory or inhibitory** at postganglionic neurons. Norepinephrine at postganglionic sympathetic terminals is **usually stimulatory**.

- Martini FH, Timmons MJ, Tallitsch RB. *Human Anatomy*. 7th ed. Benjamin-Cummings Publishing Company; 2012. p. 452.

A16 D

Note: examples of single-organ innervations are:

▸ parasympathetic only – lacrimal glands

▸ sympathetic only – adrenal medulla, arterioles in skin, viscera and kidney.

A17 B

Table 7.4 Differences between sympathetic and parasympathetic nervous systems

Characteristic	Sympathetic	Parasympathetic
Origin	Thoracolumbar (T1–L2) outflow	Cranio (CNIII, VII, IX, X) Sacral (S1,2,3) outflow
Location of ganglia	Paraverterbral, prevertebral and suprarenal medulla	Near terminal organs or intramural
Preganglionic fibres		
Length	Short	Long
Myelination	Myelinated	Myelinated
Neurotransmitter	Acetylcholine	Acetylcholine
Postganglionic fibres		
Length	Long	Short
Myelination	Unmyelinated	Unmyelinated
Neurotransmitter	Usually norepinephrine and sometimes ACh	Always ACh
Divergence and effects	Widespread 'mass action' effects	'Localised and discrete' effects
General functions	Fight or flight	Rest and repose

Note: sometimes, the postganglionic neurons of the sympathetic system may release ACh; for example, **sweat glands and smooth muscles of skin and blood vessels**.

- Martini FH, Timmons MJ, Tallitsch RB. *Human Anatomy*. 7th ed. Benjamin-Cummings Publishing Company; 2012. p. 464.

A18 C The sympathetic division has the following organisational features:

▶ Originates from thoracolumbar outflow, i.e. neurons in **lateral grey horns of T1–L2. Their** axons enter the ventral roots of spinal segments.

▶ These axons may relay in:

– **Paravertebral (or lateral) ganglia**: on either side of vertebral body. Three cervical (superior, middle and inferior), 12 thoracic, two to four lumbar, four to five sacral and one coccygeal (join in midline to form ganglion impar).

– **Prevertebral (or collateral) ganglia**: coeliac, superior mesenteric and inferior mesenteric ganglia. They form their respective plexuses.

– Suprarenal medulla: modified sympathetic ganglia. The chromaffin cells (postganglionic neurons) do not have postganglionic fibres. They are neural crest derivatives.

– **Plexus**: cardiac, pulmonary, oesophageal, hypogastric.

– They receive preganglionic fibres from the white ramus while passing on the postganglionic fibres through the grey ramus. Since the outflow is received from T1–L2, only these spinal nerves have white ramus, while others do not. **However, all spinal nerves have a grey ramus.**

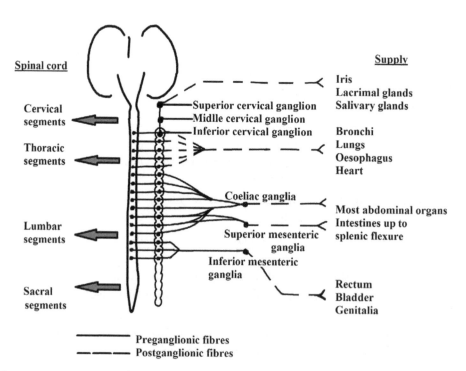

Figure 7.4 Projections of sympathetic nervous system

- Harold E. *Clinical Anatomy for Medical Students and Junior Doctors*. 11th ed. Malden, MA: Wiley-Blackwell; 2006. p. 393.

A19 D After entering the white ramus, preganglionic fibres of the sympathetic division of ANS may course along any of the following paths:

▶ Synapse in the corresponding paraverterbral ganglia. The postganglionic fibres join the spinal nerves through the **grey ramus**, to relay to the **blood vessels** of the skin and skeletal muscles, and in **sweat glands**.

▶ Ascend or descend in the sympathetic chain to relay in other paraverterbral ganglia. This is the cause for the **widespread action** of the sympathetic division.

▶ Pass through paraverterbral ganglia without relaying to synapse in the peripheral ganglia such as **prevertebral ganglia or suprarenal glands**.

- Harold E. *Clinical Anatomy for Medical Students and Junior Doctors*. 11th ed. Malden, MA: Wiley-Blackwell; 2006. p. 398.

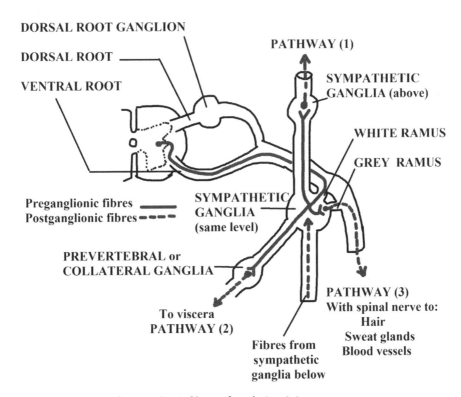

Figure 7.5 Course of sympathetic fibres after their origin

A20 A

Table 7.5 Sympathetic nerve supply of different body parts

Body part	Sympathetic supply
Head and neck	T1–T2
Upper limb	T2–T5
Thoracic viscera	T1–T4
Abdominal viscera	T4–L2
Pelvic viscera	T10–L2
Lower limb	T11–L2
Suprarenal medulla	T5–T8

Note: there is no craniosacral sympathetic outflow. Hence they derive sympathetic supply through nearest sympathetic ganglia. Cervical areas receive sympathetic supply through upper-thoracic segments, while the sacral (pelvic) areas receive same through lower thoracolumbar segments.

- Harold E. *Clinical Anatomy for Medical Students and Junior Doctors.* 11th ed. Malden, MA: Wiley-Blackwell; 2006. p. 396.

A21 C The parasympathetic system originates in the brain stem (**CNIII, VII, IX, and X**) and the sacral spinal segments (**S2–S4 – nervi erigentes**). Hence, it is often called the **craniosacral outflow**. The vagus nerve (CNX) carries 75% of the distribution of parasympathetic division. Unlike sympathetic ganglia, parasympathetic ganglia are quite distant from the brainstem and cord, often located directly on the effector organ itself. Thus the preganglionic fibres are **longer**, while the postganglionic fibres are **shorter**.

- Harold E. *Clinical Anatomy for Medical Students and Junior Doctors.* 11th ed. Malden, MA: Wiley-Blackwell; 2006. pp. 399–400.

A22 B Sensory information from the viscera travels via GVA – general visceral afferents. They are fibres that use the ANS efferents as **a conveyor belt** to send sensory information from the viscera to higher centres. They **mostly use the sympathetic** efferents, but parasympathetic efferents are also used (CNIX, X, and sacral nerves). They **do not relay** in the peripheral ganglia. We are not aware of these sensations unless they cross the **pain threshold**. This may then lead to **referred pain**.

- Harold E. *Clinical Anatomy for Medical Students and Junior Doctors.* 11th ed. Malden, MA: Wiley-Blackwell; 2006. p. 401.

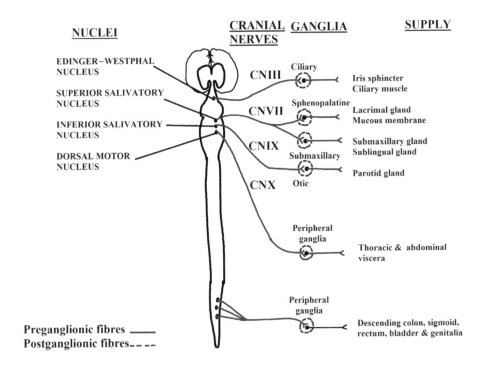

NUCLEI

CRANIAL GANGLIA
NERVES

SUPPLY

EDINGER–WESTPHAL
NUCLEUS

SUPERIOR SALIVATORY
NUCLEUS

INFERIOR SALIVATORY
NUCLEUS

DORSAL MOTOR
NUCLEUS

CNIII

Ciliary

Iris sphincter
Ciliary muscle

CNVII

Sphenopalatine

Lacrimal gland
Mucous membrane

CNIX

Submaxillary

Submaxillary gland
Sublingual gland

Parotid gland

CNX

Otic

Peripheral
ganglia

Thoracic & abdominal
viscera

Peripheral
ganglia

Descending colon, sigmoid,
rectum, bladder & genitalia

Preganglionic fibres _____
Postganglionic fibres-- --

Figure 7.6 Projections of parasympathetic nervous system

A23 A

Table 7.6 Autonomic reflexes

Sympathetic reflexes	Parasympathetic reflexes
	Distension reflexes:
	Gastric and intestinal reflex
	Defecation reflex
	Urination reflex
Cardioaccelerator reflex	Baroreceptor reflex
Vasomotor reflex	
Pupillary reflex	Direct light reflex
	Consensual light reflex
Ejaculation	Sexual arousal
	Swallowing reflex
	Vomiting reflex
	Coughing reflex

- Harold E. *Clinical Anatomy for Medical Students and Junior Doctors.* 11th ed. Malden, MA: Wiley-Blackwell; 2006. p. 465.

A24 B

▶ Cervical sympathetic ganglia are three in number: superior, middle and inferior. They communicate via grey rami with C1–C4, C5–C6 and C7–C8 spinal segments. They have no white rami. The inferior cervical ganglia are fused with upper thoracic (T1 usually) to form the stellate ganglia.

▶ The stellate ganglia lie at the level of **transverse process of the C7 vertebra**. It lies in front of vertebral artery, brachial plexus sheath and neck of the first rib. Subclavian artery lies at or above it.

▶ For a stellate ganglion block, the patient lies supine with the neck **slightly extended**. The Chassaignac tubercle (C6) is palpated between the sternocleidomastoid muscle and the trachea at cricoid level. The operator then pushes the carotid artery **laterally**. After raising a skin wheal, a 22-gauge, 5-cm needle with a 10-mL syringe attached is inserted perpendicularly until the tip contacts the C6 transverse process. The needle is then withdrawn 1–2 mm and is fixed. After careful aspiration, 10 mL of local anaesthetic solution is injected in 1-mL increments.

▶ **Signs of success**: Horner syndrome, anhidrosis, injection of the conjunctiva, nasal congestion, vasodilatation and increased skin temperature.

▶ **Complications**: haematoma, bleeding, pneumothorax, intravascular injections, seizures, spinal cord trauma, unintended nerve blocks (vagus, phrenic, brachial plexus, recurrent laryngeal), QTc alterations.

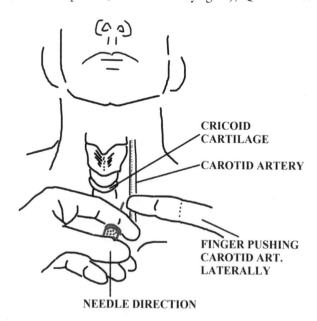

CRICOID CARTILAGE

CAROTID ARTERY

FINGER PUSHING CAROTID ART. LATERALLY

NEEDLE DIRECTION

Figure 7.7 Stellate ganglion block

Note: stellate ganglion lies at C7 (or below), but is blocked at C6 as this is safer. Vertebral artery and subclavian artery at lower levels may increase the risk at C7. Hence a high-volume injection at C6 is expected to do the job!

- Mulroy MF, Bernards CM, McDonald SB, *et al. A Practical Approach to Regional Anesthesia.* 4th ed. Philadelphia, PA: Lippincott Williams & Wilkins; 2008. p. 168.

A25 A

Table 7.7 Indications and contraindications for stellate ganglion block

Indications		Contraindications
Painful states	*Vascular insufficiency*	
Complex regional pain syndrome types I and II	Raynaud's syndrome	Coagulopathy
	Scleroderma	Recent myocardial infarction
Refractory angina	Frostbite	
Phantom limb pain	Obliterative vascular disease	Pathological bradycardia
Herpes zoster		Glaucoma
Shoulder/hand syndrome	Vasospasm	
Post-frostbite	Trauma	
Angina	Emboli	

A26 C The thoracic organs are supplied by **cardiac plexus**, the abdominal organs by **coeliac plexus**, while the pelvic organs are supplied by the **hypogastric plexus**. Of these, the coeliac is the largest. It is also known as the **solar plexus**. It supplies all abdominal organs and intestines up to the splenic flexure. The coeliac ganglia are between two and 10 (average five) in number and lie anterior to the aorta at **T12–L1** level on either side. The supra-renal glands lie lateral to celiac plexus while the stomach and pancreas are located anterior to it. The celiac plexus receives its sympathetic supply through the **greater splanchnic nerve** (T5–T6 to T9–T10), **lesser splanchnic nerve** (T10–T11) and **least splanchnic nerve** (T11–T12). The celiac plexus receives its parasympathetic supply from the left and right **vagal trunks**. The celiac plexus also transits the visceral afferents, which accounts for pain relief following celiac plexus block. The main indication for coeliac plexus block is **pancreatic cancer pain**.

A27 A Various approaches have been described for coeliac plexus:
- posterior (**most common**) – retrocrural, transcrural or transaortic
- posterior paramedian

> ▶ anterior approach
> ▶ endoscopic approach

Posterior retrocrural approach: patient is given **prone position**, and a pillow under the abdomen is used to eliminate lumbar lordosis. Then lines connecting the T12 spine with points 7–8 cm lateral at the lower edges of the 12th ribs are drawn forming a **flattened isosceles triangle**. After raising a skin wheal, a 20-G, 10–15 cm needle is inserted on the left side at 45° angle toward the body of **L1**. Bony contact should be made at an average depth of **7–9 cm** (superficial bony contact at 5–6 cm means hitting transverse process and should never be accepted). The needle is then withdrawn and redirected to slide off the tip past the vertebral body anterolaterally. It is then advanced 1.5–2 cm past this point to feel transmitted aortic pulsations along the needle (which allows the finger holding it to act as a pressure transducer). Once this depth is ascertained, the right-sided needle is inserted in a similar fashion to a depth of 1.0–1.5 cm farther than the left. After checking for blood, CSF and urine, a test dose is given. The main dose is given after this incrementally.

Note: identifying the 11th rib instead of the 12th rib significantly increases the risk of pneumothorax!

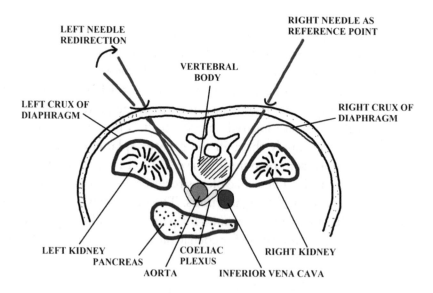

Figure 7.8 Performing a coeliac plexus block (posterior retrocrural approach)

- Mulroy MF, Bernards CM, McDonald SB, *et al. A Practical Approach to Regional Anesthesia*. 4th ed. Philadelphia, PA: Lippincott Williams & Wilkins; 2008. pp. 161–5.

A28 C

Table 7.8 Complications of celiac plexus block

Vascular	Neurological	Damage to visceral
Sympathetic block: hypotension	Lumbar plexus block, Spread to epidural space	Kidney, ureter, adrenal, bowel, stomach,
Haematoma	Intrathecal spread	Pneumothorax
Bleeding		Chylothorax
Aortic/inferior vena cava puncture		
Paraplegia (due to puncture of artery of Adamkiewicz)		

Others:

- infections
- unopposed parasympathetic: **diarrhoea**
- alcohol intoxication or acetaldehyde syndrome.
  - Cousins MJ, Bridenbaugh PO, Carr DB, *et al. Cousins and Bridenbaugh's Neural Blockade in Clinical Anesthesia and Pain Medicine*. 4th ed. Philadelphia, PA: Lippincott Williams & Wilkins; 2008. pp. 1129–31.

A29 C

Table 7.9 Indications of various blocks

Blocks	Indications
Stellate ganglion (*see* previous question)	Hyperhydrosis Limb lymphoedema
Solar plexus (coeliac)	Pancreatic cancer pain
Hypogastric plexus	Pelvic cancer pain
Lumbar sympathetic block	Complex regional pain syndrome Vascular occlusive disorders
Ganglion impar (coccyx)	Coccydynia

A30 D

Table 7.10 Definitions of some chronic pain states

Pain	An unpleasant sensory and emotional experience associated with actual or potential tissue damage, or described in terms of such damage
Allodynia	Pain due to a stimulus which does not normally provoke pain
Dysaesthesia	An unpleasant abnormal sensation, whether spontaneous or evoked
Hyperaesthesia	Increased sensitivity to stimulation, excluding the special senses
Hyperalgesia	An increased response to a stimulus which is normally painful

Note: for a full list, *see* Appendix.

A31 D

See Table 7.11.

- Coniam SW, Mendham J. *Principles of Pain Management for Anaesthetists*. 1st ed. London: Hodder Arnold Publication; 2005. pp. 30–2.

A32 C

- ❱ **Hyperalgesia** is defined as 'an increased sensitivity to pain', which may be caused by damage to nociceptors or peripheral nerves.
- ❱ **Primary hyperalgesia** describes pain sensitivity that occurs directly in the damaged tissues. This occurs by peripheral sensitisation whereby nociceptors exhibit reduction in threshold and an increase in responsiveness.
- ❱ **Secondary hyperalgesia** describes pain sensitivity that occurs in surrounding or distant undamaged tissues. This is a result of **central sensitisation** wherein there is an increase in the excitability of neurons within the central nervous system, so that normal inputs begin to produce abnormal responses.

Table 7.12 Mechanisms involved in hyperalgesia

Peripheral sensitisation	*Central sensitisation*
Abnormal nociceptor sensitivity	Short-term homosynaptic potentiation **(wind-up)**
Spontaneous neuronal activity and axonal sprouting	Long-term homosynaptic potentiation (through NMDA and AMPA receptors)
Inflammatory mediator-induced excitation of nociceptors	Changes in synaptic architecture
Sympathetically mediated pain	Loss of inhibition

- Coniam SW, Mendham J. *Principles of Pain Management for Anaesthetists*. 1st ed. London: Hodder Arnold Publication; 2005. p. 23.

Table 7.11 Pain scales for assessment of chronic pain

Multidimensional pain scales	
Global Impression Of Change Scale	Completed by both the patient and the clinician
Brief Pain Inventory	Worst, best and present pain intensity
Short Form – 36 Physical Function Scale	General measure that is intended to capture quality of life as well as whether an individual is healthy or not
Roland Morris Questionnaire	Back/leg pain
Health Assessment Questionnaire	Difficulty rating of activities

Syndrome-specific pain scales	
Galer Neuropathic Pain Score	For neuropathic pain
Oswestry Disability Questionnaire	For patients with back pain
American College of Rheumatology Response Criteria	Rheumatoid arthritis
Arthritis Impact Measurement Scale	Osteoarthritis
Western Ontario and McMaster Universities (WOMAC) Osteoarthritis Index	Osteoarthritis

Psychological assessment	
McGill Pain Questionnaire	Domains: sensory, affective, evaluative and miscellaneous *plus* a pain-intensity five-point scale
Beck's Depression Inventory	A 21-item self-rating scale that measures the severity of key symptoms associated with clinical depression but not with other psychological factors aggravating pain
Sickness Impact Profile	It is a general indicator of health status and health-related dysfunction rather than pain Best studied in the population with chronic back pain
Minnesota Multiphasic Personality Inventory	This is a self-administered true–false test The questionnaire consists of 567 items and it places patients in one of four groups: hypochondriacal, reactively depressed, 'somaticisers' and manipulators

A33 D **Glutamate receptors (AMPA and NMDA)** have been identified in spinal cord. Activation of these receptors by nociceptive inputs from periphery is involved in development of chronic pain. Hence, NMDA antagonists such as ketamine are used to treat certain chronic pain states. Persistent nociceptive stimulation of C fibres produces hyperalgesia and allodynia through **wind-up phenomena** and **central sensitisation**. Axonal sprouting and neuroma formation subsequent to nerve injury exhibit altered up-regulation of sodium channels, and down-regulation of potassium channels. The net result is increased neuronal excitability. Lastly, sensory Aβ undergo **phenotypic switching** to C fibres and start conducting pain.

- Barash PG, Cullen BF, Stoelting RK, *et al*. *Clinical Anesthesia*. 6th ed. Philadelphia, PA: Lippincott Williams & Wilkins; 2009. pp. 1506–9.
- Palazzo E, Luongo L, de Novellis V, *et al*. Moving towards supraspinal TRPV1 receptors for chronic pain relief. *Mol Pain*. 2010; **11**(6): 66.

A34 C Low-back pain is pain in the lumbosacral region arising from the spinal or paraspinal structures. Sciatica (radicular leg pain) may accompany low-back pain but is regarded as a separate entity. About **50%–80%** of adults experience low-back pain. Most backaches (85%–90%) are simple low-back pain **(mechanical back pain)** in which no particular pathology exists. Non-mechanical backaches may be due to more serious conditions like cancer, infection or inflammatory arthritis. Visceral pathologies may also lead to low-back pain.

Table 7.13 Causes of low-back pain

Mechanical	Non-mechanical (spinal pathology)
Lumbar strain or sprain	Tumours
Degenerative disease	Infection
Spondylosis	Arthritis
Spondylolysis	
Spondylolisthesis	
Disc herniation	
Facet joint arthropathy	
Spinal stenosis	
Osteoporosis	

▶ **'Red flag' signs**: non-mechanical pain, thoracic pain, history of cancer, HIV, weight loss, structural deformity, young (< 20 years) or old (> 55 years), recent trauma, osteoporosis, night pain and bladder/bowel dysfunction.

❯ **Imaging**: should be done only if the history or clinical examination is suggestive of non-mechanical back pain.

❯ **Management**: mostly early mobilisation and pain relief. Physiotherapy may be needed if progress is slow. A minority will need further evaluation and management.

Note: bed rest is not effective and may be harmful.

- Coniam SW, Mendham J. *Principles of Pain Management for Anaesthetists.* 1st ed. London: Hodder Arnold Publication: 2005. pp. 133–4.
- Wallace MS, Staats P. *Pain Medicine and Management: just the facts.* 1st ed. New York, NY: McGraw-Hill Medical; 2005. pp. 141–6.

A35 B A spinal disc herniation is a condition affecting the spine due to tear in the outer, fibrous ring (annulus fibrosus) of an intervertebral disc allowing nucleus pulposus to bulge out beyond the damaged outer rings. Tears are almost always **posterolateral** in nature owing to the presence of the posterior longitudinal ligament. This tear causes release of inflammatory chemical mediators which may directly cause severe pain, **even in the absence of nerve root compression**. They most often result due to wear and tear, and occur most frequently at **L4–L5 or L5–S1 levels**. The second most common site is lower cervical (C5–C6 or C6–C7), while it is uncommon at thoracic levels. The sitting and bending forward position (associated with desk jobs) cause the highest increases in intradiscal pressures predisposing to prolapse.

A36 B

Table 7.14 Neurology in a severe lumbar disc prolapse

Prolapse level	Motor involvement: cannot do	Sensory involvement	Reflex involvement
L2	Hip flexion (iliopsoas)	Groin	
L3	Knee extension (quadriceps)	Anterolateral thigh	Patellar reflex lost
L4	Heel walking (ankle dorsiflexors)	Medial ankle	Patellar reflex lost
L5	First-toe dorsiflexion	Dorsum of foot	
S1	Toe walking (ankle platarflexors)	Lateral foot surface	Ankle reflex lost
Cauda equina	Ankle weakness Lax anal sphincter	Paresthesia of leg and perineum	Ankle reflex lost

- Grady KM, Severn AM, Eldridge PR. *Key Topics in Chronic Pain*. 2nd ed. Oxford: BIOS Scientific Publishers Limited; 2002. p. 24.

A37 C

Table 7.15 Neurology in a severe cervical disc prolapse

Prolapse level	Motor involvement: cannot do	Sensory involvement	Reflex involvement
C5	Arm abduction (deltoid) and elbow flexion (biceps)	Shoulder area and outer upper arm	Biceps
C6	Elbow flexion (biceps) **Wrist extension**	Index finger	Brachioradialis
C7	Elbow extension (triceps) **Wrist flexion** Finger extension	Middle finger	Triceps
C8	Finger flexion and adduction	Little finger	
T1	Finger abduction	Lateral epicondyle	

- Grady KM, Severn AM, Eldridge PR. *Key Topics in Chronic Pain*. 2nd ed. Oxford: BIOS Scientific Publishers Limited; 2002. p. 25.

A38 C Facet arthropathy causes **15%–40%** of cases of low-back pain due to dysfunction or inflammation of the **facet (zygapophyseal) joints**. These joints are formed by the articulation of the articular processes of the adjacent vertebrae. They are innervated by two **medial branches of the dorsal rami** of the corresponding spinal nerves.

The patient complains of deep, achy, non-specific low-back pain localised over the **affected facet joint**. Radiation to the thigh is possible, but radiation distal to the knee is uncommon. The pain is worse with lumbar extension, extensive walking or sitting for long periods of time. The bowel and bladder are not involved. On examination, there is **pain with deep palpation** over the affected facet joint. Paraspinal muscle spasm, loss of lumbar lordosis and limited extension of spine may be noted.

However, historic or physical examination findings cannot reliably diagnose lumbar zygapophyseal joint pain. The most accepted method for diagnosing pain arising from the lumbar facet joints is with low-volume **intra-articular**

injections or medial branch blocks. Diagnostic blocks use only local anaesthetics, and analgesics (opioids) for sedation must be avoided.

- Cohen SP, Raja SN. Pathogenesis, diagnosis, and treatment of lumbar zygapophysial (facet) joint pain. *Anesthesiology*. 2007; **106**(3): 591–614.

A39 C Lumbar spinal stenosis is the narrowing of the spinal canal (transforaminal canal), resulting in nerve compression of the spinal roots laterally. It usually affects middle-age patients (> 55 years). Symptoms include leg pain, weakness, paraesthesia and radicular pain of the involved spinal root. This is similar to vascular claudication, but different in many respects, hence it is called pseudoclaudication or neurogenic claudication.

Table 7.16 Types of claudication and factors affecting them

Characteristics	Neurogenic claudication	Vascular claudication
Aggravating factors	**Extension of spine**: standing walking hyperextension of spine	Any leg exercise
Relieving factors	**Flexion of spine**: squatting/sitting bending forward when sitting walking uphill rather than on flat level lying on side rather than on back easier to cycle than to walk	Rest
Other features	**Pulse**: usually normal **Skin changes**: usually absent **Autonomic disturbances**: rare	**Vascular changes**: blood pressure decreased peripheral pulses weak or absent bruits or murmurs **Skin changes**: pallor cyanosis nail dystrophy **Autonomic**: impotence

Patients with mild to moderate symptoms are treated conservatively, while those with severe symptoms may need surgery (laminectomy) if conservative treatment fails by 3–6 months. In fact, lumbar spinal stenosis has become the most common indication for lumbar spine surgery.

- Siebert E, Prüss H, Klingebiel R, *et al.* Lumbar spinal stenosis: syndrome, diagnostics and treatment. *Nat Rev Neurol.* 2009; **5**(7): 392–403.

A40 D

▶ The sacroiliac joint (SIJ) is innervated **posteriorly** by lateral branches of the dorsal primary rami of L4–S3 and **anteriorly** by lateral branches of the dorsal primary rami of L2–S2. SIJ pain accounts for 16%–30% of cases of chronic mechanical low-back pain.

▶ SIJ pain mainly involves the **buttocks**, although it may be referred to the thigh, abdomen, groin or legs. It may also occur with systemic conditions such as ankylosing spondylitis, Crohn's disease and gout. SIJ pain is **worse in the morning** and can be exacerbated by spine flexion, prolonged sitting and weight bearing on the painful limb. Symptoms may be relieved by flexing the affected leg and weight bearing on the contralateral leg.

▶ Different provocative manoeuvres help distinguish this condition from others causing low back pain. Most commonly used is the **FABER (flexion, abduction, external rotation, and extension** of the hip to create a figure of four: elicits pain) Patrick test. This is used to increase the predictive value and establish the diagnosis. Radiological imaging is used mainly to exclude red flags.

▶ Treatment follows a multidisciplinary approach. Conservative treatments include **exercise therapy and manipulation** (address gait and posture imbalance). **Intra-articular SJ infiltrations** with local anaesthetic and corticosteroids have been found to be effective in most studies.

Note: Lasègue's sign is not seen in SIJ pain (*see* below).

- Wallace MS, Staats P. *Pain Medicine and Management: just the facts.* 1st ed. New York, NY: McGraw-Hill Medical; 2005. pp. 336–7.
- Cohen SP. Sacroiliac joint pain: a comprehensive review of anatomy, diagnosis, and treatment. *Anesth Analg.* 2005; **101**(5): 1440–53.

A41 C The piriformis is a muscle in the gluteal region of the lower limb. The piriformis muscle is part of the lateral rotators of the hip and it **externally rotates the extended thigh and abducts the flexed thigh.** In about 15% of patients, the piriformis muscle is **split** and pierced by the two components of sciatic nerve. At other times, **overuse injury** (common in cyclists, runners, tennis players, ballet dancers) of this muscle may cause symptoms. This causes sciatic compression and consequent **sciatica** (pain in the distribution of sciatic nerve). Pain worsens on squatting, climbing stairs, walking and prolonged sitting. It is **typically unilateral**.

Diagnostic tests include:
- **Pace sign**: pain and weakness on resisted abduction of flexed thigh in seated position.
- **Lasègue's sign**: pain on flexion, adduction and internal rotation of hip in a supine patient.
- **Freiberg's sign**: pain on forced internal rotation of the extended thigh.

Conservative management comprises analgesics, stretching exercises and **deep heat using ultrasound**. Fluoroscopy-guided piriformis injections using **local anaesthetics and corticosteroids** are effective. **Botulinum toxin** injections have shown more effective pain relief. **Surgical release** is the last option.
- Wallace MS, Staats P. *Pain Medicine and Management: just the facts*. 1st ed. New York, NY: McGraw-Hill Medical; 2005. pp. 331–5.

A42 C

- Intravenous drug infusion may be used to treat neuropathic pain. This uses lignocaine (Na+ channel blocker), ketamine (NMDA antagonist), magnesium (NMDA antagonist), adenosine (presynaptic antinociception by preventing release of substance P) and alfentanil (opioid).
- Phentolamine (α-blocker) infusion is used as a **diagnostic test** for sympathetic mediated pain. If positive, the patient is prescribed oral α-blocker such as doxazocin.
  - Wallace MS, Staats P. *Pain Medicine and Management: just the facts*. 1st ed. New York, NY: McGraw-Hill Medical; 2005. pp. 298, 301.

A43 D

- Fibromyalgia syndrome is a disorder characterised by **chronic generalised pain and allodynia**, a heightened and painful response to **pressure (tender points)**. Other symptoms may include fatigue, sleep disturbance, joint stiffness, bowel and bladder abnormalities, paraesthesia, depression and anxiety. It is estimated to affect 2%–4% of the population and is more common in **females** (nine times).
- The American College of Rheumatology (ACR 1990) established criteria for the diagnosis of FMS, including the presence of tenderness at 11 or more of 18 preselected sites (tender points). Additionally, the **Fibromyalgia Impact Questionnaire** is used to assess the impact of pain on a patient's life.

▶ A **multidisciplinary treatment programme** combining behavioural modification, education and physical training is effective.

- Wallace MS, Staats P. *Pain Medicine and Management: just the facts.* 1st ed. New York, NY: McGraw-Hill Medical; 2005. pp. 207–9.

A44 B Post-herpetic neuralgia is a debilitating neuralgia following an acute varicella zoster infection (usually after 6 weeks). Typically, it is confined to a **dermatomal distribution** of the skin. It is difficult to treat once established. Hence both childhood vaccination and early, aggressive treatment of acute herpes zoster infection are vital.

▶ Since it is a neuropathic pain, it is treated first with antidepressants (tricyclic antidepressants like amitryptyline) followed by anticonvulsants (**gabapentin**).

▶ **Opioids** may be needed in some (**NSAIDs are rarely useful**).

▶ **Topical local anaesthetics and capsaicin** may also relieve pain.

▶ **Intrathecal** methylprednisolone with lignocaine as repeated injection can help where non-interventional therapies fail.

- Ramamurthy S, Alanmanou E, Rogers JN. *Decision Making in Pain Management.* 2nd ed. Philadelphia, PA: Mosby; 2006. p. 76.

A45 C Diabetic neuropathies are thought to result from **microvascular injury** involving vasa nervorum, and macrovascular processes of neuronal ischaemia and infarction. Incidence increases with age, duration of diabetes and degree of hyperglycaemia.

Treatments include:
- tight glycemic control
- tricyclic antidepressants: **amitryptyline**
- selective norepinephrine reuptake inhibitors: **duloxetine**
- anticonvulsants: **gabapentine and pregabalin**
- analgesics: opioids
- topical agents: **capsaicin cream** and lignocaine patches.

Note: selective serotonin reuptake inhibitors (e.g. fluoxetine) have not been found to be as efficacious.

- Barash PG, Cullen BF, Stoelting RK, *et al. Clinical Anesthesia.* 6th ed. Philadelphia, PA: Lippincott Williams & Wilkins; 2009. p. 1517.

A46 C The neuropathic pain ladder is different from the World Health Organization pain ladder (cancer pain).
- First line: tricyclic antidepressant or antiepileptic.
- Second line: tricyclic antidepressant and antiepileptic.
- Third line: strong opioid plus above, ± invasive procedures.
  - Allen S. Pharmacotherapy of neuropathic pain. *Contin Educ Anaesth Crit Care Pain*. 2005; **5**(4): 134–7.

A47 A To make the clinical diagnosis of complex regional pain syndrome (CRPS), the following criteria (**Budapest**) must be met:
- Continuing pain, which is disproportionate to any inciting event.
- Must report at least one symptom in three of the four following categories:
  - **Sensory**: reports of hyperesthesia and/or allodynia
  - **Vasomotor**: reports of temperature asymmetry and/or skin colour changes and/or skin colour asymmetry
  - **Sudomotor/oedema**: reports of oedema and/or sweating changes and/or sweating asymmetry
  - **Motor/trophic**: reports of decreased range of motion and/or motor dysfunction (weakness, tremor, dystonia) and/or trophic changes (hair, nail, skin).
- Must display at least one sign at time of evaluation in two or more of the following categories:
  - **Sensory**: evidence of hyperalgesia (to pinprick) and/or allodynia (to light touch and/or temperature sensation and/or deep somatic pressure and/or joint movement)
  - **Vasomotor**: evidence of temperature asymmetry (> 1°C) and/or skin colour changes and/or asymmetry
  - **Sudomotor/oedema**: evidence of oedema and/or sweating changes and/or sweating asymmetry
  - **Motor/trophic**: evidence of decreased range of motion and/or motor dysfunction (weakness, tremor, dystonia) and/or trophic changes (hair, nail, skin).
- There is **no other diagnosis** that better explains the signs and symptoms.

The International Association for the Study in Pain divides CRPS into two types.
- **Type I**: formerly known as reflex sympathetic dystrophy, or Sudeck's atrophy, it does not have demonstrable nerve lesions.
- **Type II**: formerly called causalgia, it has evidence of obvious nerve damage.

pathogenesis of CRPS may include peripheral mechanisms such as **up-regulation of axonal α2 adrenoceptors**, rendering them sensitive to catecholamines (hence the term 'sympathetically mediated pain') and **denervation hypersensitivity**. Central mechanisms such as wind-up and central sensitisation play an important role. **Risk factors** for the development of CRPS include previous trauma, nerve injury, previous surgery, work-related injury and female sex. **Physical therapy** is the mainstay of management. However, pain precludes this, hence pain relief becomes vital to achieve movement. **Sympatholysis** using intravenous regional anaesthesia (lignocaine, guanethidine or bretylium) or sympathetic ganglion blocks are commonly employed to address sympathetically mediated pain. Surgical resection and radiofrequency ablation of ganglia have also been tried.

- Barash PG, Cullen BF, Stoelting RK, *et al. Clinical Anesthesia*. 6th ed. Philadelphia, PA: Lippincott Williams & Wilkins; 2009. p. 1517.
- Wilson JG, Serpell MG. Complex regional pain syndrome. *Contin Educ Anaesth Crit Care Pain*. 2007; **7**(2): 51–4.

A48 D Three phenomena occur after amputation:
- **Phantom sensation** (non-painful paraesthesias)
- **Stump pain** (pain in the stump of the amputated limb)
- **Phantom pain** (pain in the amputated limb).

Salient features of phantom pain:
- Incidence is **up to 75%** of amputees.
- May start immediately but usually starts **within first week** after amputation.
- Most complain of **intermittent pain** (few days in a month).

Pain may be shooting, cramping, burning or aching in nature.
- Pathogenesis may be related to **spinal and cortical reorganisation** of neurons.

Risk factors for development of phantom pain are pre-amputation pain, persistent stump pain, bilateral amputations and lower-limb amputations. Gender and age are not known risk factors. **Pharmacological treatment** includes antidepressants, antiepileptics and analgesics. **Non-pharmacological** methods include TENS, spinal cord stimulation and biofeedback. Recently 'Ramachandran mirror box' therapy has been used to alleviate painful spasms of phantom limb.

Note: pre-emptive regional anaesthesia has not been shown to reduce the incidence of phantom limb pain.

- Jackson MA, Simpson KH. Pain after amputation. *Contin Educ Anaesth Crit Care Pain.* 2004; **4**(1): 20–3.
- Ramachandran VS, Rogers-Ramachandran D. Synaesthesia in phantom limbs induced with mirrors. *Proc Biol Sci.* 1996; **263**(1369): 377–86.

A49 B **Melzack and Wall** proposed that the transmission of noxious information (C fibre) could be inhibited by activity in large-diameter peripheral afferents (Aβ fibre) (gate control theory of pain). In transcutaneous electrical nerve stimulation (TENS), electric current produced by a device is used to stimulate the nerves for therapeutic purposes (analgesia). Two types of TENS are used.

Table 7.17 Types of TENS

Conventional TENS	Pulsed TENS
Low intensity, high frequency	High intensity, low frequency
Mainly for nociceptive pain	Mainly for neuropathic pain
Perceived as a paraesthesia	Perceived as a muscle twitch
Relieves pain by a segmental mechanism	Works by activating extra segmental descending inhibitory pain pathways

- ▶ **Indications** include acute post-operative pain, labour pain, angina, dysmenorrhoea and chronic pain states.
- ▶ **Contraindications** include cardiac pacemakers (interference), pregnancy (can stimulate uterine contractions), bleeding diathesis and epilepsy (may induce seizures).
    - Jones I, Johnson MI. Transcutaneous electrical nerve stimulation. *Contin Educ Anaesth Crit Care Pain.* 2009; **9**(4): 130–5.

A50 D Acupuncture is a complementary therapy that originated in China. It assumes that health is achieved by maintaining a '**balanced state**' of the body, and that disease is the result of an internal imbalance. This **imbalance** leads to blockage in the flow of **qi** (vital energy) along pathways known as **meridians**. Needling increases the cerebrospinal fluid concentrations of the **endogenous opioids**. This may be the reason for the analgesia obtained. Acupuncture has been found to be effective for osteoarthritis, chronic neck pain, low-back pain, and postoperative nausea and vomiting. However, it is **not more effective** than other conventional therapies.
    - Wilkinson J, Faleiro R. Acupuncture in pain management. *Contin Educ Anaesth Crit Care Pain.* 2007; **7**(4): 135–8.

A51 D Spinal cord stimulation (SCS) is the technique of stimulation of large sensory fibres (Aβ) in dorsal column tracts to mask the pain carried by spinothalamic tracts (based on the **gate control theory of pain**). However, it may not be the only mechanism. It is not destructive, unlike cordotomy, and is **reversible**. Major indications for SCS are neuropathic states like failed back surgery (United States) and ischaemic pain (Europe). Nociceptive pain does not respond to SCS. Major psychiatric issues, drug-seeking behaviour, cardiac pacemakers and patients with secondary gain are poor candidates for this technique.

- Wallace MS, Staats P. *Pain Medicine and Management: just the facts*. 1st ed. New York, NY: McGraw-Hill Medical; 2005. pp. 285–9.

A52 C Intrathecal drug delivery systems (IDDSs) are good options for patients who have ineffective pain relief at acceptable oral or transdermal doses, or for those who have intolerable side effects. **Cancer pain (most common), chronic non-malignant pain and spasticity** are three main indications for IDDSs. Morphine is the gold-standard drug used for this. Apart from opioids, clonidine (α2 blocker), ziconitide (Ca+ channel blocker) and local anaesthetics (Na+ channel blocker) are also used. **First-line** drugs include morphine, hydromorphone and ziconitide, whereas fentanyl, clonidine and local anaesthetics are **second-line** agents.

- Intrathecal drug delivery for the management of pain and spasticity in adults; recommendations for best clinical practice (2008). The British Pain Society. Available at: www.britishpainsociety.org/book_ittd_main.pdf

A53 D Tolerance and opioid-induced hyperalgesia result from opioid therapy, but are caused by **two distinct mechanisms**.

- ▶ Opioid-induced hyperalgesia (OIH) is a phenomenon associated with the **long-term** use of opioids. Over time, individuals develop an increasing sensitivity to noxious stimuli (**hyperalgesia**), such that a non-noxious stimulus evokes a painful response (**allodynia**). Mechanisms involved in OIH are: spinal NMDA activation, spinal dynorphin release (KOP agonist) and facilitation of descending inhibitory pathways. Treatment options include:
  - reduction of opioid dose
  - opioid rotation to methadone or buprenorphine (KOP antagonist)
  - NMDA antagonists (ketamine).
- ▶ In tolerance, increasing the dose of opioid can overcome it, but doing so in opioid-induced hyperalgesia may **worsen** the patient's condition by inducing hyperalgesia while increasing physical dependence. It is

important to make a clinical distinction between **tolerance** (reduction in effect needing an increase of opioid dose to maintain pain relief) and **pseudotolerance** (request of more opioids by patient as the prevalent dose is insufficient for treating the pain).

Table 7.18 Difference between opioid tolerance and opioid-induced hyperalgesia

Opioid tolerance	Opioid-induced hyperalgesia
Due to decreased analgesic potency	Due to increased sensitivity (hyperalgesia)
Down-regulation of anti-nociceptive system	Up-regulation of pro-nociceptive system
Rightward shift of dose-response curve	Downward shift of dose-response curve
Responds to dose increase	Responds to dose decrease
Sensory testing reveals no hyperalgesia	Sensory testing reveals hyperalgesia

- Silverman SM. Opioid induced hyperalgesia: clinical implications for the pain practitioner. *Pain Physician*. 2009; **12**: 679–84.

A54 A Risk factors for the development of chronic post-surgical pain (CPSP) are:
- **Age**: decreasing incidence with increasing age
- **Preoperative attitude**: fear, anxiety or depression
- **Preoperative pain**: higher incidence of CPSP
- **Operative technique**: invasive and longer surgeries are more associated with CPSP than shorter non-invasive (laparoscopic) procedures
- **Genetic factors**
- **Severe acute post-surgical pain**
- **Anaesthesia technique**: none shown to be superior, but emphasis is on multimodal analgesia with good pain relief provision for subacute post-operative pain as well.
  - Macrae WA. Chronic post-surgical pain: 10 years on. *Br J Anaesth*. 2008; **101**(1): 77–86.

8

Complications in regional anaesthesia

Questions

Choose one best answer for each of the following questions.

Q1   Which of the following statements regarding nerve injury during peripheral nerve blocks is **incorrect**?

a. Nerve fibres with larger fascicle size are more prone to neurological damage

b. Short-bevel needles are more damaging than long-bevel on intraneural injection

c. Stretching the nerves (extremity) during nerve block is a helpful technique to minimise chances of nerve trauma

d. Peripheral nerve injury is possible even with general anaesthesia alone (without nerve block)

Q2   Which of the following is **not** a risk factor for the development of nerve damage?

a. Female sex

b. Diabetes

c. Elderly patient

d. Morbid obesity

Q3 Which of the following statements concerning the mechanisms involved in nerve injury is **false**?
  a. Lacerations due to needle trauma frequently do not lead to any long-term nerve damage
  b. Pain is the most reliable indicator of intraneuronal injection
  c. Currents less than 0.2 mA pose a risk of intraneuronal injections
  d. Motor response to nerve stimulation may be absent even when the needle is within the nerve

Q4 Injection during a peripheral nerve block should be stopped if the injection pressures exceed which of the following?
  a. 5 psi
  b. 10 psi
  c. 20 psi
  d. 40 psi

Q5 Which of the following statements regarding acute nerve injury is **correct**?
  a. Neuropraxia involves loss of axonal conduction
  b. In neuropraxia, there is loss of axonal continuity and the perineurium is damaged
  c. In axonotmesis, there is loss of axonal conduction but the endoneurium is intact
  d. In neurotmesis, there is loss of axonal conduction but the epineurium is intact

Q6 Regarding local anaesthetic-mediated neuronal cytotoxicity, which of the following statements is **correct**?
  a. Bupivacaine is more toxic than lignocaine
  b. Epinephrine may have neuroprotective effects when used as an additive
  c. Pre-existing neurological conditions do not increase the chances of local anaesthetic–mediated nerve damage
  d. Intrathecal usage is associated with greater potential of neurotoxicity than epidural or peripheral use

Q7 Which of the following regarding tourniquet neuropathy is **incorrect**?
a. Nerve damage is related to the pressures applied
b. Nerve damage is related to the duration of tourniquet time
c. Esmarch bandages are safer than pneumatic tourniquets
d. Wider tourniquets are safer than narrow tourniquets

Q8 Which of the following statements regarding the performance of nerve blocks in heavily premedicated or anaesthetised patients is **true**?
a. Risk of nerve damage may be higher because patient cannot report pain if an intraneural injection is made
b. Premedication offers protection from local anaesthetic toxicity
c. Paediatric patients, who are usually anaesthetised before doing a nerve block, have a higher risk of nerve injury
d. All of the above

Q9 Which of the following techniques may help reduce the risk of nerve damage with peripheral nerve blocks?
a. Short-bevel needle rather than long-bevel needle
b. Visualising needle tip (under ultrasound guidance) before advancing
c. Limiting injection to pressures < 20 psi
d. All of the above

Q10 For a neurological deficit still present 2 days after a peripheral nerve block, which of the following measures is/are appropriate?
a. Rule out a vascular injury
b. Electromyography helps to detect presence of a nerve lesion early
c. Nerve conduction study helps localise the lesion
d. All of the above

Q11 Study of neurological complications after regional anaesthesia has revealed:
a. Most neurological injuries after peripheral nerve block occur following lumbar plexus block
b. Complications following spinal anaesthetic are rare
c. Most of the neurological complications in peripheral nerve block occur while not using the peripheral nerve stimulator
d. All of the above

Q12 Which of the following is **not** a risk factor for the development of spontaneous haemorrhagic complications after anticoagulation?
a. Male sex
b. Increased age
c. Duration of therapy
d. Concomitant use of multiple anticoagulants/thrombolytic

Q13 Which of the following is **not** a risk factor in the development of spinal/epidural haematoma following a neuraxial anaesthetic?
a. Hepatic disease
b. Pregnancy
c. Catheter insertion
d. Preoperative anticoagulation

Q14 For a patient on heparin (unfractionated) anticoagulation, the relative risk of a spinal haematoma is maximum with which of the following options?
a. Patient on aspirin and heparin
b. Traumatic puncture
c. Neuraxial puncture after 1 hour of unfractionated heparin administration
d. Neuraxial puncture within 1 hour of unfractionated heparin administration.

Q15 Which of the following vitamin K–dependent coagulation factors has the shortest half-life?
a. Factor II
b. Factor VII
c. Factor IX
d. Factor X

Q16 A patient with a history of atrial fibrillation and a mechanical cardiac valve on lifelong warfarin therapy (5 mg daily), has presented for an elective total knee replacement. Before placing an epidural catheter for the patient, one should do all of the following **except**:
a. Determine the international normalised ratio (INR) if the last dose of warfarin was given 3 days ago
b. Use blood products to reverse the effects of warfarin
c. Start the patient on heparin after discontinuing warfarin
d. None of the above (all are correct)

Q17 Regarding the use of perioperative warfarin, which of the following is the **correct** statement?
a. Adequate levels of coagulation factors are reached when INR returns to normal range
b. The American Society of Regional Anesthesia and Pain Medicine recommends a value of INR < 2 before undertaking a neuraxial block
c. Factor levels of 20% of baseline are adequate for haemostasis
d. Higher concentrations of local anaesthetics should be used to reduce total dose needed

Q18 While performing a spinal anaesthetic, aspirin should be stopped:
a. 5 days before surgery
b. 24 hours before surgery
c. 10 days before surgery
d. It need not be stopped

Q19 A parturient patient on low-dose low molecular weight heparin for venous thromboprophylaxis may have a labour epidural for pain relief after:
a. 4 hours following last dose
b. 12 hours following last dose
c. 24 hours following last dose
d. Timing is irrelevant, as this is a low-dose therapy

Q20 Which of the following regarding epidural haematoma is **false**?
a. It is most common in the thoracic region
b. Old age increases the chances of epidural haematoma
c. Epidural haematoma usually presents itself after 6–12 hours of an epidural
d. Magnetic resonance imaging is the investigation of choice

Q21 Which of the following is/are a risk factor/s for the development of central neuraxial infections?
a. Diabetes
b. Steroid therapy
c. Chronic catheter placement
d. All of the above

Q22 Regarding meningitis after dural puncture (while doing a spinal), what is the most commonly found organism?

a. *Neisseria meningitides*

b. *Streptococcus viridians*

c. *Staphylococcus aureus*

d. *Pseudomonas aeruginosa*

Q23 Which of the following organisms is most commonly responsible for epidural abscess?

a. *Neisseria meningitides*

b. *Streptococcus viridians*

c. *Staphylococcus aureus*

d. *Pseudomonas aeruginosa*

Q24 Which of the following organisms is most frequently associated with infection following peripheral nerve blocks?

a. *Staphylococcus aureus*

b. *Pseudomonas aeruginosa*

c. *Enterococcus*

d. *Staphylococcus epidermidis*

Q25 Which of the following has not been conclusively shown to reduce infections while performing a peripheral nerve block?

a. Washing hands before procedure

b. Cleaning skin with alcohol-based antiseptic

c. Wearing sterile gloves

d. Wearing sterile gown

Q26 Local anaesthetic may cause all of the following **except**:

a. Anaphylaxis

b. Myotoxicity

c. Convulsions

d. Adhesive arachnoiditis

Q27 Regarding factors determining local anaesthetic (LA) toxicity, which of the following statements is **incorrect**?
  a. Ester LAs are less toxic than amide LAs
  b. Total dose administered is an important factor
  c. Weight of the patient correlates well with the peak plasma concentration
  d. Bigger side chains on LA increase toxicity

Q28 Systemic absorption of LA is fastest from which of the following sites?
  a. Subcutaneous
  b. Intrathecal
  c. Intercostal
  d. Caudal

Q29 Which of the following is **correct** regarding LA toxicity?
  a. Progestrone reduces sensitivity to LA in pregnancy
  b. LA toxicity is additive when different LAs are added as a mixture
  c. Acidosis and hypercarbia are protective
  d. Midazolam premedication offers no benefit

Q30 Receptors mediating LA toxicity are:
  a. Na+ channels
  b. Voltage-gated K+ channels
  c. Voltage-gated Ca+ channels
  d. All of the above

Q31 Which of the following regarding LA toxicity is **false**?
  a. Central nervous system (CNS) depression occurs first, followed by excitation at higher doses
  b. Circumoral numbness may be the first manifestation of LA toxicity
  c. Bupivacaine is more cardiotoxic than ropivacaine
  d. Bupivacaine toxicity may cause simultaneous CNS and cardiovascular system toxicity

Q32 Which of the following is **not** an accepted recommended dose of LA?
  a. Lignocaine with epinephrine 6–7 mg/kg
  b. Bupivacaine without epinephrine 2 mg/kg
  c. Ropivacaine without epinephrine 3 mg/kg
  d. Levo-bupivacaine without epinephrine 4 mg/kg

Q33 Measures minimising likelihood of LA toxicity include all except which of the following?
a. Smallest dose possible for the given procedure
b. Adequate patient monitoring
c. Fractionation of the dose while injecting
d. Use of test dose

Q34 Which of the following statements is **true** regarding treatment of LA systemic toxicity?
a. Lignocaine may be used to treat bupivacaine-induced arrhythmias
b. Amiodarone is the drug of choice for treating arrhythmias
c. Propofol may be used instead of Intralipid
d. Recovery from LA-induced circulatory arrest usually takes < 30 minutes

Q35 Which one of the following statements is **true** regarding Intralipid rescue therapy?
a. Intralipid is available as 5% lipid solution
b. There is no need to give CPR if one is using Intralipid for cardiac arrest
c. Initial dose is 1.5 mL/kg over 1 minute, followed by infusion of 0.25 mL/kg/min
d. Intralipid acts as an Na+ channel stimulant, reversing inhibition by LA

Q36 Regarding adverse reactions to LA, which is **correct**?
a. Para-amino benzoic acid (PABA)-related allergy is seen with amide LAs
b. Preservatives like methylparaben in ester LA are non-allergenic
c. Cauda equina syndrome seen with 2-chlorprocaine was attributed to sodium metabisulphite
d. Overall, amide LAs are more allergenic than ester LAs

Q37 Regarding cauda equina syndrome due to LA, which of the following statements is **correct**?
a. Associated with the use of wide-bore epidural catheters
b. Caused by maldistribution of LA in the intrathecal space
c. Emergent surgical decompression improves outcome
d. All of the above

Q38 Which of the following regarding transient neurologic symptoms is **incorrect**?
   a. Due to LA-induced neurotoxicity (neurologic)
   b. Present with aching/pain in one or both buttocks
   c. Resolve in a few days
   d. NSAIDs are useful for treatment

Answers

A1 C Regarding peripheral nerve injuries:
> ▶ Occur even with general anaesthesia (without nerve block). **Ulnar nerve injury** is the most frequent nerve injury.
> ▶ Larger fascicle size makes the nerve **more prone** to damage, as it can accommodate the tip of the needle and an intraneural injection can occur.
> ▶ Stretching the nerve during peripheral nerve block can lead to **pressure injury** (as the connective tissue may be poorly compliant).
> ▶ Shorter-bevel needles push the nerve away rather than cut it (like long-bevel needles), but should an intraneural injection occur, subsequent nerve injury can be **much worse**.
>   • Hadzic A. *Textbook of Regional Anesthesia and Acute Pain Management.* 1st ed. New York, NY: McGraw-Hill Medical; 2006. pp. 970–1.
>   • Neal JM, Rathmell JP. *Complications in Regional Anesthesia and Pain Medicine.* 1st ed. Philadelphia, PA: Saunders; 2006. pp. 127, 130–1.

A2 A Risk factors for the development of nerve damage are as follows.
> ▶ **Patient-related factors**: male sex, elderly, very thin or very obese, pre-existing diabetes or neurological damage.
> ▶ **Surgical factors**: infection, inflammation, vascular compromise, tourniquet-induced ischaemia, stretch, positional and compression injury.
> ▶ **Anaesthetic factors**: needle trauma and local anaesthetic- and adrenaline-induced neurocytotoxicity.
>   • Neal JM, Rathmell JP. *Complications in Regional Anesthesia and Pain Medicine.* 1st ed. Philadelphia, PA: Saunders; 2006. p. 126.

A3 B Mechanically, laceration due to needle trauma, stretch injury due to exaggerated positioning, and intraneuronal injections can lead to nerve damage.
> ▶ **Lacerations** by sharp needles (clear-cut wound) may be less injurious than **intrafascicular injections**, which may lead to extensive disruption of fascicular architecture.
> ▶ **Pain on injection is an unreliable indicator of intraneural injections**. Paraesthesia may not be a risk factor for nerve damage, and stopping

injection upon paraesthesia may not reduce the chances of ensuing nerve damage.

▶ Stimulating currents **less than 0.2 mA** are associated with a higher chance of needle tip lying within the nerve. Hence injections should be made within a range of **0.2–0.5 mA**.

▶ **Motor responses may not always be seen with stimulation.** They may be absent even when the needle tip is within the nerve itself! Hence nerve stimulators may not prevent nerve injuries.

- Hadzic A. *Textbook of Regional Anesthesia and Acute Pain Management.* 1st ed. New York, NY: McGraw-Hill Medical; 2006. pp. 972–3.

A4   C Intraneural injection may be of two types:

▶ **Interfascicular/extrafascicular**: when the injection is within the nerve, but between the fascicles of the nerve. This may be more common, and the developing block may be faster than usual and prolonged in duration. Neural injury may not develop secondary to interfascicular injections.

▶ **Intrafascicular**: when the injection is made within the nerve, and within a fascicle. This disrupts the fascicular architecture and leads to extensive injury. This may be accompanied by pain, paraesthesia and difficulty in injecting (pressures exceeding 20 psi).

- Hadzic A. *Textbook of Regional Anesthesia and Acute Pain Management.* 1st ed. New York, NY: McGraw-Hill Medical; 2006. p. 974.
- Neal JM, Rathmell JP. *Complications in Regional Anesthesia and Pain Medicine.* 1st ed. Philadelphia, PA: Saunders; 2006. p. 135.

A5 C

Table 8.1 Classification of acute nerve injuries

Seddon type	Sunderland class	Damaged structures	Intact structures	Functional damage
Neuropraxia	1	Myelin damage	Most	Conduction delay
Axonotmesis	2	Loss of axonal continuity	Endoneurium, perineurium and epineurium intact	No conduction
	3	Loss of axonal continuity Endoneurium damaged	Perineurium and epineurium intact	No conduction
	4	Loss of axonal continuity Endoneurium and perineurium damaged	Only epineurium intact	No conduction
Neurotmesis	5	Loss of axonal continuity Endoneurium, perineurium and epineurium damaged	No layer intact	No conduction

Note: prognosis is best in neuropraxia and worst in neurotmesis.

A6 D Local anaesthetics may have neurocytotoxic effects mediated via:
  ▶ mitochondrial damage leading to loss of adenosine triphosphate production, accumulation of intracellular calcium, activation of caspaces and ensuing apoptosis
  ▶ blockade of axonal transport
  ▶ disruption of cell membranes.

The cytotoxic potential is greater with:
  ▶ lignocaine and tetracaine than bupivacaine (although systemic toxicity is in the order tetracaine > bupivacaine > lignocaine)
  ▶ addition of epinephrine
  ▶ higher concentration of local anaesthetic
  ▶ prolonged exposure
  ▶ nerve stretching
  ▶ pre-existing neurological condition (**'double crush syndrome'**)

▶ intrathecal use rather than epidural or peripheral use.

- Hadzic A. *Textbook of Regional Anesthesia and Acute Pain Management*. 1st ed. New York, NY: McGraw-Hill Medical; 2006. pp. 976–7.
- Neal JM, Rathmell JP. *Complications in Regional Anesthesia and Pain Medicine*. 1st ed. Philadelphia, PA: Saunders; 2006. pp. 126, 133.

A7   **C** Features of '**tourniquet-induced neuropathy**':
- ▶ Incidence of 1 : 8000.
- ▶ Varies in severity from neuropraxia to permanent nerve damage.
- ▶ Associated with higher than recommended pressures.
- ▶ Duration of application should not exceed **90–120 minutes** without a 10- to 15-minute deflation period.
- ▶ Esmarch bandages may generate very high pressures immediately under the bandage (so should be avoided as sole method of tourniquet).
- ▶ Wider cuffs generate lower pressures than narrow cuffs (so are preferred).
- ▶ **Optimal cuff inflation pressure** in upper limb is 'LOP' plus 50 mmHg, while in the lower limb it is 'LOP' plus 75 mmHg.

Note: **Limb occlusion pressure (LOP)** is the minimum pressure required to stop the flow of arterial blood into the limb distal to the cuff. It may be measured by a Doppler probe.

- Hadzic A. *Textbook of Regional Anesthesia and Acute Pain Management*. 1st ed. New York, NY: McGraw-Hill Medical; 2006. p. 978.
- Murphy CG, Winter DC, Bouchier-Hayes DJ. Tourniquet injuries: pathogenesis and modalities for attenuation. *Acta Orthop Belg*. 2005; **71**(6): 635–45.

A8   **B**

Table 8.2 Nerve blocks under heavy premedication or general anaesthesia

Concern	Fact
Patients may not be able to report pain	Pain is an unreliable indicator of nerve injury
	Stopping injection after pain does not prevent the development of nerve damage
	'Pressure paraesthesia' is normal
Premedication diminishes the patient's ability to report early indicators of local anaesthetic toxicity	Premedication has anticonvulsive actions which may offer protection from local anaesthetic toxicity
	With general anaesthesia, airway is already secured, helping cardiopulmonary resuscitation should cardiovascular problems develop
Paediatric population	Are regularly anaesthetised for blocks
	Do not show greater risk of nerve damage than adults

- Hadzic A. *Textbook of Regional Anesthesia and Acute Pain Management*. 1st ed. New York, NY: McGraw-Hill Medical; 2006. pp. 981–3.

A9   D

Table 8.3 Recommendations to reduce the chance of nerve damage during a peripheral nerve block (PNB)

Equipment:	Technique:
Short-bevel/Tuohy needle less likely to enter nerves than long-bevel	Strict asepsis
Use correct-length needles	Advance needle slowly (peripheral nervous system), and only after identifying needle tip (ultrasound guidance)
Use pressure indicators (B-smart)	
Accurate peripheral nervous system	Fractionation of injections
Right probe for the given block (e.g. high frequency for superficial blocks)	Avoid rapid injections
Ultrasound guidance vs peripheral nervous system	Avoid injections when unusual high pressures are required
Echogenic vs non-echogenic needles	Avoid injection when patient complaint of pain (always ask where and what kind of pain)
	Avoid heavy premedication
	Adequately experienced operator
	Avoid repeating block
Drugs:	**Patient:**
Avoid high concentration of adrenaline (1 : 400 000 than 1 : 200 000)	Keep patient awake when you can
Lower-toxicity drugs (ropivacaine than bupivacaine)	

A10   A Regarding nerve damage after a PNB:

- It usually presents after **48 hours** of recession of the block.
- **Motor loss** is more informative than sensory loss in assessment of injury.
- First thing to do is to **exclude any vascular compromise** (arterial/venous). A Doppler may be used to do this. If such a compromise is found, surgical exploration may be needed.
- If there is no vascular compromise, then the next thing to do is to obtain an **evaluation by a neurologist**.
- Diagnostic tests may include those shown in Table 8.4.

Table 8.4 Testing following a peripheral nerve injury

Test	When and why
Nerve conduction study: measures amplitude, time for signal transmission and conduction velocity	*Why?* It helps to **detect** a nerve lesion *When?* Within 1–2 days of nerve damage *Amplitude* reduces in axonal injury *Velocity* reduces in myelin damage
Electromyography: measures muscle depolarisation	*Why?* It helps to **locate** a nerve lesion *When?* From 2 to 4 weeks after nerve injury Muscle defibrillation occurs 2–4 weeks after denervation
High-frequency ultrasound	**Morphological changes** in peripheral nerves (like nerve swelling, rupture, compression and so forth)
Magnetic resonance imaging (neurography)	Demonstrates **nerve anatomy** and can reveal nerve swelling, rupture or compression *It is the **earliest method** to detect nerve injury (24 hours)*

- Hadzic A. *Textbook of Regional Anesthesia and Acute Pain Management*. 1st ed. New York, NY: McGraw-Hill Medical; 2006. pp. 988–91.
- Neal JM, Rathmell JP. *Complications in Regional Anesthesia and Pain Medicine*. 1st ed. Philadelphia, PA: Saunders; 2006. p. 137.

A11 A A prospective French survey reported 56 major complications in 158 083 regional anaesthesia procedures performed (3.5/10 000). They noted a higher complication rate with **lumbar plexus block** than other PNBs. **Spinal anaesthetics** were more commonly associated with complications than epidurals or PNBs. Out of 12 patients with nerve damage subsequent to PNB, blocks in nine were performed using a peripheral nerve stimulator.

- Auroy Y, Benhamou D, Bargues L, *et al*. Major complications of regional anesthesia in France: the SOS Regional Anesthesia Hotline Service. *Anesthesiology*. 2002; **97**(5): 1274–80.

A12 A Risk factors for the development of **spontaneous** haemorrhagic complications after anticoagulation include:
- elderly/females/low weight (< 100 lb): higher chance of inappropriately more anticoagulation than expected because of lower metabolic capacity or lower weight

- intensity of anticoagulation
- prolonged duration of therapy
- concomitant therapy with multiple agents
- history of gastrointestinal bleed.
  - Neal JM, Rathmell JP. *Complications in Regional Anesthesia and Pain Medicine*. 1st ed. Philadelphia, PA: Saunders; 2006. p. 18.

A13 B Risk factors for development of spinal/epidural haematoma following a **neuraxial anaesthetic** include:
- **Patient factors**: elderly, females, low weight, hepatic or renal disease, congenital or acquired spinal abnormality.
- **Anaesthetic factors**: wide-gauge needles rather than finer gauge, use of spinal/epidural catheters, multiple attempts and difficulty in needle placement.
- **Drug factors**: preoperative anticoagulation, type of drug being used (maximum with thrombolytic drug), combination of drugs and early post-operative drug therapy.
  - Neal JM, Rathmell JP. *Complications in Regional Anesthesia and Pain Medicine*. 1st ed. Philadelphia, PA: Saunders; 2006. p. 20.

A14 B For a patient on heparin anticoagulation, the relative risk of a spinal haematoma is in the following increasing order:
- neuraxial puncture after 1 hour of unfractionated heparin administration – **least risk**
- neuraxial puncture within 1 hour of unfractionated heparin administration
- patient on aspirin (along with heparin)
- traumatic puncture – **maximum risk**.

Note: also *see* Appendix for recommended times before/after puncture/catheter placement/removal.
  - Neal JM, Rathmell JP. *Complications in Regional Anesthesia and Pain Medicine*. 1st ed. Philadelphia, PA: Saunders; 2006. p. 18.

A15 B

Table 8.5 Half-lives of vitamin K–dependent coagulation factors

Factor	Half-life (hours)
VII	6
IX	24
X	25–60
II	50–80

- Neal JM, Rathmell JP. *Complications in Regional Anesthesia and Pain Medicine.* 1st ed. Philadelphia, PA: Saunders; 2006. p. 24.

A16 B In a patient with atrial fibrillation and a mechanical cardiac valve on lifelong warfarin therapy (5 mg daily) for an **elective** total knee replacement, important considerations are outlined in Table 8.6.

Table 8.6 Considerations for neuraxial block in anticoagulated patient

Consideration	Interpretation	Action
Long-duration warfarin therapy	Action persists for 4–6 days after stopping warfarin (till new factors are synthesised)	**Monitor and document INR** before neuraxial block
This patient is at a **high risk** of venous thromboembolic (VTE) complications	There is a need to continue anticoagulation up to the day of surgery	**Start heparin** after stopping warfarin (unfractionated/low molecular weight)
Elective case	No indication for fresh frozen plasma	Use **only vitamin K** to reverse warfarin or postpone surgery if needed
Postoperative venous thromboprophylaxis after **major surgery** in a patient at **high risk of VTE**	Cannot give warfarin post-operatively (only used in patients with **low risk of VTE**) or Low molecular weight heparin in high therapeutic doses (only used in patients with **minor surgery**)	Use low molecular weight heparin in low doses (prophylactic)

- Horlocker TT, Wedel DJ, Rowlingson JC, *et al.* Regional anesthesia in the patient receiving antithrombotic or thrombolytic therapy. American Society of Regional Anesthesia and Pain Medicine. Evidence-Based Guidelines (Third Edition). *Reg Anesth Pain Med.* 2010; **35**(1): 64–101.

A17 **A** Regarding perioperative warfarin use:

▶ It takes **3–5 days** to achieve therapeutic anticoagulation with warfarin.

▶ Return of **INR to normal range** reflects adequate levels of anticoagulants, hence should be sought before a neuraxial block.

▶ ASRA recommends a value of **INR < 1.5** before undertaking a neuraxial block.

▶ Factor levels of **40%** of baseline are adequate for haemostasis.

▶ In those patients with an indwelling epidural catheter, if INR > 3 postoperatively, then warfarin dose should be withheld or reduced to reduce chances of neurological complications.

▶ **Dilute concentration** of local anaesthetics should be used to avoid motor block (which may interfere with neurological assessment).

- Hadzic A. *Textbook of Regional Anesthesia and Acute Pain Management.* 1st ed. New York, NY: McGraw-Hill Medical; 2006. pp. 1002–3.
- Neal JM, Rathmell JP. *Complications in Regional Anesthesia and Pain Medicine.* 1st ed. Philadelphia, PA: Saunders; 2006. p. 24.

A18 **D**

▶ Antiplatelet agents irreversibly inhibit platelet cyclooxygenase and hence prolong surgical bleeding.

▶ However, **aspirin** and **NSAIDs** have not been found to be a risk factor for bloody needle or catheter placement and they **need not be stopped** preoperatively (for a spinal anaesthetic).

▶ But **clopidogrel** and **ticlopidine** should be stopped 7 days and 10 days before spinal anaesthetic, respectively.

▶ Platelet glycoprotein **IIb/IIIa inhibitors** have to be stopped **8–48 hours** before needling.

▶ Herbal remedies like **garlic, ginkgo or ginseng** may affect platelet aggregation, but **no evidence** suggests that they need to be discontinued prior to surgery.

Note: also *see* Appendix for recommended times before/after puncture/catheter placement/removal.

- Hadzic A. *Textbook of Regional Anesthesia and Acute Pain Management.* 1st ed. New York, NY: McGraw-Hill Medical; 2006. p. 1008.

A19 **B**

▶ Unfractionated heparin (UFH) or low molecular weight heparin (LMWH) may both be used for venous thromboprophylaxis.

▶ Since doses needed for treatment are higher than the prophylactic doses, one has to wait for a longer time if treatment doses are used.

▶ If LMWH is used for **prophylaxis**, one needs to wait **12 hours** before needling/catheter placement/removal, while if used for **treatment**, the appropriate time frame is **24 hours**. The next dose of LMWH should be given **4 hours** after catheter removal.

Note: also *see* Appendix for recommended times before/after puncture/catheter placement/removal.

  • Hadzic A. *Textbook of Regional Anesthesia and Acute Pain Management.* 1st ed. New York, NY: McGraw-Hill Medical; 2006. p. 1008.

A20 C Regarding epidural haematoma:

▶ **Rare** complication after a spinal (1 : 220 000) or an epidural (1 : 150 000).

▶ Mostly associated with the use of **anticoagulants**.

▶ **Highest risk** with patients receiving **thrombolytic therapy**.

▶ **Risk factors** include old age, female sex, anticoagulant therapy and technical difficulty in performing the block.

▶ Is most common at **thoracic levels** followed by cervicothoracic levels.

▶ Presents as a severe, localised, dull back ache **24–48 hours** after the epidural block.

▶ Epidural abscess, anterior spinal artery syndrome, surgical spinal cord damage, and exacerbation of underlying neurological diseases are differentials.

▶ **Magnetic resonance imaging (MRI)** is the diagnostic imaging of choice.

▶ **Surgical decompression** is the treatment of choice. Early exploration (within **36 hours**) has a favourable outcome.

  • Hadzic A. *Textbook of Regional Anesthesia and Acute Pain Management.* 1st ed. New York, NY: McGraw-Hill Medical; 2006. pp. 1013–16.

A21 D

Table 8.7 Risk factors for the development of infectious complications after a central neuraxial block

Patient factors	Anaesthetic technique factors
Underlying sepsis	Aseptic technique
Diabetes	Chronic catheter placement
Localised bacterial infection	
Chronic steroid therapy	
Immunosupression	

Note: there are no convincing data that an infection at remote sites or lack of antibiotic prophylaxis is a risk factor for infection.

- Wedel DJ, Horlocker TT. Regional anesthesia in the febrile or infected patient. *Reg Anesth Pain Med.* 2006; **31**(4): 324–33.

A22 B Meningitis following a spinal anaesthetic (post-dural puncture meningitis – PDPM) is a rare event. It is most commonly caused by *Streptococcus viridans* (mouth commensals), followed by *Staphylococcus aureus, Pseudomonas aeruginosa* and *Enterococcus faecalis.*

Pathogenesis: a successful meningeal pathogen must be able to colonise the host mucosal epithelium, then invade the intravascular space, cross the blood–brain barrier and survive in the cerebrospinal fluid. In PDPM, it is inoculated directly in the CSF somehow and circumvents the first three obstacles. Operator role has been suggested by isolation of same bacterial types from patients having PDPM and nasal/oral cavities of the neurologists/anesthesiologists who performed the procedure.

- Baer ET. Post-dural puncture bacterial meningitis. *Anesthesiology.* 2006; **105**(2): 381–93.
- Cousins MJ, Bridenbaugh PO, Carr DB, *et al. Cousins and Bridenbaugh's Neural Blockade in Clinical Anesthesia and Pain Medicine.* 4th ed. Philadelphia, PA: Lippincott Williams & Wilkins; 2008. p. 305.

A23 C Epidural abscess following epidural anaesthetic can be a devastating complication if not recognised and treated in time. Risk factors for the development of an epidural abscess include an immunocompromised state, malignancy, localised infections near epidural site, thromboprophylaxis, and chronic catheters. *S. aureus* is the most common pathogen isolated followed by **streptococci** and **Gram-negative bacilli**. In the case of **combined spinal epidural**, meningitis is most commonly caused by *S. viridans*, while an epidural abscess is most commonly caused by *S. aureus*.

- Cousins MJ, Bridenbaugh PO, Carr DB, *et al. Cousins and Bridenbaugh's Neural Blockade in Clinical Anesthesia and Pain Medicine.* 4th ed. Philadelphia, PA: Lippincott Williams & Wilkins; 2008. p. 305.
- Wang LP, Hauerberg J, Schmidt JF. Incidence of spinal epidural abscess after epidural analgesia: a national 1-year survey. *Anesthesiology.* 1999; **91**(6): 1928.

A24 D Infections after single-injection peripheral nerve blocks are rare. Most such infections follow continuous catheter techniques. Risk factors include **catheter technique, keeping catheter for more than 48 hours, repeated changes in catheter dressings, admission to intensive care unit** and a **lack of antibiotic prophylaxis (for surgical procedure)**. Catheters at the **femoral site** have higher infection rates than axillary or popliteal catheters. *Staphylococcus epidermidis* (coagulase-negative *Staphylococcus*) is the most frequent organism in such circumstances, followed by *Enterococcus* and *Klebsiella*. Time- and concentration-dependent antibacterial activity of local anaesthetic (bupivacaine > ropivacaine) and additives (clonidine) may be protective.

- Cousins MJ, Bridenbaugh PO, Carr DB, *et al. Cousins and Bridenbaugh's Neural Blockade in Clinical Anesthesia and Pain Medicine*. 4th ed. Philadelphia, PA: Lippincott Williams & Wilkins; 2008. pp. 472–5.

A25 D

Table 8.8 Grades of recommendations for infection control while performing a peripheral nerve block

Grade A evidence:	Grade B evidence:
Hand-washing	A new face mask for each new case
Cleaning skin with alcohol-based antiseptic (chlorhexidine)	Remove jewellery before hand-washing
Wearing sterile gloves	Allow the antiseptic to dry before starting (1 minute)
	Use of bacterial filter for catheter techniques
Grade C evidence:	**Grade D evidence:**
Antibiotic prophylaxis for catheter placement	At least two disinfections of procedure site
	Wear sterile gowns for catheters
	Use sterile mixtures and minimise disconnections for top-up administration

- Hebl JR. The importance and implications of aseptic techniques during regional anesthesia. *Reg Anesth Pain Med*. 2006; **31**(4): 311–23.

A26 D Local anaesthetic toxicity includes the following:

- ▶ **Allergic response** – immediate (anaphylaxis) or delayed (urticaria)
- ▶ **Myotoxicity** – muscle damage consequent to intramuscular injection
- ▶ **Neurotrauma** – direct nerve injury or transient neurological syndromes
- ▶ **Systemic toxicity** – most severe (life-threatening); manifests as central nervous system symptoms and cardiovascular system collapse.

Response to vasoconstrictors (manifested as headache, apprehension, tachycardia and hypertension) constitutes another differential diagnosis of local anaesthetic (LA) toxicity. **Adhesive arachnoiditis** is due to contamination of LA solution with skin-prep solutions (betadine or chlorhexidine) and is not due to LA toxicity.

- Cousins MJ, Bridenbaugh PO, Carr DB, *et al. Cousins and Bridenbaugh's Neural Blockade in Clinical Anesthesia and Pain Medicine*. 4th ed. Philadelphia, PA: Lippincott Williams & Wilkins; 2008. p. 124.

A27–29 C, C, B Systemic toxicity can manifest either immediately (within minutes), because of too rapid an intravascular injection, or be delayed (after 5–15 minutes), because of toxic plasma concentrations of LA achieved over a period of time.

Note: toxicity is **additive**; mixtures may be more toxic than individual drugs.

- Barash PG, Cullen BF, Stoelting RK, *et al. Clinical Anesthesia*. 6th ed. Philadelphia, PA: Lippincott Williams & Wilkins; 2009. pp. 536–46.
- Cousins MJ, Bridenbaugh PO, Carr DB, *et al. Cousins and Bridenbaugh's Neural Blockade in Clinical Anesthesia and Pain Medicine*. 4th ed. Philadelphia, PA: Lippincott Williams & Wilkins; 2008. p. 104.
- Mulroy MF, Bernards CM, McDonald SB, *et al. A Practical Approach to Regional Anesthesia*. 4th ed. Philadelphia, PA: Lippincott Williams & Wilkins; 2008. pp. 27–33.
- Neal JM, Rathmell JP. *Complications in Regional Anesthesia and Pain Medicine*. 1st ed. Philadelphia, PA: Saunders; 2006. p. 57.

Table 8.9 Determinants of systemic toxicity

Specific agents: physicochemical properties

Amides > esters (rapidly metabolised by esterases: lower toxicity)
Hydrophobic (lipohilic) > hydrophilic (less lipophilic) agents
More potent (bigger side chains) > less potent (smaller side chains)
Vasodilators > vasoconstrictors (ropivacaine)
Protein binding: only free fraction causes toxicity
Stereospecificity: levorotatory or S/(−) stereoisomers less toxic than dextrorotatory or R/(+)
Bupivacaine > l-bupicavaine > ropivacaine > lignocaine

	Least toxic	*Most toxic*
Ester	2-Chlorprocaine	Tetracaine
Amide	Prilocaine	Dibucaine > bupivacaine

Dose

Higher dose > lower dose
High peak plasma concentration (greater than toxic levels)
*Peak plasma concentration is **not a function of body weight in adults**, and basing LA doses on body weight in adults has no scientific foundation **(except in paediatrics)***

Factors increasing systemic toxicity

Site of injection (influences rate of absorption):
intravascular > intrapleural > intercostal > caudal > epidural > brachial plexus > femorosciatic > sub-cutaneous >intra-articular > spinal
Physiological parameters:
acidosis (decreases plasma protein binding), hypercarbia, hypoxia and hyperkalaemia (increased proportion of Na+ channels in inactivated state)
Specific populations:
obstetrics (progesterone-induced sensitivity to LA)
geriatric: low dose requirements
paediatrics: lower weight and performance of blocks under sedation

Protective factors

Vasoconstrictors: may decrease rate of systemic absorption and may help reducing total dose
Hyperventilation (reduces respiratory acidosis and raises seizure threshold)
Benzodiazepine premedication (raises seizure threshold)

A30 D LAs cause toxicity by blocking the following:

▶ **Voltage-gated Na+ channels: most important.** LA blocks these channels in **open or inactivated state,** rather than in closed state. This is **a phasic or use-dependent** block. In cardiac muscle fibres, **Ca+ influx during 'plateau'** phase favours LA binding as the Na+ channels are in the inactivated state. Consequently, V_{max} (max upstroke velocity of the action potential) is reduced, causing QRS widening, and **action potential duration (APD)** is prolonged, causing QT **prolongation (leading to ventricular arrhythmias). Hypoxia, acidosis and hyperkalaemia** increase the proportion **of Na+ channels in the inactivated** state, favouring LA binding and hence toxicity.

Table 8.10 Type of sodium channel blockade by local anaesthetic

Blockade	Local anaesthetic	Toxicity
Fast in, fast out	Lignocaine	Less toxic
Slow in, slow out	Bupivacaine – lower doses	Intermediate
Fast in, slow out	Bupivacaine – high doses	More toxic

▶ **Voltage-sensitive K+ channels**: **APD** increased; QT prolongation leading to ventricular arrhythmias.

▶ **Voltage-sensitive Ca+ channels**: inhibition of myocyte Ca+ release and utilisation.

▶ **Other channels**: HERG, NMDA, nicotinic acetlycholie receptors, β-adrenergic, KATP channels and so forth.

▶ **Mitochondrial dysfunction**: uncouple oxidative phosphorylation.

  • Cousins MJ, Bridenbaugh PO, Carr DB, *et al. Cousins and Bridenbaugh's Neural Blockade in Clinical Anesthesia and Pain Medicine*. 4th ed. Philadelphia, PA: Lippincott Williams & Wilkins; 2008. pp. 117–20.

  • Finucaine BT. *Complications of Regional Anesthesia*. 2nd ed. New York, NY: Springer; 2007. p. 66.

A31 A In general, **central nervous system (CNS) signs** are first to manifest, followed by **cardiovascular system (CVS) signs**.

Table 8.11 Manifestations of local anaesthetic (LA) toxicity

CNS toxicity	CVS toxicity
Early excitement phase: perioral numbness, tinnitus tremors myoclonic jerks convulsions	Early excitement from CNS stimulation: tachycardia hypertension
Late depression phase: hypoventilation respiratory acidosis and hypoxia coma	Late CVS depression (from direct LA toxicity): arrhythmias pump failure arrest

ECG: QRS widening and QT prolongation; ventricular arrhythmias. **CVS : CNS ratio** describes ratio of dose required to cause CV toxicity to that required to cause CNS toxicity. It is **2:1** for bupivacaine and **7 : 1** for lignocaine. This implies that bupivacaine is more cardiotoxic than lignocaine. The order of toxicity (and cardiotoxicity) is:

> Bupivacaine > l-bupicavaine > ropivacaine > lignocaine.

There are clinical reports of simultaneous CNS and CVS toxicity with bupivacaine.

- Barash PG, Cullen BF, Stoelting RK, *et al. Clinical Anesthesia*. 6th ed. Philadelphia, PA: Lippincott Williams & Wilkins; 2009. pp. 540–2.
- Cousins MJ, Bridenbaugh PO, Carr DB, *et al. Cousins and Bridenbaugh's Neural Blockade in Clinical Anesthesia and Pain Medicine*. 4th ed. Philadelphia, PA: Lippincott Williams & Wilkins; 2008. pp. 120–1.

A32 D

Table 8.12 Recommended doses of common local anaesthetics (LAs)

Type of LA	Without epinephrine	With epinephrine	Toxic plasma levels
Ester			
Procaine	7	8.5	Metabolised rapidly
2-Chlorprocaine	11	14	by esterases
Amides			
Lignocaine	4	6–7	5
Mepivacaine	4	7 (not recommended)	5
Bupivacaine	2	2 (not recommended)	3
Levo-bupivacaine	2	2 (not recommended)	4
Ropivacaine	3	3	4

Table 8.12 shows the generally accepted guideline. However, maximum recommended doses by the manufacturer should be abided by. Dosages are said to be site- and block-specific rather than dependent upon weight of the patient.

Table 8.13 Dose-dependent systemic effects of lignocaine

Effect	Plasma levels (µg/mL)
Analgesia	1–5
Tinnitus, perioral numbness	5–10
Seizures	10–15
Coma and respiratory arrest	15–25
Cardiovascular depression	> 25

- Barash PG, Cullen BF, Stoelting RK, *et al. Clinical Anesthesia*. 6th ed. Philadelphia, PA: Lippincott Williams & Wilkins; 2009. pp. 539–42.
- Hadzic A. *Textbook of Regional Anesthesia and Acute Pain Management*. 1st ed. New York, NY: McGraw-Hill Medical; 2006. p. 183.

A33 B Measures to reduce LA likelihood of toxicity are:
- using smallest possible doses for the given block
- using less cardiotoxic agents
- use of vasoconstrictors to reduce systemic absorption
- fractionation of total dose
- aspiration before injection and using test doses.

Adequate patient monitoring may help to **recognise LA toxicity at an earlier stage**, but it may not reduce its likelihood.

- Neal JM, Rathmell JP. *Complications in Regional Anesthesia and Pain Medicine.* 1st ed. Philadelphia, PA: Saunders; 2006. p. 63.

A34 **B** Treatment of LA toxicity: always start with **ABC** (resuscitation).
- **Airway**:
  - Clear the airway and suction (if needed).
- **Breathing**:
  - Oxygenation and adequate ventilation to avoid hypoxia and respiratory acidosis (both potentiate LA toxicity).
  - Intubation and controlled ventilation if needed.
- **Circulation**:
  - Maintain BP: leg elevation, fluids, inotropes or vasoconstrictors.
- **Drugs**:
  - Seizures: diazepam, midazolam, thiopentone or propofol
  - Muscle relaxant: succinylcholine
  - Arrhythmias: amiodarone (best choice out of anti-arrhythmics), epinephrine (higher doses may be needed)
  - Specific therapy: Intralipid.

Note: anti-arrhythmics to be avoided in setting of LA-induced arrhythmias are **sodium valproate, phenytoin, Ca+ channel blockers, lignocaine and bretylium**. Prolonged resuscitation may be needed.

- Cousins MJ, Bridenbaugh PO, Carr DB, *et al. Cousins and Bridenbaugh's Neural Blockade in Clinical Anesthesia and Pain Medicine.* 4th ed. Philadelphia, PA: Lippincott Williams & Wilkins; 2008. p. 125.

A35 **C** Regarding Intralipid rescue therapy:
- Intralipid is available as a **10%, 20% and 30% lipid emulsion**. However, the recommended concentration to be used (lipid rescue) is 20%.
- Propofol is not an appropriate substitute.
- CPR should be continued while giving Intralipid in cardiac arrest (lipids must circulate).
- Proposed mechanism:
  - **Indirect**: acts as a **sink** for the lipid-soluble LA, drawing it back into circulation (from tissues).
  - **Direct**: the inhibition of **mitochondrial carnitine-acylcarnitine translocase** by LA is overridden by high plasma triglycerides (this

enzyme is essential for the tricarboxylic acid cycle in mitochondria, i.e. oxidative phosphorylation).

▶ **Dose used**: initially 1.5 mL/kg bolus over 1 minute followed by infusion of 0.25 mL/kg/minute. If CVS stability is not restored or adequate circulation deteriorates, give an additional two boluses at an interval of 5 minutes and continue infusion at the same or double rate (0.5 mL/kg/minute). The maximum cumulative dose should not exceed 12 mL/kg (840 mL in a 70-kg man).

- Cousins MJ, Bridenbaugh PO, Carr DB, *et al. Cousins and Bridenbaugh's Neural Blockade in Clinical Anesthesia and Pain Medicine*. 4th ed. Philadelphia, PA: Lippincott Williams & Wilkins; 2008. p. 128.
- Management of severe local anaesthetic toxicity. London: AAGBI; 2010. Available at: www.aagbi.org/sites/default/files/la_toxicity_2010_0.pdf

A36 C Ester LAs are metabolised to **PABA compounds**, which make them more allergenic than amides. PABA compounds may be present in **cosmetic products**, causing patients to react. True allergy to preservative-free amide LA is **rare**, and patients may react to **paraben** derivatives used as preservative. Reports of 'cauda equina syndrome' with unintentional intrathecal administration of high doses of 2-chloroprocaine intended for epidural use were attributed to **sodium metabisulphite** added to the solution. The present preparations for intrathecal use are free of such preservatives.

- Hadzic A. *Textbook of Regional Anesthesia and Acute Pain Management*. 1st ed. New York, NY: McGraw-Hill Medical; 2006. p. 117.
- Mulroy MF, Bernards CM, McDonald SB, *et al. A Practical Approach to Regional Anesthesia*. 4th ed. Philadelphia, PA: Lippincott Williams & Wilkins; 2008. p. 34.

A37 B Cauda equina syndrome (CES) has been reported after **unintentional intrathecal injection** of high doses of LA (mainly **lignocaine**) intended for the epidural space. In other reports, the administration of LA through continuous **spinal microcatheters** (smaller than 27 G) produced a restricted sacral block, and **repeated doses** were required to achieve adequate surgical anaesthesia. The neurotoxicity was attributed to the **maldistribution** of LA within the CSF, and subsequently the use of microcatheters was withdrawn. The addition of **vasoconstrictors** is another risk factor. The syndrome presents as **multiple-root involvement**, varying degrees of bowel and bladder dysfunction, perineal sensory loss and lower-limb motor weakness. The differentials may include **epidural haematoma or epidural abscess**, with urgent **MRI** to ascertain the cause. There is **no effective treatment**, and the patient may need considerable supportive care.

- Neal JM, Rathmell JP. *Complications in Regional Anesthesia and Pain Medicine.* 1st ed. Philadelphia, PA: Saunders; 2006. pp. 99–105.

A38 A Transient neurologic symptoms are a group of neurologic symptoms experienced by patients after spinal anaesthesia, characterised by:

- ▶ mostly aching/pain in one or both **buttocks**
- ▶ often with dysaethesia radiating into anterior or posterior **thighs**
- ▶ with **lower-back pain** in some patients
- ▶ symptoms beginning **within 24 hours** after the resolution of spinal anaesthetic
- ▶ symptoms resolving in **6 hours to 4 days**
- ▶ **no neurological finding** upon physical examination.

The name 'transient neurologic symptoms' itself is **controversial**, as it implies a neurologic aetiology that is not yet proven.

- ▶ Proposed risk factors include use of **intrathecal lignocaine, lithotomy position, outpatient surgery and obstetric patient population**, but **not** baricity and dose of LA used.
- ▶ Treatment constitutes use of NSAIDs, muscle relaxants, leg elevation, heat pads, trigger-point injections and reassurance.
- ▶ **An abnormal neurological exam** should prompt an evaluation for epidural haematoma, abscess or CES.
  - Barash PG, Cullen BF, Stoelting RK, *et al. Clinical Anesthesia.* 6th ed. Philadelphia, PA: Lippincott Williams & Wilkins; 2009. p. 545.
  - Neal JM, Rathmell JP. *Complications in Regional Anesthesia and Pain Medicine.* 1st ed. Philadelphia, PA: Saunders; 2006. pp. 119–24.

9

Statistics

Questions

Choose one best answer for each of the following questions.

Q1 Which of the following is **not** an example of categorical data?
   a. Visual analogue pain scale
   b. Three-point pain scale (mild/moderate/severe)
   c. Block outcome – success or failure
   d. Gender – male or female

Q2 Which of the following statements about the normal distribution curve is **incorrect**?
   a. It is a bell-shaped curve
   b. Mean, median and mode coincide
   c. Values are either 0 or 1
   d. The tails do not touch the baseline

Q3 Which of the following definitions is **incorrect**?
   a. Median is the middle value in the given range
   b. Mode is the most frequent value in the sample
   c. Standard deviation is the measure of dispersion of a given value around the mean
   d. Standard error of mean is the standard deviation of the sample-mean estimate of a population mean

Q4 Which of the following terms has been **correctly** defined?
   a. Reliability is the ability of the test to produce the true values of the measurements
   b. Precision is the dependability of a test (consistency and reproducibility)
   c. Validity is the extent to which the test measures what it was designed to measure
   d. Accuracy is the extent to which random variability is absent from the test

Q5 For the contingency table shown here, which of the formulae given is **incorrect**?

	Disease	
Test result	Present	Absent
Positive	A	B
Negative	C	D

   a. Sensitivity = A/(A + C)
   b. Specificity = B/(B + D)
   c. Positive predictive value = A/(A + B)
   d. Negative predictive value = D/(C + D)

Q6 To accept the occurrence of a chronic painful state, a patient must have three diagnostic criteria. Newer recommendations have added a criterion, necessitating the presence of four criteria for diagnosis. This will:
   a. Increase the sensitivity but decrease the specificity
   b. Decrease the sensitivity but increase the specificity
   c. Have no effect on both sensitivity and specificity
   d. Increase both sensitivity and specificity

Q7 For a very easy test for a given population of students, which of the following will **not** be observed?
   a. The resulting scores' data distribution will be negatively skewed
   b. Mean will be less than the median
   c. Mode is least affected
   d. Mean is more than the median

Q8 Regarding cohort study, which of the following statements is **false**?
a. It is usually a prospective study
b. It allows calculation of odds ratio
c. It gives incidence rate
d. It requires a large sample size

Q9 For the contingency table shown here, which of the following formulae is **correct**?

Risk factor	Disease	
	Present	Absent
Present	A	B
Absent	C	D

a. Odds ratio = AC/BD
b. Relative risk = A/(A+C) / B/(B+D)
c. Attributable risk = (A/(A+B)) − (C/(C+D))
d. Numbers needed to treat = 1/attributable risk

Q10 Which of the following is **false**?
a. Null hypothesis states that there is no difference between the two groups studied
b. Type I error occurs by rejecting the null hypothesis when it is true
c. Type II error occurs by missing a true difference between the groups
d. Power of the study is the probability of occurrence of type II error

Answers

A1   A

Table 9.1 Types of statistical data

Numerical data (obtained from measurements)	Categorical data (grouped data)
Continuous: can take any value in a given range (e.g. height or weight) **Discrete**: can take an integer value only (e.g. visual analogue scale) **Ratio**: a data series that has zero as its baseline, such as heart rate and temperature (degrees Kelvin) **Interval**: a data series that has zero as a point on a larger scale, such as temperature (degrees Celsius)	**Nominal (unordered)**: data comes from mutually exclusive unranked groups, e.g. procedural outcome (success or failure) and gender (male or female) **Ordinal (ordered)**: ranked groups, e.g. categorical pain rating scale (mild, moderate and severe), ASA grade (class I, II, III, IV, V)

- Smith T, Pinnock C, Lin T, *et al. Fundamentals of Anaesthesia*. 3rd ed. Cambridge: Cambridge University Press; 2009. p. 864.

A2   C Probability is the chance of occurrence of an event. It has a value between 0 and 1. The probability density curves are used to describe the distribution of data in the given population. They can be of different types: **normal (most important), binomial (value of 0 or 1) or Poisson distribution**. Characteristics of a normal distribution:

- also called the **Gaussian** distribution
- describes the distribution of **continuous variables**
- **bell-shaped** symmetrical curve
- mean, median and mode are **identical**
- tails **do not** touch the baseline
- peaks if variance (standard deviation) is low
- flattens if variance (standard deviation) is high.
    - Smith T, Pinnock C, Lin T, *et al. Fundamentals of Anaesthesia*. 3rd ed. Cambridge: Cambridge University Press; 2009. p. 866.

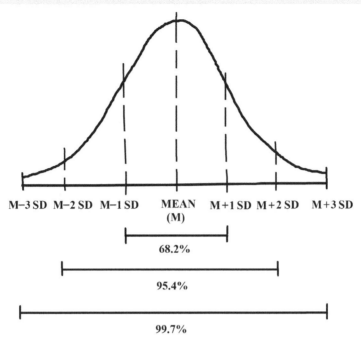

Figure 9.1 Normal distribution curve

A3   C
- **Mean**: it is the sum of all the values, divided by the number of values.
- **Median**: it is the point that has half the values above and half below.
- **Mode**: it is used when we need a label for the most frequently occurring event.
- **Standard deviation**: it indicates how much a set of values is spread around the average. It is a measure of dispersion.
- **Standard error of the mean**: it is the standard deviation of the sample-mean estimate of a population mean. It gives an idea of how closely the estimated mean value (from the sample) is likely to represent the true mean value (from the general population).

It is worth remembering that:
- ± 1 standard deviations includes **68.2%** of the data
- ± 2 standard deviations includes **95.4%** of the data
- ± 3 standard deviations includes **99.7%** of the data.
    - Smith T, Pinnock C, Lin T, *et al*. *Fundamentals of Anaesthesia*. 3rd ed. Cambridge: Cambridge University Press; 2009. p. 868–70.

A4 C

▶ **Reliability** is the dependability of a test (consistency and reproducibility).
▶ **Precision** is the extent to which random variability is absent from the test. Reliability of a test is dependent upon its precision.
▶ **Validity** is the extent to which the test measures what it was designed to measure. It has two components: sensitivity and specificity.
▶ **Accuracy** is the ability of the test to produce the true values of the measurements.

A5 B

	Disease	
Test result	Present	Absent
Positive	A	B
Negative	C	D

A = true positive, B = false positive, C = false negative, D = true negative.

Table 9.2 Statistical definitions

Term	Definition	Formulae
Sensitivity	The ability of a test to correctly identify the individuals **who have the condition**	$A/(A + C)$
Specificity	The ability of a test to correctly identify the individuals **who do not have the condition**	$D/(B + D)$
False-positive rate	Proportion of **false positives** in the non-diseased population	$B/(B + D)$ or (1 – specificity)
False-negative rate	Proportion of **false negatives** in the diseased population	$C/(A + C)$ Or (1 – sensitivity)
Positive predictive value	Proportion of true positives among all positives	$A/(A + B)$
Negative predictive value	Proportion of true negatives among all negatives	$D/(C + D)$
Accuracy	Proportion of true results (true positive and true negative) among all results	$(A + B)/(A + B + C + D)$

• Lalkhen AG, McCluskey A. Clinical tests: sensitivity and specificity. *Contin Educ Anaesth Crit Care Pain*. 2008; **8**(6): 221–3.

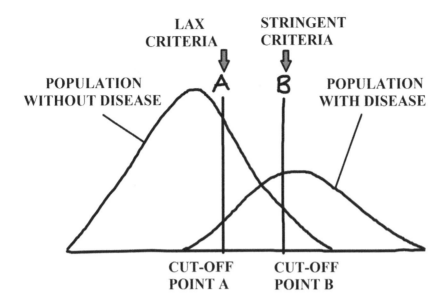

Figure 9.2 Relationship between cut-off criteria, sensitivity and specificity

A6 B Look at the contingency table in the previous question to understand the explanation better.

As can be seen above, having a **lax criteria (three criteria – Point A)** for diagnosis leads to:
- more total positives and less total negatives
- high true positive (high sensitivity)
- high false positive (low specificity)
- low false negative
- low true negative.

On the other hand, using **stringent criteria (four criteria – Point B)** for diagnosis means:
- less total positives and more total negatives
- low true positive (low sensitivity)
- low false positive (high specificity)
- high false negative
- high true negative.

Hence adding another criterion as a requirement for diagnosis will lead to lower true-positive rate (low sensitivity), but a lower false-negative rate as well (higher specificity). The former situation is desirable in a **screening test** (high sensitivity), while the latter is desirable in a **confirmatory test** (high specificity).

A7 D Not all data are normally distributed. Some may be skewed. **Skewed data are named according to the direction of the tail.**

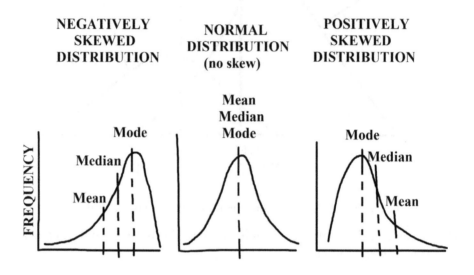

NEGATIVELY SKEWED DISTRIBUTION	NORMAL DISTRIBUTION (no skew)	POSITIVELY SKEWED DISTRIBUTION

Figure 9.3 Spread of mean, median and mode in various types of distributions

Table 9.3 Types of skewed data

Negatively skewed data	Positively skewed data
Most of the values are positive, tail points negatively (left)	Most of the values are negative, tail points positive (right)
Mode is least changed, while mean the most	Mode is least changed, while mean the most
Mean < Median < Mode	Mean > Median > Mode
Example: a very easy test will be high-scoring, so it will be negatively skewed	Example: a very difficult test will be poor-scoring, so it will be positively skewed

A8 B

Table 9.4 Comparison of case-control and cohort study

Case-control study	Cohort study
Example: study of a group of chronic obstructive pulmonary disease patients (case) and without chronic obstructive pulmonary disease (control) to identify risk factors (smoking)	Example: follow-up of smokers (cohort) and non-smokers (another cohort) and the development of chronic obstructive pulmonary disease in each cohort
Retrospective study	Prospective study
Outcome is measured before exposure	Outcome is measured after exposure
Inexpensive, easier, hospital-based	Expensive, harder, community-based
Needs small sample size	Needs large sample size
Allows estimation of odds risk only	Allows determination of incidence and relative risk
Used to study relatively rare conditions	Used to study common conditions
Selection bias more likely	Selection bias less likely

Cross-sectional study (prevalence study): studies present cases, allowing estimation of prevalence and risk factors at the same time. It is easy and inexpensive.

Randomised clinical trial: is a prospective study with randomised study groups. It may be blinded to reduce selection bias.

A9 C

	Disease	
Risk factor	Present	Absent
Present	A	B
Absent	C	D

Here, if risk factor is smoking and the disease is cancer, then:

Risk of disease in exposed population   = A/(A + B)

Risk of disease in non-exposed population = C/(C + D)

Table 9.5 Statistical definitions

Term	Formula
Relative risk is a **ratio** of the probability of the event (disease) occurring in the exposed group versus a non-exposed group	$RR = \dfrac{A/(A+B)}{C/(C+D)}$
Attributable risk is the **difference** in rate of a condition between an exposed population and an unexposed population	$AR = \left(\dfrac{A}{A+B}\right) - \left(\dfrac{C}{C+D}\right)$
The **odds ratio** is the ratio of the odds of an event occurring in one group to the odds of it occurring in another group	$OR = \dfrac{AD}{BC}$
Absolute risk reduction is the reduction in risk associated with treatment (or removal of risk factor) as compared with placebo	$ARR = \dfrac{1}{NNT}$

Number needed to treat is the average number of patients who need to be treated to prevent one additional bad outcome.

▶ *It is the inverse of absolute risk reduction.*

▶ Example: number of children we need to vaccinate to prevent one case of disease.

▶ **The lower the number needed to treat, the more effective the intervention is.**

Number needed to harm is the number of patients that need to be exposed to a risk factor over a specific period to cause harm in one additional patient.

▶ *It is the inverse of the attributable risk.*

▶ Example: number of adults that need to be exposed to smoking to have one more case of lung cancer.

▶ **The lower the number needed to harm, the worse the risk factor.**

A10 D **Null hypothesis** states that there is **no difference** between the two groups being studied. It provides a starting point for the study. Then, if no difference is found, it is accepted and there is no statistical difference noted. However, if a difference is noted, it is rejected and the result is ascribed a statistical significance. The level of statistical significance is called the *P*-value **(usually 0.05)** and is the **probability of occurrence of a type I error** (α).

	Truth	
Decision	H_0 true	H_0 false
Accept	Correct	Type II error
Reject	Type I error	Correct

Table 9.6 Types of error

Type I error	Type II error
Cause: rejecting null hypothesis when it is true	Cause: accepting null hypothesis when it is false
Inference: finding a false difference between groups when none exists	Inference: missing a true difference between groups
Propability of type I error is α	Probability of type II error is β

Power of a study is described as its ability to detect a difference between groups. It may be described as the probability of not obtaining a type II error (β). Hence, **power = (1 – β)**. For a good study, Power should be 0.8 or more.

- Smith T, Pinnock C, Lin T, *et al*. *Fundamentals of Anaesthesia*. 3rd ed. Cambridge: Cambridge University Press; 2009. p. 872.

Appendix

Table A.1 Dosage for upper- or lower-limb blocks

Duration (hours)	Single injection in adults
Short (3–4)	Lignocaine 1.5%
	Mepivacaine 1%–1.5%
Intermediate (4–5)	Lignocaine 2% (+ adrenaline)
	Mepivacaine 1%–1.5%
Long (10–14)	Bupivacaine 0.5%
	Ropivacaine 0.5%

Continuous blocks:
   bupivacaine 0.0625%–0.125% or ropivacaine 0.1%–0.2%
   @ 6–8 mL/hour with 2–3 mL bolus.
For analgesia only:
   0.2 % ropivacaine or 0.25% bupivacaine.
Additives:
   adrenaline: 1 : 400000–1 : 200000
   clonidine: 75–150 mcg (additional 4 hours' analgesia)
   bicarbonate: 1 mL/10 mL lignocaine
   buprenorphine: 300 mcg prolongs analgesia.
Volumes for upper limb used:
   traditional peripheral nervous system blocks: 30–40 mL
   ultrasound-guided blocks: 10–20 mL.

Table A.2 Volumes for lower limb used (approximate guides)

Block	Traditional peripheral nervous system blocks (mL)	Ultrasound-guided blocks (mL)
Lumbar plexus	40	
Femoral	20–30	10–20
Fascia iliaca/femoral three-in-one	30	
Obturator block	10–15	
Lateral femoral cutaneous nerve block	10	
Sciatic block proximal	30–40	
Popliteal block	25	
Saphenous block	10	
Ankle block	Up to 25	

Overall, ultrasound guidance reduces total volume needed to block any nerve.

Table A.3 Anatomical landmarks for blocks

Block	Structure
Interscalene block	At interscalene groove at C6
Supraclavicular	Lateral to subclavian artery
Infraclavicular	Medial to coracoid process (peripheral nervous system) or axillary artery (ultrasound guidance)
Axillary	Around axillary artery
Median nerve	Medial to brachial artery
Radial nerve	Between brachioradialis and biceps tendon
Ulnar nerve	Above medial epicondyle
Lumbar plexus	Transverse process of L4/L5
Femoral	Lateral to femoral artery
Lateral femoral cutaneous nerve	Medio-inferior to anterior superior iliac spine
Ilioinguinal	Medio-superior to anterior superior iliac spine
Obturator	Medial to pubic tubercle
Saphenous	Adductor canal Descending genicular artery (ultrasound guidance)
Sciatic (parasacral)	Posterior superior iliac spine and ischial tuberosity
Sciatic (Labat)	Posterior superior iliac spine, greater trochanter, sacral hiatus Inferior gluteal artery (ultrasound guidance)
Infragluteal	Greater trochanter and ischial tuberosity
Sciatic (popliteal)	Semimebranosus (medially) and biceps femoris (laterally) Popliteal artery (ultrasound guidance)
Ankle: posterior tibial block	Posterior to posterior tibial artery
Ankle: deep peroneal	Lateral to extensor hallucis longus Anterior tibial artery (ultrasound guidance)
Ankle: sural nerve	Deep to Achilles tendon
Ankle: saphenous	Above medial malleolus
Ankle: superficial peroneal	Above lateral malleolus

Table A.4 Trigeminal nerve branches and foramen

Branch	Exit cranium through	Associated foramen
Ophthalmic nerve	Superior orbital fissure	Supraorbital notch
Maxillary nerve	Foramen rotundum	Inferior orbital fissure
		Infraorbital foramen
Mandibular nerve	Foramen ovale	Mental foramen

Table A.5 Branches of ophthalmic division of trigeminal nerve (V$_1$)

Frontal nerve *(largest branch of V$_1$)*

Branches	Innervation	Useful blocks
Supraorbital nerve: exits skull through the supraorbital notch	Upper lid and the scalp up to the lambdoid suture	At the **supraorbital notch** in the middle of the upper margin of orbit
Supratrochlear nerve: emerges from the upper medial quadrant of the orbit	Medial eyelid and medial forehead	A single injection in the midline **between the eyebrows** to block nerves from both sides

Lacrimal nerve
Passes in the **lateral part of the superior orbital fissure**
Supplies the lacrimal gland, conjunctiva and upper lid

Nasociliary nerve
Passes in the **central part of the superior orbital fissure**

Branch	Innervation	Block
Anterior ethmoid nerve	Frontal and anterior ethmoid sinuses	
Posterior ethmoid nerves	Posterior ethmoid and sphenoid sinuses	
Internal nasal branch	Anterior part of the septum and lateral nasal wall	**Nasal pellets with local anaesthetic**
External nasal branches	Skin of the nasal tip	
2–3 long ciliary nerves	Iris and cornea	**Topical anaesthesia**

Table A.6 Branches of maxillary division of trigeminal nerve (V$_2$)

Nerve	Sub-branches	Supply	Useful blocks
In the cranium			
Middle meningeal		Dura	n/a
In the pterygopalatine fossa			
Zygomatic	Zygomaticofacial	Skin of cheek	At the cheek
	Zygomaticotemporal	Skin of temples	At the **zygomatic arch**
Sphenopalatine nerve	Nerves to the orbit	Orbital periorsteum (floor)	
	Nasal branches	Nasal cavity	**Nasal pellets** with local anaesthetic (described later)
	Nasopalatine (exits through incisive foramen)	Premaxillary palatal mucosa	Midline behind the **upper incisors** on inner side
	Greater palatine (anterior) (exits through greater palatine canal)	Hard and soft palate	At junction between **second and third maxillary molar** on **inner side**
	Lesser palatine (middle and posterior)	Hard and soft palate	
	Pharyngeal br.	Soft palate and tonsillar mucosa	
Posterior superior alveolar branches		Alveolus, maxillary sinus mucosa and cheeks	Mucobuccal fold over maxillary **second molar**
In the infraorbital canal			
Infraorbital nerve	Middle alveolar nerve	Middle upper alveolus	Mucobuccal fold over maxillary **second premolar**
	Anterior alveolar nerve	Anterior upper alveolus	**Infraorbital nerve block** at the infraorbital foramen
On the face			
Infraorbital nerve (exits through the **infraorbital foramen**)	Inferior palpebral	Lower eyelid (skin)	**Infraorbital nerve block** at the infraorbital foramen
	Lateral nasal	Lateral aspect of nose (skin)	
	Superior labial	Upper lip (skin and mucoa)	

Table A.7 Branches of mandibular division of trigeminal nerve (V₃)

The mandibular nerve (V₃) is the **largest** branch of the trigeminal nerve; its sensory and motor roots exit through the **foramen ovale** and unite to form the main trunk

Part	Nerves	Useful blocks
Main trunk	Nervus spinosus (meningeal branch) Medial pterygoid nerve Nerve to tensor tympani Nerve to tensor veli palatini	None
Anterior division	Masseteric nerve Deep temporal nerves (anterior and posterior) Buccal nerve (a sensory nerve) Lateral pterygoid nerve	None
Posterior division	**Auriculotemporal nerve** Lingual nerve **Inferior alveolar nerve** Mylohyoid nerve	**Scalp block** **Mental nerve block**

Table A.8 Nerves exiting through various foramina of the cranium

Foramina	Nerves
Foramina of cribriform plate	Olfactory nerve bundles (I)
Optic canal	Optic nerve (II)
Superior orbital fissure	Oculomotor nerve (III) Trochlear nerve (IV) Lacrimal, frontal and nasociliary branches of ophthalmic nerve (V₁) Abducens nerve (VI)
Foramen rotundum	Maxillary nerve (V₂)
Foramen ovale	Mandibular nerve (V₃)
Stylomastoid foramen	Facial nerve (VII)
Internal acoustic meatus	Facial nerve (VII), vestibulocochlear nerve (VIII)
Jugular foramen	Glossopharyngeal nerve (IX), vagus nerve (X), accessory nerve (XI)
Hypoglossal canal	Hypoglossal nerve (XII)
Foramen lacerum	Nerve of pterygoid canal
Foramen magnum	Medulla oblongata
Supraorbital foramen	Supraorbital nerve
Anterior ethmoidal foramen	Anterior ethmoidal nerve
Posterior ethmoidal foramen	Posterior ethmoidal nerve
Infraorbital foramen	Infraorbital nerve
Mental foramen	Mental nerve

Table A.9 Parasympathetic nerve supply

Nerve	Origin	Relay	Innervates	Action
CNIII	Edinger–Westphal nucleus (an accessory nucleus of III) in tegmentum	Ciliary ganglion	Sphincter muscles of the iris	Control pupillary diameter
		Episcleral ganglion	Ciliary muscle	Curvature of the lens
CNVII	Superior salivatory nucleus in the pons	Sphenopalatine ganglion	Lacrimal gland and mucous membranes	Lacrimal and other secretions
		Submandibular ganglion	Submandibular and sublingual salivary glands	Salivary secretions
CNIX	Inferior salivatory nucleus at the pontomedullary border	Otic ganglion	Parotid gland	Salivary secretions
CNX	Dorsal motor nucleus of X in the medulla	Peripheral ganglia	Thoracic and abdominal organs, glands and some blood vessels	Multiple
Nervi ergentes	S2–S4 spinal segments (lamina VII)	Hypogastric plexus	Pelvic organs	Multiple

Table A.10 Referred pain

Body organ of origin	Body part of referred pain
Heart	Chest and left arm
Lung and diaphragm	Left neck and trapezius
Liver and gall bladder	Right neck and trapezius Right hypochondrium Right shoulder tip
Stomach	Epigastrium
Small intestine	Periumbilical area
Appendix	Right iliac fossa
Ovary, sigmoid	Left iliac fossa
Kidneys	Loin and thighs
Ureters	Groin (inguinal) area

Table A.11 Definition of pain and associated terms, from the International Association for the Study of Pain

Term	Definition
Pain	An unpleasant sensory and emotional experience associated with actual or potential tissue damage, or described in terms of such damage
Analgesia	Absence of pain in response to stimulation which would normally be painful
Allodynia	Pain due to a stimulus which does not normally provoke pain
Paraesthesia	An abnormal sensation, whether spontaneous or evoked
Dysaesthesia	An unpleasant abnormal sensation, whether spontaneous or evoked
Hyperaesthesia	Increased sensitivity to stimulation, excluding the special senses
Hypoaesthesia	Decreased sensitivity to stimulation, excluding the special senses
Hyperalgesia	An increased response to a stimulus which is normally painful
Hypoalgesia	Diminished pain in response to a normally painful stimulus
Hyperpathia	A painful syndrome characterised by an abnormally painful reaction to a stimulus, especially a repetitive stimulus, as well as an increased threshold
Nociceptor	A receptor preferentially sensitive to a noxious stimulus or to a stimulus which would become noxious if prolonged
Noxious stimulus	A noxious stimulus is one that is damaging to normal tissues
Neuralgia	Pain in the distribution of a nerve or nerves
Neuritis	Inflammation of a nerve or nerves
Neuropathy	A disturbance of function or pathological change in a nerve: mononeuropathy, mononeuropathy multiplex or polyneuropathy
Neuropathic pain	Pain initiated or caused by a primary lesion or dysfunction in the nervous system
Central pain	Pain initiated or caused by a primary lesion or dysfunction in the central nervous system
Peripheral neuropathic pain	Pain initiated or caused by a primary lesion or dysfunction in the peripheral nervous system
Pain threshold	The least experience of pain which a subject can recognise
Pain tolerance level	The greatest level of pain which a subject is prepared to tolerate
Complex Regional Pain Syndrome I	CRPS I, formerly known as reflex sympathetic dystrophy, consists of continuous pain (allodynia or hyperalgesia) in part of an extremity after trauma, including fractures

(continued)

Table A.11 Definition of pain and associated terms, from the International Association for the Study of Pain (*continued*)

Term	Definition
Complex Regional Pain Syndrome II	CRPS II, formerly known as causalgia, consists of burning pain in the distribution of a partially damaged peripheral nerve (most commonly median, ulnar or sciatic)
Anaesthesia dolorosa	Pain in an area or region which is anaesthetic

Table A.12 Mechanism of action of some drugs used in chronic pain

Drug	Action	Use
Ketamine	NMDA antagonist	Chronic pain (complex regional pain syndrome)
Tricyclic antidepressants	Monoamine reuptake inhibition	Diabetic neuropathy and post-herpetic neuralgia
Bisphosphonates	Inhibit osteoclast medicated bone resportion	Osteoporotic pain, bone pain in cancers
Amantadine	NMDA antagonist	Neuropathic pain
Carbamazepine	Potentiate GABA action	Trigeminal neuralgia
Gabapentin	Calcium channel inhibition	Diabetic neuropathy
Pregabalin	Calcium channel inhibition	Diabetic neuropathy
Lamotrigene	Sodium channel blocker	Resistant trigeminal neuralgia
Topiramate	Modulated sodium and calcium channels; potentiates GABA and blocks glutamate	Neuropathic pain
Baclofen	$GABA_B$ potentiation	Spasticity
Botulinum toxin	Inhibition of ACh release at neuromuscular junction	Myofascial pains, dystonia, contractures

Table A.13 Potency of commonly used opioids

Drug	Potency ratio (compared with morphine)	One ampoule contains
Sufentanil	1000 : 1	10 mcg
Fentanyl	100 : 1	100 mcg
Remifentanil	50 : 1 (approx)	1/2/5 mg (only infusion)
Buprenorphine	30 : 1	300 mcg
Alfentanyl	10 : 1	1/2 mg
Butorphanol	5 : 1	2 mg
Hydromorphone	5 : 1	2 mg
Diamorphine	2 : 1	5/10/30 mg
Morphine	1 : 1	10 mg
Pethidine	1 : 10	100 mg
Tramadol	1 : 10	100 mg
Codeine	1 : 20	Only oral

Table A.14 Opioid misuse and associated terms

Term	Definition
Tolerance	Neuroadaptation through receptor desensitisation resulting in reduced drug effects
Pharmacological tolerance	Decrease in the number of opioid-binding sites *or* an acute depletion of the neurotransmitter released by the drug *or* decreased activity in intracellular second-messenger systems
Behavioural tolerance	Patient learns to compensate for the expected pharmacological effects of the drug over time
Pseudotolerance/ pseudoaddiction	Medication-seeking behaviour due to insufficiently treated pain
Withdrawal	Constellation of psychological and physical s/s seen when opioid is stopped or rapidly tapered, or when an opioid antagonist is given
Addiction	It is the process whereby physical plus or minus psychological dependence develops to opioids; it is characterised by impaired control and compulsive use of the drug, continued use despite harm and craving
Opioid-induced hyperalgesia	Development of hyperalgesia or allodynia secondary to chronic opioid use
Opioid rotation	Switching to a different opioid than that used by the patient, to reduce tolerance or address opioid-induced hyperalgesia
Diversion	Transfer of prescribed opioids for unlawful use
Opiophobia	Reluctance of prescribers to use opioid medication for fear of inducing addiction or toxicity

Table A.15 Statistics: definitions and formulae

Term	Definition	Formula
Mean	It is the sum of all the values, divided by the number of values	$\bar{X} = \dfrac{\sum x}{n}$
Median	It is the point that has half the values above and half below	$\left(\dfrac{n}{2}\right)^{\text{'th}}$ if even & $\left(\dfrac{n+1}{2}\right)^{\text{'th}}$ if odd
Mode	It is used when we need a label for the most frequently occurring event	
Standard deviation	It indicates how much a set of values is spread around the average; it is a measure of dispersion	$SD = \sqrt{\dfrac{(x - \bar{X})^2}{n - 1}}$
Standard error of mean	It is the standard deviation of the sample-mean estimate of a population mean; it gives an idea of how closely the estimated mean value (from the sample) is likely to represent the true mean value (from the general population)	$SE = \dfrac{SD}{\sqrt{n}}$

Table A.16 Statistical definitions Part 1

Test result	Disease		
	Present	Absent	
Positive	A (true positive)	B (false positive)	A + B (total positives)
Negative	C (false negative)	D (true negative)	C + D (total negatives)
	A + C	B + D	

Term	Definition	Formula
Sensitivity	The ability of a test to correctly identify the individuals **who have the condition**	$A/(A + C)$
Specificity	The ability of a test to correctly identify the individuals **who do not have the condition**	$D/(B + D)$
False positive rate	Proportion of **false positives** in the non-diseased population	$B/(B + D)$ or (1 – specificity)
False negative rate	Proportion of **false negatives** in the diseased population	$C/(A + C)$ or (1 – sensitivity)
Positive predictive value	Proportion of true positives among all positives	$A/(A + B)$
Negative predictive value	Proportion of true negatives among all negatives	$D/(C + D)$
Accuracy	Proportion of true results (true positive and true negative) among all results	$(A + B)/(A + B + C + D)$

Table A.17 Statistical definitions Part 2

	Disease	
Risk factor	Present	Absent
Present	A	B
Absent	C	D

Term	*Formula*
Relative risk is a **ratio** of the probability of the event (disease) occurring in the exposed group versus a non-exposed group	$RR = \dfrac{A/(A+B)}{C/(C+D)}$
Attributable risk is the **difference** in rate of a condition between an exposed population and an unexposed population	$AR = \left(\dfrac{A}{A+B}\right) - \left(\dfrac{C}{C+D}\right)$
The **odds ratio** is the ratio of the odds of an event occurring in one group to the odds of it occurring in another group	$OR = \dfrac{AD}{BC}$
Absolute risk reduction is the reduction in risk associated with treatment (or removal of risk factor) as compared with placebo	$ARR = \dfrac{1}{NNT}$
Number needed to treat is the average number of patients who need to be treated to prevent one additional bad outcome	$NNT = \dfrac{1}{Absolute\ risk\ reduction}$
Number needed to harm is the number of patients that need to be exposed to a risk factor over a specific period to cause harm in one additional patient	$NNH = \dfrac{1}{Attributable\ risk}$

Table A.18 Recommended time intervals before and after neuraxial puncture or catheter removal (for commonly used anticoagulants)

Drug	Time before puncture/ catheter removal	Time after puncture/ catheter removal
Heparins		
unfractionated heparin (for prophylaxis, ≤15 000 IU/ day)	4–6 hours	1 hour
unfractionated heparin (for treatment)	4–6 hours, intravenous 8–12 hours, subcutaneous	1 hour
low molecular weight heparin (prolonged effect in renal failure) (for prophylaxis)	12 hours	4 hours
low molecular weight heparin (for treatment)	24 hours	4 hours
Coumarins		
warfarin	INR < 1.4	After catheter removal
Antiplatelets		
acetylsalicylic acid	None	None
clopidogrel	7 days	After catheter removal
ticlopidine	10 days	After catheter removal
non-steroidal anti-inflammatory drugs	None	None
Platelet glycoprotein IIb/IIIa inhibitors	8 hours (eptifibtide/ tirofiban) 48 hours (abciximab)	–

Index

Please note: Page numbers are given in the following format Q/A where Q = 'Question' and A = 'Answer'

T - #0624 - 101024 - C0 - 246/174/20 - PB - 9781846199714 - Gloss Lamination